T0319103

Anti-VEGF
USE IN OPHTHALMOLOGY

Editors

Jay S. Duker, MD
Director, New England Eye Center
Professor and Chairman, Department of Ophthalmology
Tufts Medical Center
Tufts University School of Medicine
Boston, Massachusetts

Michelle C. Liang, MD
Assistant Professor of Ophthalmology
New England Eye Center
Tufts Medical Center
Tufts University School of Medicine
Boston, Massachusetts

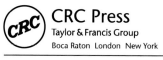

CRC Press is an imprint of the
Taylor & Francis Group, an **informa** business

First published 2017 by SLACK Incorporated

Published 2024 by CRC Press
2385 NW Executive Center Drive, Suite 320, Boca Raton FL 33431

and by CRC Press
4 Park Square, Milton Park, Abingdon, Oxon, OX14 4RN

CRC Press is an imprint of Taylor & Francis Group, LLC

Library of Congress Cataloging-in-Publication Data

Names: Duker, Jay S., 1958- editor. | Liang, Michelle C., 1983- editor.
Title: Anti-VEGF use in ophthalmology / editors, Jay S. Duker, Michelle C. Liang.
Other titles: Anti-vascular endothelial growth factor use in ophthalmology
Description: Thorofare, NJ : SLACK Incorporated, [2017] | Includes bibliographical references and index.
Identifiers: LCCN 2017010954| ISBN 9781630913212 (paperback : alk. paper) |
Subjects: | MESH: Eye Diseases--drug therapy | Vascular Endothelial Growth Factor A--antagonists & inhibitors | Angiogenesis Inhibitors--therapeutic use | Neovascularization, Pathologic--drug therapy
Classification: LCC RE991 | NLM WW 166 | DDC 617.7/061--dc23 LC record available at https://lccn.loc.gov/2017010954

ISBN: 9781630913212 (pbk)
ISBN: 9781003522577 (ebk)

DOI: 10.1201/9781003522577

Dedication

To the doctors, staff, and patients of the New England Eye Center who are a constant inspiration to disseminate knowledge and drive our field forward.

—Jay S. Duker, MD

To my loving husband, Brian, and my adorable baby boy, Ethan. Your unconditional love and support helped make this book possible.

—Michelle C. Liang, MD

Contents

About the Editors

Jay S. Duker, MD, is Professor and Chairman of Ophthalmology at the Tufts Medical Center and Tufts University School of Medicine and Director of the New England Eye Center in Boston, Massachusetts. Dr. Duker graduated from Jefferson Medical College and completed ophthalmology and retina training at the Wills Eye Hospital. His research and clinical interests are focused on the posterior segment ranging from macular degeneration, diabetic retinopathy, and retinal vascular diseases, as well as uveitis and intraocular tumors. He has published more than 280 journal articles and has been lead editor on six books and dozens of book chapters. Dr. Duker is the co-editor of the *International Journal of Retina and Vitreous.*

Michelle C. Liang, MD, is Assistant Professor of Ophthalmology at the Tufts University School of Medicine and a vitreoretinal specialist at the New England Eye Center in Boston, Massachusetts. She graduated with honors from Johns Hopkins University with a degree in Biology and earned her medical degree from the University at Buffalo School of Medicine and Biomedical Sciences. She performed her residency in ophthalmology at the New England Eye Center at Tufts Medical Center and went on to complete a vitreoretinal surgery fellowship at the New England Eye Center and Ophthalmic Consultants of Boston.

Dr. Liang has authored numerous scientific papers and book chapters and has presented at several national meetings. She treats all conditions of the retina and vitreous, including macular degeneration, vitreomacular disorders, diabetic retinopathy, retinal vascular disorders, retinal detachment, and cataract complications. Her research interests include retinal imaging and new therapies for macular degeneration, diabetic macular edema, and other diseases. Dr. Liang is a board-certified member of the American Board of Ophthalmology and a member of the American Academy of Ophthalmology and American Society of Retinal Specialists.

Contributing Authors

Alessandro Abbouda, MD (Chapter 17)
Cornea Service
New England Eye Center
Department of Ophthalmology
Tufts Medical Center
Tufts University School of Medicine
Center for Translational Ocular
Immunology
Boston, Massachusetts

Sophie J. Bakri, MD (Chapter 2)
Department of Ophthalmology
Mayo Clinic
Rochester, Minnesota

Caroline R. Baumal, MD (Chapter 11)
New England Eye Center
Department of Vitreoretinal Surgery
Tufts University School of Medicine
Boston, Massachusetts

Audina M. Berrocal, MD (Chapter 13)
Department of Ophthalmology
Bascom Palmer Eye Institute
Miller School of Medicine
University of Miami Health System
Miami, Florida

David M. Brown, MD, FACS (Chapter 3)
Retina Consultants of Houston
Blanton Eye Institute
The Methodist Hospital
Houston, Texas

Michael N. Cohen, MD (Chapter 6)
New England Eye Center
Tufts University School of Medicine
Ophthalmic Consultants of Boston
Boston, Massachusetts

Emily D. Cole, BS (Chapter 9)
Tufts University School of Medicine
Boston, Massachusetts

Sabin Dang, MD (Chapter 10)
Vitreoretinal Surgical Fellow
Ophthalmic Consultants of Boston
New England Eye Center
Boston, Massachusetts

Shilpa Desai, MD (Chapter 11)
New England Eye Center
Department of Vitreoretinal Surgery
Tufts University School of Medicine
Boston, Massachusetts

Manik Goel, MD (Chapter 15)
Assistant Professor
Marshall University
Joan C. Edwards School of Medicine
Huntington, West Virginia

Darin R. Goldman, MD (Chapter 8)
Partner, Retina Group of Florida
Affiliate Associate Professor
Charles E. Schmidt College of Medicine
Florida Atlantic University
Boca Raton, Florida

Pedram Hamrah, MD, FRCS (Chapter 17)
Cornea Service
New England Eye Center
Department of Ophthalmology
Tufts Medical Center
Tufts University School of Medicine
Center for Translational Ocular
Immunology
Boston, Massachusettss

Jeffrey S. Heier, MD (Chapter 6)
Ophthalmic Consultants of Boston
Boston, Massachusetts

Anthony Joseph, MD (Chapters 1, 4)
Vitreoretinal Surgery and
Disease Specialist
Ophthalmic Consultants of Boston
Boston, Massachusetts

Bijan Khaksari, BA (Chapter 17)
Center for Translational Ocular
Immunology
Boston, Massachusetts

Kendra Klein, MD (Chapter 5)
Clinical Associate of Ophthalmology
Tufts University School of Medicine
Boston, Massachusetts

Nikisha A. Kothari, MD (Chapter 13)
Department of Ophthalmology
Bascom Palmer Eye Institute
Miller School of Medicine
University of Miami Health System
Miami, Florida

Michael D. Lewen, MD (Chapter 7)
New England Eye Center
Department of Ophthalmology
Tufts Medical Center
Boston, Massachusetts

Maya H. Maloney, MD (Chapter 2)
Department of Ophthalmology
Mayo Clinic
Rochester, Minnesota

*Angeline Mariani Derham, MD
(Chapter 3)*
Retina Consultants of Houston
Blanton Eye Institute
The Methodist Hospital
Houston, Texas

Cynthia Mattox, MD (Chapter 16)
New England Eye Center
Tufts University School of Medicine
Boston, Massachusetts

Jessica J. Moon, MD (Chapter 16)
New England Eye Center
Tufts University School of Medicine
Boston, Massachusetts

Nora Muakkassa, MD (Chapter 5)
Assistant Professor of Ophthalmology
Tufts University School of Medicine
Boston, Massachusetts

Eduardo A. Novais, MD (Chapter 9)
Retina Specialist
Universidade Federal de São Paulo
São Paulo, Brazil

Ehsan Rahimy, MD (Chapters 1, 4)
Department of Ophthalmology
Palo Alto Medical Foundation
Palo Alto, California

Elham Rahimy, BS (Chapter 4)
Yale School of Medicine
New Haven, Connecticut

Elias Reichel, MD (Chapter 5)
New England Eye Center
Tufts University School of Medicine
Boston, Massachusetts

Lana M. Rifkin, MD (Chapter 12)
Uveitis Specialist
Ophthalmic Consultants of Boston
New England Eye Center
Assistant Professor of Ophthalmology
Tufts University School of Medicine
Boston, Massachusetts

Joel S. Schuman, MD, FACS (Chapter 15)
Professor and Chairman of
Ophthalmology
NYU Langone Medical Center
NYU School of Medicine
New York, New York

Chirag P. Shah, MD, MPH
(Chapters 6, 10)
Attending Vitreoretinal Surgeon
Ophthalmic Consultants of Boston
Vitreoretinal Surgery Fellowship
Co-Director
Assistant Professor
Tufts Medical Center
Boston, Massachusetts

Michael D. Tibbetts, MD (Chapter 14)
Director of Retina Services at Tyson Eye
Cape Coral, Florida

Nadia K. Waheed, MD, MPH (Chapter 9)
Associate Professor
Tufts University School of Medicine
Director
Boston Image Reading Center
Boston, Massacheusetts

Andre J. Witkin, MD (Chapter 7)
New England Eye Center
Department of Ophthalmology
Tufts Medical Center
Boston, Massachusetts

Introduction

A variety of pathologic ocular conditions are associated with leakage from normal blood vessels and pathologic blood vessel growth. Vascular endothelial growth factor (VEGF) is the key component in ocular angiogenesis and microvascular permeability that contributes to such vision loss.

The introduction of anti-VEGF agents approximately a decade ago has revolutionized therapy for a host of ocular disorders. We sought to create a detailed, up-to-date, clinically relevant, all-inclusive reference on the current use of anti-VEGF agents in the treatment of all ocular conditions.

As the use of anti-VEGF has widely increased over the years, it is important for eye care providers to be familiar with up-to-date aspects of the medications and indications for use. The first section of this book provides the history of VEGF and the development of anti-VEGF agents. It also goes into the current and future therapies of anti-VEGF and its administration. Section two delves into the use of anti-VEGF agents in numerous ocular diseases, from the anterior segment including cornea and glaucoma, to uveitis and various retinal and choroidal diseases. Each chapter summarizes the disease process(es) and uses high-quality ocular imaging to help demonstrate the therapeutic use of various anti-VEGF agents.

We hope this book becomes a useful reference for a wide range of eye care professionals, including optometrists, ophthalmologists-in-training, comprehensive ophthalmologists and those who specialize from the anterior segment to pediatrics to vitreoretinal disease.

We extend a special thank you to the experts in the field that contributed to the writing of this book and to the editors at SLACK Incorporated who made this book possible.

Jay S. Duker, MD
Michelle C. Liang, MD

SECTION I

OVERVIEW OF ANTI-VASCULAR ENDOTHELIAL GROWTH FACTOR AGENTS

1

VASCULAR ENDOTHELIAL GROWTH FACTOR

BACKGROUND AND HISTORY

Anthony Joseph, MD and Ehsan Rahimy, MD

Early Research

Vascular endothelial growth factor (VEGF) was officially discovered in 1983 as vascular permeability factor (VPF) by Senger and colleagues at Beth Israel Hospital in Boston.[1] However, the notion of such a biologic mediator and the significance of angiogenesis existed long before its physical isolation. As far back as the late 1800s, several German pathologists, including the renowned Rudolph Virchow, observed increased vascularity in some human tumors, suggesting that new vessels played a role in these cancers.[2] Over the ensuing decades, scientists continued to describe the varying vascular patterns of different tumors[3] until 1939, when Gordon Ide and colleagues noted the correlation between tumor growth and blood vessel formation using a rabbit model and transplanted carcinoma.[4] Their observation of a marked angiogenic response associated with tumor transplantation led them to hypothesize the existence of a vascular growth factor produced by tumor cells. Algire and a group at the National Cancer Institute built on this work in 1945, demonstrating that transplanted tumor tissue in rats led to increased vessel formation while transplanted normal tissue did not. This finding again suggested the presence of a vascular growth factor associated with tumor tissue.[5]

Some time passed for these postulations on angiogenic factors to translate into experimental evidence of their existence. In 1968, two different groups published research supporting the release of these factors. Both Greenblatt and Shubi[6] as well as Ehrmann and Knoth[7] showed that melanoma and choriocarcinoma cells in a hamster model stimulated the growth of blood vessels in a host even when filter paper physically separated the tumor cells from the host. These findings strongly suggested the presence of a diffusible factor promoting vascular proliferation produced by tumor cells.

Duker JS, Liang MC, eds.
*Anti-VEGF Use in
Ophthalmology* (pp. 3-10).
© 2017 Taylor & Francis Group.

As interest continued to grow in the role of angiogenesis factors in cancer, Judah Folkman published his seminal work on the topic in 1971 with the novel idea that vascular proliferation was instrumental for tumor progression, and accordingly, that inhibition of angiogenesis could provide a potential approach to treating malignancy.[8] Along with his colleagues, he also began work to isolate a tumor angiogenesis factor (TAF) from human and animal tumors that would incite blood vessel proliferation in a rat model.[8,9] He coined the term *anti-angiogenesis* referring to prevention of vascular proliferation into early tumors through inhibition of such angiogenesis factors, giving rise to a new field of research into therapies for cancer and eventually vascular diseases of the eye.

In the decade following Folkman's report, research accelerated to isolate and identify different angiogenesis factors. Even so, after isolating a specific biologic mediator, progress was limited by the time required to purify and subsequently reproduce sufficient amounts of the compound, a task that could take years in the era before gene sequencing.[2] Once again, Folkman's group provided a stimulus to the field with their description of a method for the production of pure capillary endothelial cells.[10] These cells could be used to study angiogenesis factors in vitro, and as a result, many researchers began to study the effects of different biologic factors on endothelial cell proliferation. Epidermal growth factor, transforming growth factor (-α and-β), tumor necrosis factor, and angiogenin were shown to stimulate endothelial cell proliferation either directly or indirectly through the action of inflammatory cells.[2,11] Special consideration was also given to acidic fibroblast growth factor (aFGF) identified by Maciag and colleagues in 1979[12] and basic fibroblast growth factor (bFGF) identified by Gospodarowicz in 1974[13] as they were shown to stimulate both endothelial cells and a variety of other cell types. Even so, early trials to correlate FGF with tumor angiogenesis yielded negative results.[2] More recently, antibodies against bFGF were not found to hinder tumor growth in mouse models,[14] and mouse models with both defective aFGF and bFGF genes did not demonstrate vascular defects. In the meantime, researchers continued to hunt for angiogenesis factors more directly related to tumorigenesis.

Isolation of Vascular Endothelial Growth Factor

In 1983, more than a decade after Folkman published his research on the therapeutic implications of tumor angiogenesis, Senger and Dvorak, along with their colleagues at Beth Israel Hospital, found that ascites fluid associated with tumors in guinea pigs, hamsters, and mice had activity that increased microvascular permeability. They partially purified the active protein from a guinea pig line and referred to this mediator as VPF.[1] The authors recognized that VPF appeared to play a role in the hyper-permeability of tumor vasculature, but they were seemingly unaware of its angiogenic properties. Furthermore, since the protein was not completely purified and sequenced, its identity remained unknown for several years.

Then, in 1989, two groups simultaneously reported findings on VEGF and VPF in back-to-back articles in the same issue of *Science*.[15,16] Napoleone Ferrara and his group at Genentech used a media conditioned by bovine pituitary follicular cells to purify a biologic factor that induced angiogenesis in vivo.[16] The isolated protein was termed *vascular endothelial growth factor,* and given its great angiogenic activity, the authors hypothesized that it was a secreted factor different from aFGF, bFGF, and platelet-derived growth factor (PDGF), which were stored factors previously shown to exist in the same cells.[17] Indeed, N-terminal amino acid sequencing conclusively showed that VEGF was a unique protein not described in any database.[18]

At the same time, Connolly and his group at Monsanto Company had worked to purify and sequence human VPF,[15] building on Senger's previous work. They found the protein to be active in increasing blood vessel permeability as well as endothelial cell growth and angiogenesis. In their research, Ferrara's group had identified complementary DNA (cDNA) clones encoding for 3 different molecular species of VEGF containing 121, 165, and 189 amino acids. As it turned out, the cDNA clone identified by Connolly's group encoded a protein identical to $VEGF_{189}$, revealing that VEGF and VPF were indeed the same factor, even though the former was isolated because of its angiogenic activity while the latter was isolated through its propensity to stimulate vascular permeability. Full sequencing of the gene encoding for VEGF demonstrated that it and PDGF shared similar genetic characteristics as well.[2] Additionally, around the same time, various groups purified factors in other species that stimulated endothelial cell proliferation. These factors, such as vasculotropin in mice[19] and VPF in guinea pigs,[20] were found to be orthologues of VEGF, thus demonstrating the conservation of VEGF across species.[2]

Further examination of VEGF in the succeeding years demonstrated varied molecular properties of the different isoforms. $VEGF_{165}$, a diffusible heparin-binding variant, was found to be the most abundant form.[21] $VEGF_{121}$ was noted to be freely diffusible while $VEGF_{189}$ was largely bound to the cell surface and extracellular matrix.[22,23] Consequently, VEGF could be directly secreted as its shorter isoforms or released by protease activation and cleavage of longer isoforms.[2]

In the following years, VEGF was found to play a role in many human physiologic processes. VEGF actually encompasses 5 major subtypes: VEGF-A, VEGF-B, VEGF-C, VEGF-D, and placental growth factor (PlGF). The original VEGF was later termed VEGF-A as the other family members were discovered. As described above, VEGF-A plays a prominent role in angiogenesis and vascular permeability, often with respect to tumor proliferation. Additionally, VEGF-A affects other angiogenic processes such as wound healing, ovulation, menstruation, and pregnancy.[24] VEGF-B is less well understood, but is highly expressed in striated muscle, myocardium, and brown fat. Research suggests it plays a role in embryonic angiogenesis, especially with respect to the heart.[25] VEGF-C is produced as a precursor protein and induces selective lymphangiogenesis without accompanying angiogenesis.[26] It appears to play a role in lymphatic invasion of tumors and lymphatic metastasis.[27] VEGF-D is closely related to VEGF-C and also plays a pivotal role in tumor lymphangiogenesis and lymphatic metastasis as well as angiogenesis.[28] Finally, PlGF was originally discovered in the placenta but is also expressed in the heart and lungs.[29] Loss of PlGF impairs angiogenesis in ischemia, wound healing, inflammation, and cancer.[30] Other VEGF derivatives have also been discovered, including VEGF-E encoded by the Orf virus genome[31] and VEGF-F identified from viper snake venom,[32] which may have therapeutic implications down the road. Undoubtedly, the VEGF family of proteins plays a broad and significant role in human pathophysiology, a role eventually found to extend to ocular conditions as well.

Vascular Endothelial
Growth Factor in the Eye

Just as the notion of a tumor-related angiogenesis factor existed long before its actual identification, eye researchers independently theorized the idea of VEGF decades before it was discovered. As early as 1948, Michaelson proposed the existence of a diffusible factor responsible for retinal vascular growth in various developmental and disease processes.[33] This unknown factor would come to be known as Factor X, and George Wise later elaborated on the topic in his 1956 thesis suggesting that retinal neovascularization was stimulated by retinal tissue factor x, a mediator presumed to be related to tissue anoxia.[34] Clinicians recognized the correlation between retinal injury and new blood vessel growth elsewhere in the eye, but it would be decades before Judah Folkman published his seminal paper on TAF, research that coincidentally relied on eye models in many cases.[8,35]

In 1980, just before Senger and Dvorak published their work on VPF, Glaser and D'Amore, along with their colleagues at Johns Hopkins University, recognized that the retina and vitreous might be potential sources of vasoproliferative factors in the eye.[36-38] In another parallel to the search for a TAF, aFGF[39] and later bFGF[40] were suggested as possible candidates for Factor X after being identified as angiogenic mediators in the eye. But these compounds were not secreted, so the search for Factor X continued.[35]

In the meantime, Ferrara's team and Connolly's team had independently isolated VEGF,[15,16] which soon became a leading candidate for Factor X. Studies using a glioblastoma tumor model confirmed that VEGF expression correlated with vascular proliferation and was induced by hypoxia.[41,42] These findings were consistent with the suspected mechanism of neovascularization in various retinopathies and coincided with the original postulations about Factor X. Additionally, VEGF stimulated vascular permeability, another common feature in retinal vascular disorders in which Factor X was suspected to play a role.[35,43]

With these implications in mind, researchers began to investigate the potential role of VEGF in ocular disease. Adamis and Shima, along with D'Amore and Folkman, used in vitro experiments to demonstrate that human retinal pigment epithelial cells could synthesize VEGF.[44] Shima and colleagues went on to establish that expression of VEGF by retinal cells was promoted by hypoxia[45] and correlated spatially and temporally with the onset of angiogenesis in the eye.[46] These findings suggested that induction of VEGF by hypoxia mediated the neovascular response to retinal ischemia seen in various retinal vascular conditions.

At the same time, Miller and collaborators at the Massachusetts Eye and Ear Infirmary became the first to confirm this hypothesis in vivo using aqueous samples collected from monkey eyes with laser-induced vein occlusion. The resultant retinal ischemia induced iris neovascularization, which was consistent with the presence of a diffusible molecule. Additionally, aqueous samples revealed that levels of VEGF and its associate messenger RNA (mRNA) were elevated both synchronously and proportionally to the extent of new blood vessel growth in the iris.[47] The same monkey model was later used to establish that production of VEGF occurred in the inner retina with expression of the secreted $VEGF_{121}$ and $VEGF_{165}$ variants.[48] These findings pushed VEGF to the front as the likely candidate for a retinal-derived vascular permeability and angiogenic factor.

The next step was to translate in vitro and animal model findings to humans. Aiello and collaborators measured the concentration of VEGF in aqueous or vitreous from patients undergoing intraocular surgery. They found VEGF was more prevalent in patients with ischemic retinal disease including diabetic retinopathy and retinal vein occlusions compared to those with no neovascular disorders.[49] Adamis's group had similar findings using vitreous samples from patients with proliferative diabetic retinopathy.[50] These studies provided some of the most direct evidence yet regarding a key role for VEGF in neovascular eye disease.

Up until this point, researchers had correlated the presence and level of VEGF with ischemic eye disease and proliferative changes. They now looked to show a more causative link by establishing whether VEGF was sufficient to incite neovascularization in the eye. Using the primate model described previously, Miller and Tolentino demonstrated that intravitreal injections of recombinant human VEGF$_{165}$ produced iris neovascularization with prolonged exposure leading to ectropion uveae and neovascular glaucoma.[51] They used the same technique to further show that VEGF was sufficient to produce retinal ischemia and microangiopathy in normal eyes with VEGF$_{165}$ injections leading to the development of hemorrhage, edema, venous beading, microaneurysms, capillary occlusion with ischemia, and vascular proliferation.[52]

At the same time, researchers examined VEGF inhibition to solidify the role of VEGF in ischemic ocular disease. Aiello and company used a soluble VEGF-receptor protein to suppress retinal neovascularization in vivo in animals with an oxygen-induced ischemic retinopathy.[53] Robinson and Smith then used an anti-VEGF aptamer in a murine model of proliferative retinopathy to inhibit retinal neovascularization.[54] Meanwhile, Adamis and Miller used their primate model to establish that injections of a monoclonal antibody to VEGF prevented iris neovascularization in eyes with retinal ischemia secondary to laser-induced vein occlusion.[55] This antibody was the precursor to bevacizumab.[35] It was 1996 by this time, and the clinical potential for VEGF inhibition in neovascular eye disease was evident. It would still be years before pharmaceutical companies would put the resources toward ophthalmic clinical trials necessary to bring anti-VEGF therapy to everyday practice, but this marked the beginning of a new era in treating previously blinding retinal disease.

References

1. Senger DR, Galli SJ, Dvorak AM, Perruzzi CA, Harvey VS, Dvorak HF. Tumor cells secrete a vascular permeability factor that promotes accumulation of ascites fluid. *Science*. 1983;219(4587):983-985.
2. Ferrara N. VEGF and the quest for tumour angiogenesis factors. *Nat Rev Cancer*. 2002;2(10):795-803.
3. Lewis WH. The vascular pattern of tumors. *Johns Hopkins Hosp Bull*. 1927;41:156-162.
4. Ide AG, Baker NH, Warren SL. Vascularization of the Brown Pearce rabbit epithelioma transplant as seen in the transparent ear chamber. *Am J Roentgenol*. 1939;42:891-899.
5. Algire GH, Chalkley HW. Vascular reactions of normal and malignant tissues in vivo. I. Vascular reactions of mice to wounds and to normal and neoplastic transplants. *J Natl Cancer Inst*. 1945;6:73-85.
6. Greenblatt M, Shubi P. Tumor angiogenesis: transfilter diffusion studies in the hamster by the transparent chamber technique. *J Natl Cancer Inst*. 1968;41(1):111-124.
7. Ehrmann RL, Knoth M. Choriocarcinoma. Transfilter stimulation of vasoproliferation in the hamster cheek pouch. Studied by light and electron microscopy. *J Natl Cancer Inst*. 1968;41(6):1329-1341.

8. Folkman J. Tumor angiogenesis: therapeutic implications. *N Engl J Med*. 1971;285(21):1182-1186.

9. Folkman J, Merler E, Abernathy C, Williams G. Isolation of a tumor factor responsible for angiogenesis. *J Exp Med*. 1971;133(2):275-288.

10. Folkman J, Haudenschild CC, Zetter BR. Long-term culture of capillary endothelial cells. *Proc Natl Acad Sci U S A*. 1979;76(10):5217-5221.

11. Folkman J, Klagsbrun M. Angiogenic factors. *Science*. 1987;235(4787):442-447.

12. Maciag T, Cerundolo J, Ilsley S, Kelley PR, Forand R. An endothelial cell growth factor from bovine hypothalamus: identification and partial characterization. *Proc Natl Acad Sci U S A*. 1979;76(11):5674-5678.

13. Gospodarowicz D. Localisation of a fibroblast growth factor and its effect alone and with hydrocortisone on 3T3 cell growth. *Nature*. 1974;249(453):123-127.

14. Dennis PA, Rifkin DB. Studies on the role of basic fibroblast growth factor in vivo: inability of neutralizing antibodies to block tumor growth. *J Cell Physiol*. 1990;144(1):84-98.

15. Keck PJ, Hauser SD, Krivi G, et al. Vascular permeability factor, an endothelial cell mitogen related to PDGF. *Science*. 1989;246(4935):1309-1312.

16. Leung DW, Cachianes G, Kuang WJ, Goeddel DV, Ferrara N. Vascular endothelial growth factor is a secreted angiogenic mitogen. *Science*. 1989;246(4935):1306-1309.

17. Ferrara N, Schweigerer L, Neufeld G, Mitchell R, Gospodarowicz D. Pituitary follicular cells produce basic fibroblast growth factor. *Proc Natl Acad Sci U S A*. 1987;84(16):5773-5777.

18. Ferrara N, Henzel WJ. Pituitary follicular cells secrete a novel heparin-binding growth factor specific for vascular endothelial cells. *Biochem Biophys Res Commun*. 1989;161(2):851-858.

19. Plouët J, Schilling J, Gospodarowicz D. Isolation and characterization of a newly identified endothelial cell mitogen produced by AtT-20 cells. *EMBO J*. 1989;8(12):3801-3806.

20. Senger DR, Connolly DT, Van de Water L, Feder J, Dvorak HF. Purification and NH2-terminal amino acid sequence of guinea pig tumor-secreted vascular permeability factor. *Cancer Res*. 1990;50(6):1774-1778.

21. Houck KA, Ferrara N, Winer J, Cachianes G, Li B, Leung DW. The vascular endothelial growth factor family: identification of a fourth molecular species and characterization of alternative splicing of RNA. *Mol Endocrinol*. 1991;5(12):1806-1814.

22. Park JE, Keller GA, Ferrara N. The vascular endothelial growth factor (VEGF) isoforms: differential deposition into the subepithelial extracellular matrix and bioactivity of extracellular matrixbound VEGF. *Mol Biol Cell*. 1993;4(12):1317-1326.

23. Houck KA, Leung DW, Rowland AM, Winer J, Ferrara N. Dual regulation of vascular endothelial growth factor bioavailability by genetic and proteolytic mechanisms. *J Biol Chem*. 1992;267(36):26031-26037.

24. Otrock ZK, Makarem JA, Shamseddine AI. Vascular endothelial growth factor family of ligands and receptors: review. *Blood Cells Mol Dis*. 2007;38(3):258-268.

25. Claesson-Welsh L. VEGF-B taken to our hearts: specific effect of VEGF-B in myocardial ischemia. *Arterioscler Thromb Vasc Biol*. 2008;28(9):1575-1576.

26. Jeltsch M, Kaipainen A, Joukov V, et al. Hyperplasia of lymphatic vessels in VEGF-C transgenic mice. *Science*. 1997;276(5317):1423-1425.

27. Fujimoto J, Toyoki H, Sato E, Sakaguchi H, Tamaya T. Clinical implication of expression of vascular endothelial growth factor-C in metastatic lymph nodes of uterine cervical cancers. *Br J Cancer*. 2004;91(3):466-469.

28. Stacker SA, Caesar C, Baldwin ME, et al. VEGF-D promotes the metastatic spread of tumor cells via the lymphatics. *Nat Med*. 2001;7(2):186-191.

29. Persico MG, Vincenti V, DiPalma T. Structure, expression and receptor-binding properties of placenta growth factor (PlGF). *Curr Top Microbiol Immunol*. 1999;237:31-40.

30. Carmeliet P, Moons L, Luttun A, et al. Synergism between vascular endothelial growth factor and placental growth factor contributes to angiogenesis and plasma extravasation in pathological conditions. *Nat Med*. 2001;7(5):575-583.

31. Lyttle DJ, Fraser KM, Fleming SB, Mercer AA, Robinson AJ. Homologs of vascular endothelial growth factor are encoded by the poxvirus orf virus. *J Virol*. 1994;68(1):84-92.

32. Suto K, Yamazaki Y, Morita T, Mizuno H. Crystal structures of novel vascular endothelial growth factors (VEGF) from snake venoms: insight into selective VEGF binding to kinase insert domain-containing receptor but not to fms-like tyrosine kinase-1. *J Biol Chem*. 2005;280(3):2126-2131.

33. Michaelson IC. The mode of development of the vascular system of the retina, with some observations on its significance for certain retinal diseases. *Trans Ophthalmol Soc U K*. 1948;68:137-180.

34. Wise GN. Retinal neovascularization. *Trans Am Ophthalmol Soc*. 1956;54:729-826.

35. Miller JW. The Harvard angiogenesis story. *Surv Ophthalmol*. 2014;59(3):361-364.

36. Glaser BM, D'Amore PA, Lutty GA, Fenselau AH, Michels RG, Patz A. Chemical mediators of intraocular neovascularization. *Trans Ophthalmol Soc U K*. 1980;100(3):369-373.

37. Glaser BM, D'Amore PA, Michels RG, et al. The demonstration of angiogenic activity from ocular tissues. Preliminary report. *Ophthalmology*. 1980;87(5):440-446.

38. Glaser BM, D'Amore PA, Michels RG, Patz A, Fenselau A. Demonstration of vasoproliferative activity from mammalian retina. *J Cell Biol*. 1980;84(2):298-304.

39. D'Amore PA, Glaser BM, Brunson SK, Fenselau AH. Angiogenic activity from bovine retina: partial purification and characterization. *Proc Natl Acad Sci U S A*. 1981;78(5):3068-3072.

40. Sivalingam A, Kenney J, Brown GC, Benson WE, Donoso L. Basic fibroblast growth factor levels in the vitreous of patients with proliferative diabetic retinopathy. *Arch Ophthalmol*. 1990;108(6):869-872.

41. Plate KH, Breier G, Welch HA, Risau W. Vascular endothelial growth factor is a potential tumour angiogenesis factor in human gliomas in vivo. *Nature*. 1992;359(6398):845-848.

42. Shweiki D, Itin A, Soffer D, Keshet E. Vascular endothelial growth factor induced by hypoxia may mediate hypoxia-initiated angiogenesis. *Nature*. 1992;359(6398):843-845.

43. Kim LA, D'Amore PA. A brief history of anti-VEGF for the treatment of ocular angiogenesis. *Am J Pathol*. 2012;181(2):376-379.

44. Adamis AP, Shima DT, Yeo KT, et al. Synthesis and secretion of vascular permeability factor/ vascular endothelial growth factor by human retinal pigment epithelial cells. *Biochem Biophys Res Commun*. 1993;193(2):631-638.

45. Shima DT, Deutsch U, D'Amore, PA. Hypoxic induction of vascular endothelial growth factor (VEGF) in human epithelial cells is mediated by increases in mRNA stability. *FEBS Lett*. 1995;370(3):203-208.

46. Shima DT, Adamis AP, Ferrara N, et al. Hypoxic induction of endothelial cell growth factors in retinal cells: identification and characterization of vascular endothelial growth factor (VEGF) as the mitogen. *Mol Med*. 1995;1(2):182-193.

47. Miller JW, Adamis AP, Shima DT, et al. Vascular endothelial growth factor/vascular permeability factor is temporally and spatially correlated with ocular angiogenesis in a primate model. *Am J Pathol*. 1994;145(3):574-584.

48. Shima DT, Gougos A, Miller JW, et al. Cloning and mRNA expression of vascular endothelial growth factor in ischemic retinas of Macaca fascicularis. *Invest Ophthalmol Vis Sci*. 1996;37(7):1334-1340.

49. Aiello LP, Avery RL, Arrigg PG, et al. Vascular endothelial growth factor in ocular fluid of patients with diabetic retinopathy and other retinal disorders. *N Engl J Med*. 1994;31(22):1480-1487.

50. Adamis AP, Miller JW, Bernal MT, et al. Increased vascular endothelial growth factor levels in the vitreous of eyes with proliferative diabetic retinopathy. *Am J Ophthalmol*. 1994;118(4):445-450.

51. Tolentino MJ, Miller JW, Gragoudas ES, Chatzistefanou K, Ferrara N, Adamis AP. Vascular endothelial growth factor is sufficient to produce iris neovascularization and neovascular glaucoma in a nonhuman primate. *Arch Ophthalmol*. 1996;114(8):964-970.

52. Tolentino MJ, Miller JW, Gragoudas ES, et al. Intravitreous injections of vascular endothelial growth factor produce retinal ischemia and microangiopathy in an adult primate. *Ophthalmology*. 1996;103(11):1820-1828.

53. Aiello LP, Pierce EA, Foley ED, et al. Suppression of retinal neovascularization in vivo by inhibition of vascular endothelial growth factor (VEGF) using soluble VEGF-receptor chimeric proteins. *Proc Natl Acad Sci U S A*. 1995;92(23):10457-10461.

54. Robinson GS, Pierce EA, Rook SL, Foley E, Webb R, Smith LE. Oligodeoxynucleotides inhibit retinal neovascularization in a murine model of proliferative retinopathy. *Proc Natl Acad Sci U S A*. 1996;93(10):4851-4856.

55. Adamis AP, Shima DT, Tolentino MJ, et al. Inhibition of vascular endothelial growth factor prevents retinal ischemia-associated iris neovascularization in a nonhuman primate. *Arch Ophthalmol*. 1996;114(1):66-71.

2

Development of Anti-Vascular Endothelial Growth Factor Agents

Maya H. Maloney, MD and Sophie J. Bakri, MD

As vascular endothelial growth factor (VEGF) was identified as a regulator of tumor angiogenesis, it was also identified as a mediator of angiogenesis in the eye. VEGF was suggested to play a role in neovascularization secondary to ischemic retinal disorders, such as active proliferative diabetic retinopathy, ischemic central retinal vein occlusion, and retinopathy of prematurity.[1,2] Later, the importance of VEGF in choroidal neovascularization, and therefore age-related macular degeneration (AMD), was also recognized.[3,4] During this time, multiple animal models helped shed light on ocular angiogenesis. Occlusion of retinal veins by laser in a cynomolgus monkey stimulated rubeosis iridis and showed increases in aqueous VEGF levels proportional to the severity of iris neovascularization.[5] Subsequent studies demonstrated that intravitreal injection of VEGF was sufficient to produce iris neovascularization and injection of anti-VEGF antibodies prevented such neovascularization.[6,7] Mouse models of ischemia-induced proliferative retinopathy showed similar results of suppressed neovascularization by inhibition of VEGF with VEGF receptor chimeric proteins and antisense oligodeoxynucleotides.[8,9] As we learned that the inhibition of VEGF action could have therapeutic applications, further strategies were developed and honed to inhibit VEGF production, neutralize free VEGF, block VEGF receptors, and interfere with the endothelial cell response to VEGF.[10]

Pegaptanib

Pharmacology

Pegaptanib (Macugen) is an RNA aptamer that binds the heparin-binding site of the $VEGF_{165}$ isoform, thereby preventing it from binding to VEGF receptors. Aptamers (from the Latin *aptus,* to fit, and the Greek *meros*, part or region) are RNA or DNA oligonucleotide ligands that can bind extracellular target molecules with high affinity and specificity. Unlike monoclonal antibodies, they are easily produced and non-immunogenic.

Duker JS, Liang MC, eds.
Anti-VEGF Use in
Ophthalmology (pp. 11-18).
© 2017 Taylor & Francis Group.

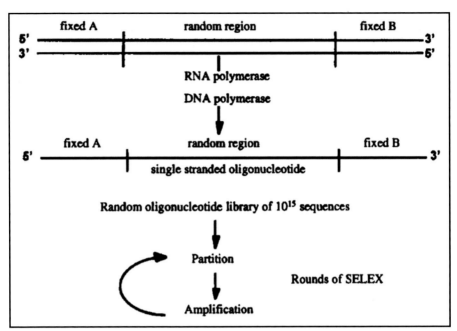

Figure 2-1. A diagram of systematic evolution of ligands by exponential enrichment (SELEX). A library of random oligonucleotide sequences are flanked by fixed regions, labeled A and B, that allow for enzyme binding and other chemical reactions. Sequences are selected during repeated rounds of partitioning and amplification. (Adapted from Eaton BE, Gold L, Hicke BJ, et al. Post-SELEX combinatorial optimization of aptamers. *Bioorg Med Chem.* 1997;5(6):1087-1096. Used with permission of Mayo Foundation for Medical Education and Research. All rights reserved.)

Aptamers are selected during systematic evolution of ligands by exponential enrichment (Figure 2-1). In this process, up to 10^{15} random oligomer sequences are flanked by binding sites for reverse transcriptase and polymerase chain reaction primers, promoter sequences for T7 RNA polymerase, and restriction endonuclease sites. These 20 to 40 nucleotide-long regions that bind targets are selected, amplified, and reselected. In the case of anti-VEGF aptamer development, iterations of the systematic evolution of ligands by exponential enrichment process identified ligands that were subsequently modified for improved stability and nuclease resistance.[11] The VEGF antagonist that was ultimately chosen for development, and became known as pegaptanib is shown in Figure 2-2. It significantly reduced VEGF-induced vascular permeability in adult guinea pigs compared to its counterparts.[12] Pegaptanib was developed specifically to antagonize the pathologic 165 isoform of VEGF because of concern that inhibition of all VEGF isoforms would interfere with physiologic angiogenesis in addition to antagonizing pathologic neovascularization. It became the first aptamer successfully developed as a therapeutic for human use when the United States Food and Drug Administration (FDA) approved it for the treatment of neovascular AMD in 2004.[11]

Prior to clinical trials, studies were conducted to better characterize the aptamer. Pegaptanib was stable after 18 hours of incubation at ambient temperature. The half-life was 9.3 hours in monkeys after intravenous administration. In another study using a monkey model, biologically active pegaptanib remained in the vitreous for at least 28 days

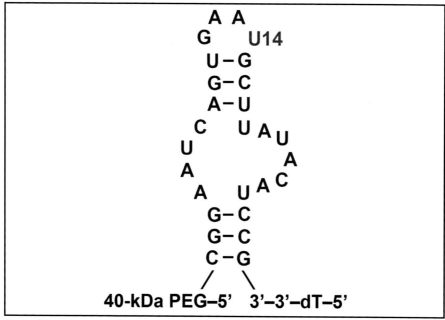

Figure 2-2. Structure of pegaptanib. Sequence of modified nucleotides in pegaptanib. Uridine-14 (pink) interacts with the heparin-binding domain of VEGF$_{165}$. There is a 40 kDa polyethylene glycol moiety at the 5′ end and a 3′-terminal deoxythymidine at the 3′ end. (Adapted from Ng EW, Shima DT, Calias P, Cunningham ET Jr, Guyer DR, Adamis AP. Pegaptanib, a targeted anti-VEGF aptamer for ocular vascular disease. *Nat Rev Drug Discov.* 2006;5(2):123-132. Used with permission of Mayo Foundation for Medical Education and Research. All rights reserved.)

following a single 0.5 mg intravitreal injection.[11] Other preclinical studies confirmed the anti-angiogenic effects of pegaptanib with its inhibition of corneal neovascularization in rats and of retinal neovascularization in the rat model of retinopathy of prematurity.[13] Pegaptanib is cleared by the kidneys[11] and has been shown not to elicit an immunogenic response.[14] Previous studies supported that it was the 165 isoform of VEGF, and not other isoforms like VEGF$_{121}$, that was responsible for pathological ocular neovascularization, and further research suggested that pegaptanib inhibited VEGF$_{165}$ by binding a residue in the heparin-binding domain of VEGF$_{165}$ that is not found in VEGF$_{121}$.[11] With these results, this targeted anti-VEGF agent entered preliminary clinical trials.

Therapeutic Efficacy

In phase Ia and II trials, pegaptanib was administered to small groups for evaluation of safety and efficacy. In the phase Ia trial, patients with poor vision from neovascular AMD received intravitreal injections of varying doses of pegaptanib to establish a safe dosage range. No serious side effects were noted, and vision stabilized or improved in 80% of patients at 3 months.[13] The phase II trial involving 21 patients compared the use of pegaptanib alone to pegaptanib treatment with concomitant photodynamic therapy. Eight patients completed the 3-month course of monthly intravitreal injection of pegaptanib alone; 7 had stabilization or improvement of their vision.[15] This encouraging preliminary data led to larger-scale studies.

Pegaptanib was subsequently tested in pivotal clinical trials for the treatment of neo-vascular AMD and diabetic macular edema (DME). In the phase III VEGF Inhibition Study in Ocular Neovascularization (VISION) trials, intravitreal injection of pegaptanib was compared to sham injection at 1 and 2 years. Results demonstrated that pegaptanib was both safe and effective, reducing vision loss in patients when compared to sham injection. Another phase II trial was also conducted to investigate the efficacy of pegap-tanib in the treatment of DME and similarly showed improved visual acuity outcomes in treated patients.[11] These trials supported the successful development of a therapeutic aptamer targeted at VEGF and pathologic ocular neovascularization, a novel treatment not dependent on the classification of neovascularization by fluorescein angiogram like the previously available therapies.

Bevacizumab

Pharmacology

Bevacizumab (Avastin) was developed to inhibit VEGF for the treatment of metastatic colorectal cancer and FDA approved for this use in 2004. The original mouse anti-human VEGF antibody, A.4.6.1, was produced by mice immunized with $VEGF_{165}$ but recognized all VEGF-A isoforms. This full-length monoclonal antibody was later humanized by transferring the VEGF-binding regions of A.4.6.1 to a human antibody framework (Figure 2-3); the final product contains 93% human amino acid sequence. Large quantities are produced in Chinese hamster ovary cells using expression plasmids.[16]

Initial preclinical work with bevacizumab was focused on tumor anti-angiogenesis. Further research regarding intravitreal injection and ocular use was performed only after the medication was already in active use off-label for ocular indications. As with pegaptanib, safety studies were performed in cynomolgus monkeys as VEGF isoforms were found to be identical between the *Macaca fascicularis* and humans.[17] In rabbits receiving the 1.25 mg dose that is commonly administered today, the half-life of intra-vitreal bevacizumab was 4.32 days, compared to 2.88 days for 0.5 mg ranibizumab.[18,19] Interestingly, bevacizumab can be found in the vitreous of the contralateral eye after intravitreal injection[18,19] and has been shown to penetrate throughout the retina on con-focal immunohistochemistry.[20]

Therapeutic Efficacy

Phase I trials started in 1997 for systemic administration and showed that the addi-tion of bevacizumab to standard chemotherapy regimens was safe. Multiple phase II trials were then conducted to study the role of bevacizumab in the treatment of different cancers, including colorectal cancer, renal cell cancer, and non-small cell lung cancer, among others. These oncology trials suggested that adverse events such as thrombosis, bleeding, and hypertension may be systemic adverse events related to bevacizumab administration.[17] Results from the Systemic Avastin for Neovascular AMD trial support-ed the hypothesis that systemic bevacizumab improved vision in affected patients.[21,22] Later, larger-scale phase III studies to assess the efficacy of intravitreal bevacizumab in the treatment of neovascular AMD were initiated, such as the Avastin for Treatment of Choroidal Neovascularization (ABC) trial and the Comparison of Age-Related

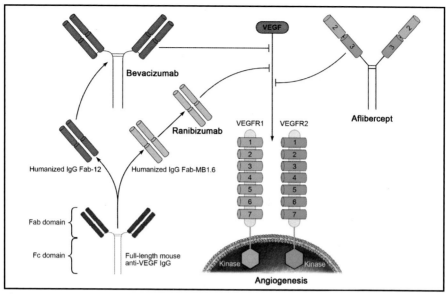

Figure 2-3. Structures and roles of bevacizumab, ranibizumab, and aflibercept. Bevacizumab and ranibizumab were both developed from a mouse immunoglobulin G. Bevacizumab is a humanized full-length monoclonal antibody and ranibizumab is a humanized Fab fragment. Aflibercept is a fusion protein comprised of ligand-binding domains 2 and 3 of VEGFR1 and VEGFR2, respectively, attached to the Fc region of a human immunoglobulin G. Fab = fragment antigen binding; Fc = fragment crystallizable; VEGFR1 = vascular endothelial growth factor receptor 1; VEGFR2 = vascular endothelial growth factor receptor 2. (Adapted from Au A, Singh RP. A multimodal approach to diabetic macular edema. *J Diabetes Complications.* 2016;30(3):545-553. Used with permission of Mayo Foundation for Medical Education and Research. All rights reserved.)

Macular Degeneration (CATT) trial. Internationally, there have now been multiple comparative treatment trials, including the Inhibition of VEGF in Age-Related Choroidal Neovascularisation (IVAN), the Multicentre Anti-VEGF Trial in Austria (MANTA), the Avastin Versus Lucentis for Neovascular AMD (GEFAL), and others.

Ranibizumab

Pharmacology

Ranibizumab (Lucentis) is an antibody fragment targeted against all VEGF isoforms (Figure 2-3). Although immunohistochemistry shows that bevacizumab penetrates all layers of the retina, it was initially thought that a smaller antibody fragment would be more effectively distributed. This fragment antibody also has a shorter systemic half-life, addressing concerns regarding the long half-life of full-length antibodies such as bevacizumab in systemic VEGF inhibition. Ranibizumab was developed for enhanced binding affinity to VEGF from a different humanized anti-VEGF antibody than A.4.6.1 and is produced in *Escherichia coli.* Unlike bevacizumab, which has 2 antigen-binding

Property	Antibody	
	Bevacizumab	Ranibizumab
Development intention	Oncology	Wet AMD
Parent molecule	Mouse mAb	Mouse mAb
Produced in	CHO cells	*Escherichia coli*
Target	All human VEGF-A isoforms	All human VEGF-A isoforms
Final structure	Full-Length IgG antibody	IgG antigen-binding fragment
Fc domain	Yes	No
Molecular weight	149 kDa	48 kDa

Table 2-1. Comparison of Bevacizumab and Ranibizumab

Adapted from Meyer CH, Holz FG. Preclinical aspects of anti-VEGF agents for the treatment of wet AMD: ranibizumab and bevacizumab. *Eye (Lond).* 2011;25(6):661-672. Used with permission of Mayo Foundation for Medical Education and Research. All rights reserved.

domains, ranibizumab has only 1 such domain.[23] Other differences between the two agents are described in Table 2-1.

Therapeutic Efficacy

Ranibizumab was approved by the FDA in 2006 for the treatment of neovascular AMD after publication of the Minimally Classic/Occult Trial of the Anti-VEGF Antibody Ranibizumab in the Treatment of Neovascular AMD (MARINA) and Anti-VEGF Antibody for the Treatment of Predominantly Classic Choroidal Neovascularization in AMD (ANCHOR) trials. The 2-year HORIZON extension supported continued use. Ranibizumab has since been approved for the treatment of DME after the Diabetic Retinopathy Clinical Research (DRCR) and RESTORE studies, and for retinal vein occlusions with macular edema after the Central Retinal Vein Occlusion Study: Evaluation of Efficacy and Safety (CRUISE) and Branch Retinal Vein Occlusion: Evaluation of Efficacy and Safety (BRAVO) trials.[23]

Aflibercept

Pharmacology

Aflibercept (Eylea), also known as VEGF Trap for systemic use and VEGF Trap-Eye for ocular use, is a fusion protein that combines the fragment crystallizable constant region of human immunoglobulin G to extracellular ligand-binding domains of VEGF receptor 1 and VEGF receptor 2 (Figure 2-3). Like bevacizumab and ranibizumab, it binds all isoforms of VEGF-A but also binds VEGF-B and placental growth factors 1 and 2. It is of intermediate molecular weight (heavier than ranibizumab and lighter than bevacizumab). Aflibercept is produced in Chinese hamster ovary cells, penetrates all layers of the retina, and has low immunogenicity with a long half-life.[23]

Therapeutic Efficacy

Multiple animal models support the use of aflibercept in the treatment of choroidal neovascularization. In mice with laser-induced ruptures of Bruch's membrane, aflibercept inhibited choroidal neovascularization. Comparable results came from a similar experiment in cynomolgus monkeys. Multiple studies also support the efficacy of aflibercept in maintaining the blood-retinal barrier.[23] Phase III trials of aflibercept, VEGF Trap-Eye: Investigation of Efficacy and Safety in Wet Age-Related Macular Degeneration 1 and 2 (VIEW trials 1 and 2), showed noninferiority of visual acuity outcomes in patients treated with aflibercept compared to ranibizumab at 1 year.[24] Controlled Phase III Evaluation of Repeated Intravitreal Administration of VEGF Trap-Eye in Central Retinal Vein Occlusion (COPERNICUS) and General Assessment Limiting Infiltration of Exudates in Central Retinal Vein Occlusion with VEGF Trap-Eye (GALILEO), with more recent Protocol T results from the DRCR Network, also support the use of aflibercept in the treatment of macular edema secondary to retinal vein occlusions and diabetic macular edema.[23]

Conclusion

Identification of VEGF as a target to affect pathologic angiogenesis led to a paradigm shift in the treatment of ocular neovascularization. Anti-VEGF agents are now administered to millions of patients by intravitreal injection to treat the anterior and posterior segment. Some of these medications were developed with this intent, while others were repurposed when promise was recognized. Available anti-VEGF agents have provided us with the ability to protect and preserve vision. The need for repeated administration of these ophthalmic drugs has led to research pursuing longer-acting therapeutics and intraocular drug delivery systems. Still, further work focuses on the development of medications that can be administered topically. As we await the next dramatic advance in treatment, we continue to study medications currently in use to better assess their safety characteristics and make more informed recommendations regarding therapeutic options.

References

1. Adamis AP, Miller JW, Bernal MT, et al. Increased vascular endothelial growth factor levels in the vitreous of eyes with proliferative diabetic retinopathy. *Am J Ophthalmol.* 1994;118(4):445-450.
2. Aiello LP, Avery RL, Arrigg PG, et al. Vascular endothelial growth factor in ocular fluid of patients with diabetic retinopathy and other retinal disorders. *N Engl J Med.* 1994;331(22):1480-1487.
3. Kvanta A, Algvere PV, Berglin L, Seregard S. Subfoveal fibrovascular membranes in age-related macular degeneration express vascular endothelial growth factor. *Invest Ophthalmol Vis Sci.* 1996;37(9):1929-1934.
4. Lopez PF, Sippy BD, Lambert HM, Thach AB, Hinton DR. Transdifferentiated retinal pigment epithelial cells are immunoreactive for vascular endothelial growth factor in surgically excised age-related macular degeneration-related choroidal neovascular membranes. *Invest Ophthalmol Vis Sci.* 1996;37(5):855-868.
5. Miller JW, Adamis AP, Shima DT, et al. Vascular endothelial growth factor/vascular permeability factor is temporally and spatially correlated with ocular angiogenesis in a primate model. *Am J Pathol.* 1994;145(3):574-584.

6. Tolentino MJ, Miller JW, Gragoudas ES, Chatzistefanou K, Ferrara N, Adamis AP. Vascular endothelial growth factor is sufficient to produce iris neovascularization and neovascular glaucoma in a nonhuman primate. *Arch Ophthalmol.* 1996;114(8):964-970.

7. Adamis AP, Shima DT, Tolentino MJ, et al. Inhibition of vascular endothelial growth factor prevents retinal ischemia-associated iris neovascularization in a nonhuman primate. *Arch Ophthalmol.* 1996;114(1):66-71.

8. Aiello LP, Pierce EA, Foley ED, et al. Suppression of retinal neovascularization in vivo by inhibition of vascular endothelial growth factor (VEGF) using soluble VEGF-receptor chimeric proteins. *Proc Natl Acad Sci U S A.* 1995;92(23):10457-10461.

9. Robinson GS, Pierce EA, Rook SL, Foley E, Webb R, Smith LE. Oligodeoxynucleotides inhibit retinal neovascularization in a murine model of proliferative retinopathy. *Proc Natl Acad Sci U S A.* 1996;93(10):4851-4856.

10. Schlingemann RO, van Hinsbergh VW. Role of vascular permeability factor/vascular endothelial growth factor in eye disease. *Br J Ophthalmol.* 1997;81(6):501-512.

11. Ng EW, Shima DT, Calias P, Cunningham ET Jr, Guyer DR, Adamis AP. Pegaptanib, a targeted anti-VEGF aptamer for ocular vascular disease. *Nat Rev Drug Discov.* 2006;5(2):123-132.

12. Ruckman J, Green LS, Beeson J, et al. 2'-Fluoropyrimidine RNA-based aptamers to the 165-amino acid form of vascular endothelial growth factor (VEGF165). Inhibition of receptor binding and VEGF-induced vascular permeability through interactions requiring the exon 7-encoded domain. *J Biol Chem.* 1998;273(32):20556-20567.

13. Eyetech Study Group. Preclinical and phase 1A clinical evaluation of an anti-VEGF pegylated aptamer (EYE001) for the treatment of exudative age-related macular degeneration. *Retina.* 2002;22(2):143-152.

14. Macugen AMD Study Group, Apte RS, Modi M, et al. Pegaptanib 1-year systemic safety results from a safety-pharmacokinetic trial in patients with neovascular age-related macular degeneration. *Ophthalmology.* 2007;114(9):1702-1712.

15. Eyetech Study Group. Anti-vascular endothelial growth factor therapy for subfoveal choroidal neovascularization secondary to age-related macular degeneration: phase II study results. *Ophthalmology.* 2003;110(5):979-986.

16. Meyer CH, Holz FG. Preclinical aspects of anti-VEGF agents for the treatment of wet AMD: ranibizumab and bevacizumab. *Eye (Lond).* 2011;25(6):661-672.

17. Ferrara N, Hillan KJ, Gerber HP, Novotny W. Discovery and development of bevacizumab, an anti-VEGF antibody for treating cancer. *Nat Rev Drug Discov.* 2004;3(5):391-400.

18. Bakri SJ, Snyder MR, Reid JM, Pulido JS, Singh RJ. Pharmacokinetics of intravitreal bevacizumab (Avastin). *Ophthalmology.* 2007;114(5):855-859.

19. Bakri SJ, Snyder MR, Reid JM, Pulido JS, Ezzat MK, Singh RJ. Pharmacokinetics of intravitreal ranibizumab (Lucentis). *Ophthalmology.* 2007;114(12):2179-2182.

20. Shahar J, Avery RL, Heilweil G, et al. Electrophysiologic and retinal penetration studies following intravitreal injection of bevacizumab (Avastin). *Retina.* 2006;26(3):262-269.

21. Michels S, Rosenfeld PJ, Puliafito CA, Marcus EN, Venkatraman AS. Systemic bevacizumab (Avastin) therapy for neovascular age-related macular degeneration twelve-week results of an uncontrolled open-label clinical study. *Ophthalmology.* 2005;112(6):1035-1047.

22. Moshfeghi AA, Rosenfeld PJ, Puliafito CA, et al. Systemic bevacizumab (Avastin) therapy for neovascular age-related macular degeneration: twenty-four-week results of an uncontrolled open-label clinical study. *Ophthalmology.* 2006;113(11):2002-2011.e2

23. Keane PA, Sadda SR. Development of anti-VEGF therapies for intraocular use: a guide for clinicians. *J Ophthalmol.* 2012;2012:483034.

24. Heier JS, Brown DM, Chong V, et al. Intravitreal aflibercept (VEGF trap-eye) in wet age-related macular degeneration. *Ophthalmology.* 2012;119(12):2537-2548.

3

Available Anti-Vascular Endothelial Growth Factor Agents

Angeline Mariani Derham, MD and
David M. Brown, MD, FACS

Pegaptanib

Pharmacology

Pegaptanib sodium (Macugen) is a 50 kDa pegylated modified oligonucleotide aptamer that adopts a 3-dimensional shape to selectively inhibit extracellular vascular endothelial growth factor $(VEGF)_{165}$, the major VEGF-A isoform in the eye.[1] Aptamers are single-stranded nucleotides that bind with high affinity and specificity to predetermined target molecules such as proteins and peptides.[2] These aptamers are selected in vitro using the systematic evolution of ligands by exponential enrichment technique to isolate oligonucleotide ligands that bind to a variety of proteins.[3] Because VEGF is a secreted protein that binds to and activates receptors located predominantly on the surface of vascular endothelial cells, a selective antagonist in the form of a modified aptamer mitigates VEGF-induced angiogenesis, vascular permeability, and inflammation.[4]

Therapeutic Efficacy

Pegaptanib, approved by the United States (US) Food and Drug Administration (FDA) in 2004, was the first anti-VEGF agent approved for ocular use. It is currently approved for the treatment of neovascular age-related macular degeneration (AMD) as a 0.3 mg intravitreal injection every 6 weeks.[1]

The first preclinical and phase Ia evaluation of the pegylated aptamer was conducted by the Eyetech Study Group in 2002. They found that patients with neovascular AMD had no adverse outcomes related to the drug and 80% of patients experienced stable or improved vision 3 months after the injection.[5] A larger subsequent trial involving 1186

Duker JS, Liang MC, eds.
*Anti-VEGF Use in
Ophthalmology (pp. 19-27).*
© 2017 Taylor & Francis Group.

patients with neovascular AMD proved efficacy of pegaptanib across 3 dosages, 0.3 mg, 1.0 mg, and 3.0 mg, compared to sham injection, but were unable to find a dose-response relationship.[6] Various randomized trials have since been conducted displaying therapeutic benefits from pegaptanib in patients with macular edema secondary to retinal vein occlusions, Von Hippel-Lindau disease, diabetic macular edema, and diabetic retinopathy.[7-10]

Despite its early advantage, the emergence of additional anti-VEGF agents with wider isoform antagonism has limited the use of pegaptanib. More recent clinical trials focus on pegaptanib as a supplemental therapy, such as preoperative injection to improve surgical outcomes of patients with proliferative diabetic retinopathy. The concept behind this use is that the selectivity of pegaptanib may result in regression of neovascularization with a diminished tractional response compared with pan-anti-VEGF agents that can result in a "crunch" tractional retinal detachment phenomenon.[11]

Conclusions

The first intravitreal anti-VEGF agent to be approved by the FDA, pegaptanib was a monumental discovery in the treatment of AMD. It was quickly replaced with newer, broader-acting anti-VEGF agents; however, there is continued interest in using pegaptanib as a supplemental treatment.

Ranibizumab

Pharmacology

Ranibizumab (Lucentis), the first VEGF inhibitor designed specifically for ocular use, is a 48 kDa recombinant humanized immunoglobulin G1 kappa monoclonal antibody fragment that binds to and inhibits VEGF-A.[12] Its lack of a fragment crystallizable region results in a more rapid systemic clearance.[13] It is produced by an *Escherichia coli* expression system in a growth medium containing tetracycline. The advantage of protein expression in *E coli* is the ability to express and purify a desired recombinant protein in large quantities.[14]

Therapeutic Efficacy

Approved by the FDA in 2006, ranibizumab was the second anti-VEGF agent approved for ocular use. It is currently approved for the treatment of neovascular AMD, diabetic macular edema, diabetic retinopathy, macular edema following retinal vein occlusion, and more recently, choroidal neovascularization secondary to pathologic myopia.

For patients with neovascular AMD, ranibizumab is approved as a monthly 0.5 mg intravitreal injection, with less frequent injections allowable after the first 3 or 4 months.[12] There were 4 large, randomized phase III studies evaluating the safety and efficacy of ranibizumab in neovascular AMD. In Study AMD-1 (Minimally Classic/Occult Trial of the Anti-VEGF Antibody Ranibizumab in the Treatment of Neovascular AMD [MARINA]) and Study AMD-2 (Anti-VEGF Antibody for the Treatment of Predominantly Classic Choroidal Neovascularization in AMD [ANCHOR]), patients received monthly 0.3 mg ranibizumab, 0.5 mg ranibizumab, sham injections, or verteporfin (photodynamic therapy, PDT) for 2 years. MARINA patients had minimally classic or occult neovascularization, whereas ANCHOR patients had predominantly classic neovascularization. Both studies showed ranibizumab to be effective and safe in neovascular AMD patients with differing anatomically categorized disease.[15,16] In Study AMD-3 (PIER), patients received 0.3 mg ranibizumab, 0.5 mg ranibizumab, or sham injections monthly for 3 consecutive doses, followed by a mandated dose every 3 months for a total of 24 months. This study treated a wider variety of lesion subtypes and also showed an improvement in ranibizumab-treated patients compared to sham.[17,18] These trials advocated for the use of ranibizumab in all angiographic subtypes of neovascular AMD and across lesions of all sizes.[15-18] Study AMD-4 (HARBOR) was a dose-response study in which 1098 patients received monthly or pro re nata (PRN) ranibizumab injections of either 0.5 mg or 2.0 mg following 3 initial monthly injections. Although all groups experienced visual improvement, the 2.0 mg monthly group did not meet the prespecified superiority comparison and the 0.5 mg and 2.0 mg PRN groups did not meet the prespecified noninferiority comparison. This study confirmed that 0.5 mg doses of ranibizumab monthly provides the best results in patients with neovascular AMD.[19-20]

For patients with diabetic macular edema or diabetic retinopathy, ranibizumab is approved for a monthly 0.3 mg intravitreal injection.[12] This indication was evaluated in 2 pivotal parallel trials (RISE and RIDE) in which 759 patients were assigned to monthly ranibizumab 0.3 mg or 0.5 mg or sham injection for 24 months.[21] All outcome measures were superior in ranibizumab-treated patients as compared to sham, and these benefits were maintained at 36 months.[22]

For patients with choroidal neovascularization secondary to pathologic myopia, ranibizumab was recently approved as a 0.5 mg intravitreal injection with allowable repeated treatment at monthly intervals.[12] The clinical benefit of ranibizumab in these patients was demonstrated in a randomized phase III trial known as RADIANCE. In this trial, intravitreal ranibizumab was found to be superior to intravenous verteporfin plus PDT. Improvements in vision were sustained for up to 12 months in ranibizumab recipients and were mirrored by improvements in anatomic outcomes.[23]

For patients with macular edema following retinal vein occlusion, ranibizumab is approved as a monthly 0.5 mg intravitreal injection.[12] Study RVO-1 (Branch Retinal Vein Occlusion: Evaluation of Efficacy and Safety [BRAVO]) and Study RVO-2 (Central Retinal Vein Occlusion Study: Evaluation of Efficacy and Safety [CRUISE]) were parallel studies that analyzed the use of ranibizumab for patients with center-involved macular edema following branch (397 patients) and central (392 patients) retinal vein occlusions, respectively. Both studies had a treatment period of 6 months of monthly 0.3 mg or 0.5 mg ranibizumab or sham injection followed by a 6-month observation period. Results demonstrated a greater improvement in best-corrected visual acuity (BCVA) in both treatment groups compared to sham.[24-27]

Conclusions

Ranibizumab is a safe treatment strategy for a variety of retinal diseases, including neovascular AMD, diabetic macular edema, diabetic retinopathy, choroidal neovascularization secondary to pathologic myopia, and macular edema following retinal vein occlusion. It was the first anti-VEGF agent designed and approved for ocular use. Ongoing research focuses on adjusting dosing regimen and treatment schedule.

Bevacizumab

Pharmacology

Bevacizumab (Avastin) is a 140 kDa recombinant humanized monoclonal antibody that binds to VEGF-A.[28] It is a much larger molecule than ranibizumab, which theoretically may limit efficacy and contribute to a weaker binding affinity. Nevertheless, it has been proven to penetrate the retina[29] and comparative trials have showed near equivalence in clinical efficacy.[30,31]

Therapeutic Efficacy

Bevacizumab, initially designed for non-ocular use, was approved by the FDA in 2004 for metastatic colorectal cancer.[32] It is currently approved for treating a range of cancers, including angiosarcoma, cervical cancer, endometrial cancer, ovarian cancer, glioblastoma, renal cell carcinoma, colorectal cancer, and small-cell lung cancer, and is used off-label for metastatic breast cancer and a variety of ocular diseases including neovascular AMD.[28,33] Because no industry-sponsored ophthalmology trials were conducted, ocular use of bevacizumab is strictly off-label. As it is less expensive than both ranibizumab and aflibercept, it is an appealing alternative to the FDA-approved medications, especially in patients undergoing monthly injections in one or both eyes.

Postinjection endophthalmitis is a risk for any intravitreal injection, but because bevacizumab is not provided as an individual dose, it must be compounded by a local pharmacy into ready-to-use syringes. For this reason, publicized outbreaks of endophthalmitis have been caused by contamination at the time of compounding.[34] Nevertheless, studies have shown that after controlling for age, race, sex, injection-related diagnosis, and year of injection, there is no significant association with development of endophthalmitis after an injection of bevacizumab compared to ranibizumab.[35]

With regard to systemic adverse events, a meta-analysis of 9 studies found no difference in adverse events between bevacizumab and ranibizumab in the first 2 years of treatment, but did find a higher risk of gastrointestinal disorders in patients treated with bevacizumab in their secondary analysis.[36] In the United Kingdom-based Age-Related Choroidal Neovascularization (IVAN) trial, fewer patients in the bevacizumab group experienced arteriothrombotic events or heart failure than in the ranibizumab group. Another interesting finding was that patient median serum VEGF concentrations at one year were lower for bevacizumab than for ranibizumab.[37]

A large multicenter study, the Comparison of Age-related Macular Degeneration Treatments Trials (CATT), aimed to elucidate whether bevacizumab and ranibizumab were clinically equivalent and whether monthly vs as-needed treatments were clinically equivalent. After the 2-year endpoint, CATT found that visual outcomes between the 2 groups were statistically insignificant but that anatomic markers for dry eyes as measured by optical coherence tomography were more common in eyes treated with ranibizumab.[30]

Conclusions

Bevacizumab is an off-label alternative to the other anti-VEGF agents. It is a much cheaper therapeutic regimen and, despite initial safety and efficacy concerns, has proven to be an effective way to treat many ocular diseases.

Aflibercept

Pharmacology

Aflibercept (Eylea) is a 115 kDa glycosylated dimeric human VEGF receptor fusion protein created with Trap technology in which portions of 2 receptors (extracellular domains of VEGF-R1 and VEGF-R2) are fused with the immunoglobulin constant region of human immunoglobulin G1.[38,39] This creates a soluble decoy receptor with a ligand-binding affinity more potent than the individual native endogenous receptors. Aflibercept binds to VEGF-A, VEGF-B, and placental growth factor and demonstrates higher binding affinity for VEGF-A when compared to previously designed anti-VEGF agents.[40]

Therapeutic Efficacy

Aflibercept was approved by the FDA for the treatment of neovascular AMD in 2011. Since then, it has also been approved for macular edema following retinal vein occlusion, diabetic macular edema, and diabetic retinopathy on different scheduled regimens. In addition, it has been approved in various countries outside the US for the treatment of choroidal neovascularization secondary to myopia.

For patients with neovascular AMD, aflibercept is approved as a 2 mg intravitreal injection every 2 months following 3 initial monthly injections.[39] The phase I and II Clinical Evaluation of Anti-Angiogenesis in the Retina (CLEAR) trials examined the safety, pharmacokinetics, and biological activity of aflibercept in neovascular AMD patients[41-43] and the CLEAR IT 2 trial refined the dosing regimens for the subsequent VIEW trials.[42] The VEGF Trap-Eye: Investigation of Efficacy and Safety in Wet AMD (VIEW 1 and VIEW 2) trials were large, randomized, controlled phase III trials, enrolling 1217 and 1240 patients, respectively. VIEW 1 was conducted in the US and Canada, and VIEW 2 was conducted across Europe, Middle East, Asia-Pacific, and Latin America. Both trials were similarly designed to compare 3 different dosing regimens of aflibercept (0.5 mg every 4 weeks, 2 mg every 4 weeks, and 2 mg every 8 weeks after 3 initial monthly doses) compared to 0.5 mg ranibizumab every 4 weeks. They found all 3 dosing groups of aflibercept to be noninferior and clinically equivalent to ranibizumab at 52 weeks.[44] In the second year of the VIEW trials, all groups were found to be equally effective in improving BCVA and preventing BCVA loss at 96 weeks.[45]

For patients with macular edema following retinal vein occlusion, aflibercept is approved as a 2 mg intravitreal injection administered monthly.[39] The parallel trials General Assessment Limiting Infiltration of Exudates in Central Retinal Vein Occlusion with VEGF Trap-Eye (GALILEO) (Europe and Asia-Pacific) and Controlled Phase III Evaluation of Repeated Intravitreal Administration of VEGF Trap-Eye in Central Retinal Vein Occlusion (COPERNICUS) (US, Canada, Columbia, India, and Israel) proved monthly 2 mg aflibercept injections followed by PRN treatment superior to sham injection in 365 patients with macular edema secondary to central retinal vein occlusion.[46,47] The phase III VIBRANT trial (North America and Japan) randomized 183 eyes with macular edema following branch retinal vein occlusion to 2 mg aflibercept group or laser photocoagulation and sham groups. Patients in the aflibercept group received a 2 mg injection every 4 weeks through week 20, followed by every 8 weeks through week 48. Significantly greater visual and anatomic improvements in the aflibercept group were maintained by week 52.[48]

For patients with diabetic macular edema, aflibercept is approved as a 2 mg intravitreal injection every 2 months following 5 initial monthly injections.[39] The VISTA (US) and VIVID (Europe, Japan, and Australia) studies randomized 872 patients with center-involved diabetic macular edema to aflibercept 2 mg every 4 weeks, 2 mg every 8 weeks after 5 initial monthly doses, or laser photocoagulation. Visual and anatomic gains were found to be superior in both aflibercept groups as compared to the laser group for both studies at 52 weeks[49] and maintained through week 100.[50] The Diabetic Retinopathy Clinical Research Network-led Protocol T trial was the first trial comparing 3 of the most widely used anti-VEGF agents for center-involved diabetic macular edema. A total of 660 patients were randomized to arms with 2 mg aflibercept, 0.3 mg ranibizumab, or 1.25 mg bevacizumab.[51] Patients treated with aflibercept had significantly greater BCVA gains from baseline (13.3 letters) compared with those treated with either ranibizumab (11.2 letters, $P = .03$) or bevacizumab (9.7 letters, $P < .001$) at 1 year, required 1 fewer injection, and had a lower proportion of patients requiring rescue treatment with laser compared with the other 2 groups. At 2 years, treatment benefits observed in year 1 were maintained across all 3 treatment groups.[52]

There is evidence to suggest that aflibercept is also a promising intervention for patients with recalcitrant disease. Small retrospective studies have shown that aflibercept therapy might be helpful for AMD patients exhibiting recurrent or resistant leakage despite prior anti-VEGF treatment.[53-55]

Conclusions

Aflibercept has been shown to improve both visual and anatomic outcomes with an acceptable safety profile in patients with neovascular AMD, macular edema following retinal vein occlusion, diabetic macular edema, and choroidal neovascularization in myopia. It is the first anti-VEGF agent demonstrating similar results whether given every 8 weeks following a loading dose or dosed monthly in patients with neovascular AMD and diabetic macular edema. Although it provides an alternative treatment regimen, the high cost of this newest anti-VEGF agent may be prohibitive for some patients but potentially worthwhile if treatment intervals can be extended.

References

1. Macugen [package insert]. Bridgewater, NJ: Bausch & Lomb Incorporated; 2004.
2. Hernandez LI, Machado I, Schafer T, Hernandez FJ. Aptamers overview: selection, features and applications. *Curr Top Med Chem.* 2015;15(12):1066-1081.
3. Trujillo CA, Nery AA, Alves JM, Martins AH, Ulrich H. Development of the anti-VEGF aptamer to a therapeutic agent for clinical ophthalmology. *Clin Ophthalmol.* 2007;1(4):393-402.
4. Leung DW, Cachianes G, Kuang WJ, Goeddel DV, Ferrara N. Vascular endothelial growth factor is a secreted angiogenic mitogen. *Science.* 1989;246(4935):1306-1309.

5. Eyetech Study Group. Preclinical and Phase 1A clinical evaluation of an anti-VEGF pegylated aptamer (EYE001) for the treatment of exudative age-related macular degeneration. *Retina.* 2002;22:143-152.

6. Gragoudas ES, Adamis AP, Cunningham ET Jr, Feinsod M, Guyer DR for the VEGF Inhibition Study in Ocular Neovascularization Clinical Trial Group. Pegaptanib for neovascular age-related macular degeneration. *N Engl J Med.* 2004;351(27):2805-2816.

7. Wroblewski JJ, Wells JA 3rd, Gonzales CR. Pegaptanib sodium for macular edema secondary to branch retinal vein occlusion. *Am J Ophthalmol.* 2010;149(1):147-154.

8. Wroblewski JJ, Wells JA 3rd, Adamis AP, et al. Pegaptanib sodium for macular edema secondary to central retinal vein occlusion. *Arch Ophthalmol.* 2009;127(4):374-380.

9. Dahr SS, Cusick M, Rodriguez-Coleman H, et al. Intravitreal anti-vascular endothelial growth factor therapy with pegaptanib for advanced von Hippel-Lindau disease of the retina. *Retina.* 2007;27(2):150-158.

10. Cunningham ET Jr, Adamis AP, Altaweel M, et al. A phase II randomized double-masked trial of pegaptanib, an anti-vascular endothelial growth factor aptamer, for diabetic macular edema. *Ophthalmology.* 2005;112(10):1747-1757.

11. Oellers P, Mahmoud TH. Surgery for proliferative diabetic retinopathy: new tips and tricks. *J Ophthalmic Vis Res.* 2016;11(1):93-99.

12. Lucentis [package insert]. San Francisco, CA: Genentech; 2006.

13. Ferrara N, Damico L, Shams N, et al. Development of ranibizumab, an anti-vascular endothelial growth factor antigen binding fragment, as therapy for neovascular age-related macular degeneration. *Retina.* 2006;26(8):859-870.

14. Rosano GL, Ceccarelli EA. Recombinant protein expression in Escherichia coli: advances and challenges. *Front Microbiol.* 2014;5:172.

15. Rosenfeld PJ, Brown DM, Heier JS, et al. Ranibizumab for neovascular age-related macular degeneration. *N Engl J Med.* 2006;355(14):1419-1431.

16. Boyer DS, Antoszyk AN, Awh CC, et al. Subgroup analysis of the MARINA study of ranibizumab in neovascular age-related macular degeneration. *Ophthalmology.* 2007;114(2):246-252.

17. Regillo CD, Brown DM, Abraham P, et al. Randomized, double-masked, sham-controlled trial of ranibizumab for neovascular age-related macular degeneration: PIER study year 1. *Am J Ophthalmol.* 2008;145:239-248.

18. Abraham P, Yue H, Wilson L. Randomized, double-masked, sham-controlled trial of ranibizumab for neovascular age-related macular degeneration: PIER study year 2. *Am J Ophthalmol.* 2010;150(3):315-324.e1.

19. Busbee BG, Ho AC, Brown DM, et al. Twelve-month efficacy and safety of 0.5 mg or 2.0 mg ranibizumab in patients with subfoveal neovascular age-related macular degeneration. *Ophthalmology.* 2013;120(5):1046-1056.

20. Ho AC, Busbee BG, Regillo CD, et al. Twenty-four-month efficacy and safety of 0.5 mg or 2.0 mg ranibizumab in patients with subfoveal neovascular age-related macular degeneration. *Ophthalmology.* 2014;121(11):2181-2192.

21. Nguyen QD, Brown DM, Marcus DM, et al. Ranibizumab for diabetic macular edema: results from 2 phase III randomized trials: RISE and RIDE. *Ophthalmology.* 2012;119(4):789-801.

22. Brown DM, Nguyen QD, Marcus DM, et al. Long-term outcomes of ranibizumab therapy for diabetic macular edema: the 36-month results from two phase III trials: RISE and RIDE. *Ophthalmology.* 2013;120(10):2013-2022.

23. Wolf S, Balciuniene VJ, Laganovska G, et al. RADIANCE: a randomized controlled study of ranibizumab in patients with choroidal neovascularization secondary to pathologic myopia. *Ophthalmology.* 2014;121(3):682-692.

24. Campochiaro PA, Heier JS, Feiner L, et al. Ranibizumab for macular edema following branch retinal vein occlusion: six-month primary endpoint results of a phase III study. *Ophthalmology.* 2010;117:1102-1112.

25. Brown DM, Campochiaro PA, Bhisitkul RB, et al. Sustained benefits from ranibizumab for macular edema following branch retinal vein occlusion: 12-month outcomes of a Phase III study. *Ophthalmology.* 2011;118:1594-1602.

26. Brown DM, Campochiaro PA, Singh RP, et al. Ranibizumab for macular edema following central retinal vein occlusion: six-month primary end point results of a Phase III study. *Ophthalmology.* 2010;117:1124-1133.e1.

27. Campochiaro PA, Brown DM, Awh CC, et al. Sustained benefits from ranibizumab for macular edema following central retinal vein occlusion: twelve-month outcomes of a Phase III study. *Ophthalmology.* 2011;118:2041-2049.

28. Avastin® [package insert]. South San Francisco, CA, USA: Genentech. 2004.

29. Heiduschka P, Fietz H, Hofmeister S, et al. Penetration of bevacizumab through the retina after intravitreal injection in the monkey. *Invest Ophthalmol Vis Sci.* 2007;48(6):2814-2823.

30. CATT Research Group, Martin DF, Maguire MG, et al. Ranibizumab and bevacizumab for neovascular age-related macular degeneration. *N Engl J Med.* 2011;364(20):1897-1908.

31. Ruiz-Moreno JM, Montero JA, Araiz J, et al. Intravitreal anti-vascular endothelial growth factor therapy for choroidal neovascularization secondary to pathologic myopia: six years outcome. *Retina.* 2015;35(12):2450-2456.

32. Hurwitz H, Fehrenbacher L, Novotny W, et al. Bevacizumab plus irinotecan, fluorouracil, and leucovorin for metastatic colorectal cancer. *N Engl J Med.* 2004;350:2335-2342.

33. Avery RL, Pieramici DJ, Rabena MD, et al. Intravitreal bevacizumab (Avastin) for neovascular age-related macular degeneration. *Ophthalmology.* 2006;113:363-372.

34. Sigford DK, Reddy S, Mollineaux C, Schaal S. Global reported endophthalmitis risk following intravitreal injections of anti-VEGF: a literature review and analysis. *Clin Ophthalmol.* 2015;9:773-781.

35. VanderBeek BL, Bonaffini SG, Ma L. Association of compounded bevacizumab with postinjection endophthalmitis. *JAMA Ophthalmol.* 2015;133(10):1159-1164.

36. Moja L, Lucenteforte E, Kwag KH, et al. Systemic safety of bevacizumab versus ranibizumab for neovascular age-related macular degeneration. *Cochrane Database Syst Rev.* 2014;9:CD011230.

37. IVAN Study Investigators, Chakravarthy U, Harding SP, et al. Ranibizumab versus bevacizumab to treat neovascular age-related macular degeneration: one-year findings from the IVAN randomized trial. *Ophthalmology.* 2012;119(7):1399-1411.

38. Holash J, Davis S, Papadopoulos N, et al. VEGF-Trap: a VEGF blocker with potent antitumor effects. *Proc Natl Acad Sci U S A.* 2002;99:11393-11398.

39. Eylea® [package insert]. Tarrytown, NY, USA: Regeneron. 2011.

40. Papadopoulos N, Martin J, Ruan Q, et al. Binding and neutralization of vascular endothelial growth factor (VEGF) and related ligands by VEGF Trap, ranibizumab and bevacizumab. *Angiogenesis.* 2012;15:171-185.

41. Nguyen QD, Shah SM, Hafiz G, et al. A phase I trial of an IV-administered vascular endothelial growth factor trap for treatment in patients with choroidal neovascularization due to age-related macular degeneration. *Ophthalmology.* 2006;113(9):1522.e1-1522.e14.

42. Heier JS, Boyer D, Nguyen QD, et al. The 1-year results of CLEAR-IT 2, a phase 2 study of vascular endothelial growth factor trap-eye dosed as-needed after 12-week fixed dosing. *Ophthalmology.* 2011;118:1098-1106.

43. Nguyen QD, Campochiaro PA, Shah SM, et al. Evaluation of very high- and very low-dose intravitreal aflibercept in patients with neovascular age-related macular degeneration. *J Ocul Pharmacol Ther.* 2012;28(6):581-588.

44. Heier JS, Brown DM, Chong V, et al. Intravitreal aflibercept (VEGF trap-eye) in wet age-related macular degeneration. *Ophthalmology.* 2012;119:2537-2548.

45. Schmidt-Erfurth U, Kaiser PK, Korobelnik JF, et al. Intravitreal aflibercept injection for neovascular age-related macular degeneration: ninety-six-week results of the VIEW studies. *Ophthalmology.* 2014;121(1):193-201.

46. Ogura Y, Roider J, Korobelnik JF, et al. Intravitreal aflibercept for macular edema secondary to central retinal vein occlusion: 18-month results of the phase 3 GALILEO study. *Am J Ophthalmol.* 2014;158:1032-1038.

47. Heier JS, Clark WL, Boyer DS, et al. Intravitreal aflibercept injection for macular edema due to central retinal vein occlusion: two-year results from the COPERNICUS study. *Ophthalmology.* 2014;121(7):1414-1420.e1.

48. Clark WL, Boyer DS, Heier JS, et al. Intravitreal aflibercept for macular edema following branch retinal vein occlusion: 52-week results of the VIBRANT Study. *Ophthalmology.* 2016;123(2):330-336.

49. Korobelnik JF, Do DV, Schmidt-Erfurth U, et al. Intravitreal aflibercept for diabetic macular edema. *Ophthalmology.* 2014;121:2247-2254.

50. Brown DM, Schmidt-Erfurth U, Do DV, et al. Intravitreal aflibercept for diabetic macular edema: 100-week results from the VISTA and VIVID Studies. *Ophthalmology.* 2015;122(10):2044-2052.

51. Diabetic Retinopathy Clinical Research Network, Wells JA, Glassman AR, et al. Aflibercept, bevacizumab, or ranibizumab for diabetic macular edema. *N Engl J Med.* 2015;372(13):1193-1203.

52. Wells JA, Glassman AR, Ayala AR, et al. Aflibercept, bevacizumab, or ranibizumab for diabetic macular edema: two-year results from a comparative effectiveness randomized clinical trial. *Ophthalmology.* 2016;123(6):1351-1359.

53. Grewal DS, Gill MK, Sarezky D, Lyon AT, Mirza RG. Visual and anatomical outcomes following intravitreal aflibercept in eyes with recalcitrant neovascular age-related macular degeneration: 12-month results. *Eye (Lond).* 2014;28(7):895-899.

54. Wykoff CC, Brown DM, Maldonado ME, Croft DE. Aflibercept treatment for patients with exudative age-related macular degeneration who were incomplete responders to multiple ranibizumab injections (TURF trial). *Br J Ophthalmol.* 2014;98(7):951-955.

55. Major JC, Wykoff CC, Croft DE, et al. Aflibercept for pigment epithelial detachment for previously treated neovascular age-related macular degeneration. *Can J Ophthalmol.* 2015;50(5):373-377.

4

AGENTS UNDER STUDY

Ehsan Rahimy, MD; Elham Rahimy, BS; and
Anthony Joseph, MD

The advent of intravitreal anti-vascular endothelial growth factor (VEGF) therapy has undoubtedly revolutionized the field of ophthalmology and how physicians manage many potentially debilitating retinal conditions. In the recently published 5-year outcomes with anti-VEGF therapy from the Comparison of Age-Related Macular Degeneration Treatment Trials, a remarkable 50% of follow-up participants had visual acuity of 20/40 or better; however, 20% of individuals had acuity of 20/200 or worse.[1] While this represents a significant improvement over previous natural history studies prior to the commencement of the anti-VEGF era, it is a reminder that much work remains to be accomplished.

In an effort to reduce the overall treatment burden of serial anti-VEGF injections on retinal specialists, patients, caregivers, and society at large, numerous targeted therapies are under investigation to further improve patient outcomes and decrease overall costs of treatment to the health care system. This chapter will serve to summarize some of the most pertinent programs in development, and is broken down based on the different routes of drug delivery: gene therapy, intravitreal injections, systemic therapy, and topical treatment.

Gene Therapy

The goal of gene therapy is to provide continual expression of a protein(s) of interest involved in the pathogenesis of a disease for sustained therapeutic benefit. Gene therapy for retinal degenerative diseases is a field receiving significant research and developmental focus recently, as a number of therapies are progressing to human clinical trials. In these individuals, a viral vector is used to carry the desired genetic information encoding a protein(s) of interest into the target cells. Successfully transduced vectors then use the host cell's machinery to express the particular protein(s). Two main categories of vectors are being investigated: integrating vectors and nonintegrating vectors. Integrating

Duker JS, Liang MC, eds.
*Anti-VEGF Use in
Ophthalmology (pp. 29-45).*
© 2017 Taylor & Francis Group.

vectors (ie, lentiviral vectors) insert themselves into the recipient's genome, whereas nonintegrating vectors (ie, adeno-associated virus [AAV]) usually form an extrachromosomal genetic element.

Intravitreal Adeno-Associated Virus 2-sFLT01

The secreted extracellular domain of sFlt-1 is a soluble isoform of the VEGF receptor 1 and a naturally occurring protein antagonist of VEGF. Adeno-associated virus type 2 (AAV2)-sFLT01 (Genzyme) is a replication-deficient AAV vector with a plasmid that expresses a portion of the sFlt1 receptor termed *sFlt01*.[2] The viral vector is injected intravitreally, after which it transfects native cells to produce the modified protein. It has been shown to be well tolerated in monkeys.[3] Intravitreal AAV2-*sFLT01* is currently being studied in phase I clinical trials in humans with neovascular age-related macular degeneration (AMD).[4]

Subretinal AVA-101 and Intravitreal AVA-102

Like Genzyme's lead candidate, AAV2-sFLT01, Avalanche Biotechnologies developed a similar replication-deficient AAV2 vector containing the sFLT-1 plasmid (AVA-101). However, in contrast to the intravitreal approach, AVA-101 is injected into the subretinal space, requiring concurrent vitrectomy surgery.

Phase I studies demonstrated AVA-101 to be well tolerated in the 6 study participants with no significant drug-related safety concerns.[5] Topline results from a phase IIa study involving 32 patients with advanced AMD became available in 2015.[6] Patients were randomized to the AVA-101 treatment group ($n = 21$) or control ($n = 11$). Participants in both arms received 2 initial ranibizumab (Lucentis) injections at day 0 and week 4, followed by ranibizumab rescue therapy as early as week 8, according to prespecified criteria. Twenty-nine of 32 individuals received prior anti-VEGF therapy (average of 10 prior injections). The reported data met the primary endpoint in terms of ophthalmic and systemic safety measures; however, secondary endpoints assessing functional and anatomic outcomes were not as clear. In terms of visual improvement, the mean change from baseline showed a difference of 11.5 letters between the treatment (2.2 letters gained) and the ranibizumab control (9.3 letters lost) groups. The degree of vision loss in the control group was uncharacteristic, but was attributed to the refractory nature of disease displayed by many of the study's participants as they received extensive previous anti-VEGF treatment prior to enrollment. A significant number of AVA-101-treated patients (43%) improved or maintained stable vision with 2 or fewer rescue injections, compared with individuals in the control group (9%). With regards to anatomic changes, the treatment group demonstrated a mean increase of 25 μm over baseline in central retinal thickness measurements on optical coherence tomography (OCT) compared to a mean decrease of 56 μm in the control group.[6]

Avalanche reported in late 2015 that it will not proceed with a phase IIb trial on AVA-101 and its focus has shifted toward developing its next-generation candidate, AVA-201. In contrast to AVA-101, which uses a wild-type AAV2 vector, AVA-201 employs a novel vector that has been optimized for delivery via intravitreal injection. Because of the less-invasive route of administration and potential for 1-time dosing, the company is exploring AVA-201 as a potential prevention therapy for patients with high risk of progression from non-neovascular to neovascular AMD.[7]

Subretinal RetinoStat

RetinoStat (Oxford BioMedica) is an equine infectious anemia viral lentiviral vector expressing the genes of 2 naturally occurring inhibitors of angiogenesis, endostatin and angiostatin. Subretinal injection of RetinoStat in monkey and rabbit models have been shown to be capable of persistent, localized gene expression.[8,9] On the basis of preclinical data, it is anticipated that RetinoStat may require only a single administration if it proves to be safe and effective in human trials.

A phase I clinical trial enrolling 21 patients with advanced neovascular AMD to receive escalating doses of subretinally injected RetinoStat was recently completed.[10] The study met the primary endpoints of safety and tolerability at 6-month postsurgical transfection.[11] In addition, patients showed signs of clinical benefit, with stabilization of vision and an anatomic reduction in vascular leakage. Successful retinal transduction was demonstrated by a substantial increase in expression and secretion of endostatin and angiostatin proteins, as measured in the anterior chamber of the study's eyes.[11] Longer-term protein expression has been sustained for up to one year post-treatment, and preliminary data show a dose response, with the higher dose levels yielding a proportional increase in average protein expression.[11]

Intravitreal Therapy

RTH258

RTH258 (formerly ESBA1008) is a novel, humanized single-chain antibody fragment that inhibits all isoforms of VEGF-A. With a molecular weight of 26 kDa, RTH258 is smaller than any of the commercially available VEGF inhibitors. For comparison, the molecular weights of ranibizumab, aflibercept, and bevacizumab are 48 kDa, 115 kDa, and 150 kDa, respectively.[12] The smaller size of RTH258 may offer the following several potential advantages:

- Greater drug penetration into the desired ocular tissue[13]
- Delivery of a higher molar dose of medication in a given volume (RTH258 can be concentrated up to 120 mg/ml, allowing the administration of 6 mg in a single 50 μl intravitreal injection)[12,13]
- Formulation within a sustained release platform in the future
- Reduced risk of systemic side effects owing to the rapid systemic clearance[12,13]

The phase II OSPREY trial was a randomized, double-masked, controlled study that enrolled 89 patients with neovascular AMD to receive repeated doses of 6 mg RTH258 or aflibercept.[14] Both therapies were dosed upfront every 8 weeks through week 32, and then the dosing interval was increased to 12 weeks, with follow-up continuing to week 56. Throughout the course of the study, patients were reassessed monthly and could receive rescue treatment injections as needed. The results demonstrated promising visual acuity gains as well as fluid reduction in the RTH258 group that were noninferior to aflibercept, meeting the study's primary endpoint. Additionally, after the treatment interval was switched to every 12 weeks, patients in the RTH258 group continued to require fewer rescue treatments (60 vs 94 in the aflibercept arm), potentially leading to a reduced overall treatment burden (approximately half of patients in the RTH258 arm were successfully maintained on quarterly injections). Both treatments were well tolerated with no new safety concerns reported during the study.

On the heels of these positive phase II results, Alcon initiated a large phase III clinical study (HAWK) to evaluate the efficacy and safety of RTH258 vs aflibercept in neovascular AMD.[15] A target enrollment is set at approximately 1700 patients and is due for completion in 2018. The primary objective of the phase III study is to compare the efficacy of RTH258 (3 mg and 6 mg doses) vs aflibercept, with the mean visual change from baseline to week 48 as the primary endpoint. Participants will be dosed every 3 months with RTH258, while a bimonthly dosing regimen will be followed for those patients considered unsuitable for a quarterly dosing schedule because of their level of disease activity.

An implantable, refillable Posterior MicroPump is also being developed to allow for pulsatile intravitreal drug delivery of RTH258 over many months, which may help significantly reduce injection burden. In a separate phase II microvolume study evaluating RTH258 administered via Posterior MicroPump, clinical outcomes were compared in 13 patients randomly assigned to 1.2 mg of a 10-μL injection of RTH258 and 13 patients treated with an infusion of 1 mg in 8.3 μL RTH258.[16] For the primary endpoint, patients had to meet at least 3 of the following 4 criteria: a gain in best-corrected visual acuity (BCVA) of at least 4 letters at day 14 or at day 28, and a decrease in central subfield foveal thickness of at least 80 μm at day 14 or at day 28. This was met by 70% of patients in the injection group and 60% in the infusion group. The results of the microvolume study showed promise that a small volume of RTH258 can be successfully delivered via micropump. Further development is ongoing.

Abicipar

Another potential anti-VEGF agent under development is based on designed ankyrin repeat proteins, or DARPins for short. DARPins are genetically engineered proteins, typically with high-affinity binding to their respective target sites, that can be made into custom-designed therapeutics with optimized properties: small molecular size, high stability, high solubility, and low immunogenicity. Compared to monoclonal antibodies, DARPins appear to bind with similar high affinity and specificity to their targets, but in addition, show increased potency and longer ocular pharmacokinetics.[17]

The lead candidate in this class is abicipar pegol (previously MP0112, Allergan, and Molecular Partners), a small-molecular weight (34 kDa) DARPin with highly potent activity against all VEGF-A isoforms. In a rabbit model of VEGF-induced vasculopathy, abicipar demonstrated a higher binding affinity and longer vitreous half-life compared with ranibizumab, and provided superior duration of action compared with ranibizumab in equimolar dosages.[17,18]

A phase II clinical study of abicipar for the treatment of neovascular AMD (REACH) assessed the safety and treatment effects of 2 different doses of abicipar every 4 weeks in treatment-naïve patients. Sixty-four patients in total were randomized to 2 mg abicipar ($n = 23$), 1 mg abicipar ($n = 25$), or ranibizumab ($n = 16$) and were followed for 20 weeks.[19]All patients received intravitreal injections at day 1, week 4, and week 8. Patients in the ranibizumab arm of the study received additional doses at weeks 12 and 16. The results demonstrated that after 16 weeks (8 weeks after the last abicipar injection), mean visual acuity improvement from baseline was 8.2 letters for abicipar 2 mg, 6.3 letters for abicipar 1 mg, and 5.3 letters for ranibizumab. After 20 weeks (12 weeks after the last abicipar injection and 4 weeks after the last ranibizumab injection), mean visual acuity improvement from baseline was 9.0 letters for abicipar 2 mg, 7.1 letters for abicipar 1 mg, and 4.7 letters for ranibizumab. Anatomic improvements on OCT imaging were also supportive of the functional visual gains. While the study was not powered to show statistically significant differences between treatment groups, the data suggested that abicipar was at least as effective as monthly ranibizumab, with a longer duration of action.

Of note, during preclinical and early clinical studies, episodes of intraocular inflammation (uveitis, vitritis, choroiditis) related to abicipar were encountered.[17] Specifically, during the REACH trial, inflammatory events occurred in 2 patients treated with abicipar 2 mg, in 3 patients treated with abicipar 1 mg, and none receiving ranibizumab.[19] Believing this adverse event to be due to the purification process, Allergan has since reformulated abicipar to remove potential proinflammatory impurities.

A large phase III program for abicipar in the treatment of neovascular AMD is underway, composed of 2 trials (Colour Contrast Sensitivity for the Early Detection of Wet Age-Related Macular Degeneration [CEDAR] and Safety and Efficacy of Abicipar Pegol [AGN-150998] in Patients With Neovascular Age-Related Macular Degeneration [SEQUOIA]), with each expected to recruit 900 patients.[20] Beyond the indications for AMD, abicipar is also in development for diabetic macular edema (DME), with a phase II study ongoing. Furthermore, Allegan and Molecular Partners are collaborating on a combination VEGF and platelet-derived growth factor (PDGF) DARPin for neovascular AMD that is currently in preclinical testing.

OPT-302

Currently available VEGF inhibitors target VEGF-A; however, OPT-302 (formerly VGX-300, Opthea, South Yarra) is a soluble form of human VEGF receptor-3 (VEGFR-3) that specifically functions by trapping VEGF-C and VEGF-D. VEGF-C and VEGF-D can stimulate angiogenesis and leakage either through the same pathway as VEGF-A (via VEGFR-2) or through an alternative mechanism independent of VEGF-A (via VEGFR-3). VEGF-C levels have additionally been demonstrated to be significantly elevated in the plasma of AMD individuals compared to healthy controls, potentially implicating this isoform in the pathogenesis of the disease process.[21]

In a preclinical mouse model of neovascular AMD, OPT-302 was able to significantly inhibit choroidal neovascularization (CNV) and vascular leakage to a comparable extent as aflibercept.[21-23] When used in combination in the same model, an additive benefit was observed, with more effective inhibition of CNV lesions than using either agent alone.[21-23] This observed synergistic effect may be due to a more complete and effective blockade of the VEGF family of molecules.

In a phase I study that enrolled 20 patients with neovascular AMD, OPT-302 administered by intravitreal injection as a monotherapy (2.0 mg) or at 3 escalating doses (0.3, 1.0, or 2.0 mg) in combination with ranibizumab was safe and well tolerated at all dose levels.[24,25] A phase IIa study is currently ongoing.

PF582

PF582 (Pfenex) is a humanized monoclonal antibody fragment targeted against VEGF-A that is biologically similar to ranibizumab. Referred to as biosimilars, these agents are comparable to generic drugs, and are intended to be a more affordable and cost-effective alternative to their United States Food and Drug Administration

(FDA)-licensed reference counterparts.[26] The difference from generics is that they are derived from biologics (ie, monoclonal antibodies) rather than pharmaceuticals, which are made from synthetic chemicals. A phase I/II trial in New Zealand is comparing 3 monthly intravitreal injections of PF582 to ranibizumab in patients with neovascular AMD to demonstrate equal safety and efficacy of PF582 over a 12-month period.[27]

DE-120

DE-120 (Santen Pharmaceuticals) is a dual tyrosine kinase receptor inhibitor of VEGF and PDGF. Currently, patients with treatment-naïve neovascular AMD are being recruited to participate in a multicenter, randomized, open-label, phase IIa study (VAPOR1) assessing the efficacy, safety, and the duration of effect of intravitreal injections of DE-120 as monotherapy and with a single aflibercept injection.[28]

Fovista (Pegpleranib)

In addition to VEGF, a key modulator in the pathogenesis of neovascular AMD is PDGF. Through the oncology literature, the role of PDGF in the proliferation and maturation of new vessels has become better elucidated, and these findings are now being extrapolated to retinovascular diseases. Chronic anti-VEGF therapy for neovascular AMD is known to induce CNV remodeling whereby it becomes covered and protected by pericytes as new vessels form and mature within the complex. These pericytes provide VEGF and other proliferative factors to the endothelial cells in which they house.[29-31] Sprout cells, also known as "tip" cells, lead the growth of the CNV membrane, and are the only endothelial cells associated with the neovascular complex not covered by pericytes. Therefore, it is believed that the tip cells are the most vulnerable to anti-VEGF therapy, while the remainder of the CNV tissue is conferred relative resistance to current treatments by the pericytes.[32,33]

The recruitment of pericytes is driven by locally produced PDGF.[34-36] Furthermore, VEGF antagonism causes upregulation of PDGF, so that more pericytes are recruited and the CNV membrane undergoes maturation.[37] Essentially, serial anti-VEGF injections prune off the exposed tip cells and mature the underlying neovascular tissue. It is postulated that an anti-PDGF agent would be able to strip the pericyte armor from the neovascular lesion, exposing the underlying endothelial cells to the effects of subsequent anti-VEGF therapy. In this regard, combination treatment with both anti-VEGF and anti-PDGF injections holds significant promise to potentially induce CNV regression and prevent fibrosis.[38]

Numerous companies are working on anti-PDGF agents, but the one furthest along is Fovista (pegpleranib, formerly E10030, Ophthotech). In the largest phase IIb trial conducted in retina to date (449 patients), participants were randomized to receive 1 of the following treatment regimens administered every 4 weeks for 24 weeks:

- 0.3 mg Fovista in combination with 0.5 mg ranibizumab
- 1.5 mg Fovista in combination with 0.5 mg ranibizumab
- Sham in combination with 0.5 mg ranibizumab[39,40]

The primary endpoint was mean change in visual acuity from baseline to week 24. The results showed that the combination arm with the higher dose of Fovista led to statistically significant greater visual improvements than ranibizumab alone. At the higher Fovista dose, BCVA improved by 62% more from baseline (10.6 letters gained) than with ranibizumab monotherapy (6.5 letters gained), with a classic dose-response curve that continued to outpace monotherapy over the 6-month course.[39,40] There were no concerning safety events reported.

In addition to fluid reduction on OCT imaging, an area of particular interest was the significant regression of subretinal hyperreflective material (SRHM) present, thought to represent the neovascular lesion itself. Resolution of SRHM at week 24 demonstrated a clear dose-related response.[39,40] This effect on SRHM has not been previously described in clinical trials of anti-VEGF therapy. The dose-response effect was also seen in patients who gained 3 lines of visual acuity or more. Furthermore, for patients who lost vision in the study, eyes treated with ranibizumab monotherapy had developed fibrosis and disciform scarring, whereas eyes receiving combination therapy showed little, if any, scarring.[39,40] Because PDGF is a potent fibrotic agent, it is feasible that its blockade has a direct impact on the degree of fibrosis and scar formation, as seen in this subgroup.

Unfortunately, preliminary phase III results released in 2016 demonstrated that Fovista (1.5 mg) in combination therapy with ranibizumab did not result in any added visual acuity benefit compared to ranibizumab monotherapy alone after 12 months, failing to meet the study's primary endpoint. In the combined analysis from the two studies, patients receiving combination therapy with Fovista gained a mean of 10.24 ETDRS letters compared to 10.01 letters on ranibizumab monotherapy, which did not achieve statistical significance. Ophthotech is further analyzing this data to better understand the results and the pathophysiology of neovascular AMD.[41]

REGN2176-3

REGN2176-3 (Regeneron Pharmaceuticals) is a combination product comprising an antibody to PDGF receptor-b (rinucumab) co-formulated together with aflibercept. In a phase I study, 4 cohorts of 3 patients each received REGN2176-3 at baseline and at 4 weeks. Visual acuity remained stable or increased in the majority of patients, and the central retinal thickness on OCT decreased in all 4 cohorts. No dose-limiting toxicities, intraocular inflammation, or treatment-related serious adverse events were encountered.[42]

A phase II, multicenter, double-masked, randomized controlled study (CAPELLA) evaluating 4 different dosing regimens of REGN2176-3 is ongoing to investigate its efficacy and safety compared to aflibercept monotherapy in patients with neovascular AMD.[43]

Nesvacumab

Angiopoietin-2 (Ang2) belongs to a family of proangiogenic factors selectively expressed during the angiogenesis process, and is an antagonistic ligand for the vascular endothelial cell receptor tyrosine kinase, Tie2.[44,45] Unlike some of the damage-inducing pathways in retinovascular diseases that are targeted by most pharmacotherapy agents, Tie2 is protective and improves the stability of retinal vasculature. Drugs that interfere with Ang2/Tie2 signaling may help regulate vascular permeability, which may be of particular interest in treating conditions such as diabetic retinopathy and DME. Nesvacumab (REGN910-3, Regeneron Pharmaceuticals) is a fully human immunoglobulin G1 (IgG1) monoclonal antibody that selectively binds Ang2 with high affinity and blocks it from binding to the Tie2 receptor.

Two separate phase II clinical studies are underway to assess combination therapy of nesvacumab plus aflibercept as a co-formulated single intravitreal injection in patients with neovascular AMD (ONYX, Anti-angiOpoeitin 2 Plus Anti-vascular eNdothelial Growth Factor as a therapY for Neovascular Age Related Macular Degeneration: Evaluation of a fiXed Combination Intravitreal Injection)[46] and DME (RUBY, Anti-vasculaR Endothelial Growth Factor plUs Anti-angiopoietin 2 in Fixed comBination therapY: Evaluation for the Treatment of Diabetic Macular Edema).[47]

RG7716

RG7716 (Hoffmann-La Roche) is a unique bispecific monoclonal antibody that targets both VEGF and Ang2. In a phase I study evaluating RG7716 in patients with neovascular AMD who demonstrated suboptimal therapeutic response after multiple previous anti-VEGF injections, promising improvements in BCVA and key OCT parameters were observed.[48] Additionally, investigators found RG7716 to be well tolerated and exhibiting an overall favorable safety profile. Larger phase II studies are currently underway to evaluate RG7716's potential to further enhance anti-VEGF monotherapy efficacy and safety.

ICON-1

ICON-1 (formerly hI-con1, Iconic Therapeutics) belongs to a class of novel human immunoconjugate proteins. It is a 160 kDa chimeric, IgG-like homodimeric protein composed of a targeting domain (mutated, inactive factor VIIa) fused to an effector domain (fragment crystallizable portion of IgG) with an intact hinge region.[49] ICON-1 targets tissue factor (TF), which is a promoter of inflammation and angiogenesis.[50] A positive feedback loop exists between VEGF and TF such that TF can induce angiogenesis by upregulating VEGF and increased VEGF can, in turn, increase TF expression.[50] By binding to cells that aberrantly overexpress TF (ie, in CNV tissue) the effector domain of ICON-1 triggers the immune destruction of these targeted cells, inducing natural killer cell-mediated cytotoxicity of the CNV complex.[51,52]

The results of a multicenter phase I study evaluating a single intravitreal injection of 60 mg, 150 mg, or 300 mg ICON-1 in 18 eyes with neovascular AMD (6 eyes per cohort) revealed the therapy to be well tolerated and led to increased visual acuity, reduced retinal thickness, and CNV regression.[53] Furthermore, no drug-related serious ocular or systemic adverse events were observed. In 2015, Iconic initiated a phase II randomized, double-masked, multicenter, active-controlled study (EMERGE) to evaluate the safety and biological activity of repeated intravitreal administration of ICON-1 in patients with CNV secondary to AMD. Three treatment arms are being investigated in the 6-month study: ICON-1 monotherapy, ICON-1 with ranibizumab, and ranibizumab alone as a comparator.

Luminate

Integrins are cell surface receptors involved in angiogenesis and inflammation, acting both upstream and downstream of the VEGF pathway. There are 27 types of integrin receptors; however, there are no anti-integrin drugs currently available for commercial ophthalmic use.[54] Luminate (formerly ALG-1001, Allegro Ophthalmics) is an integrin

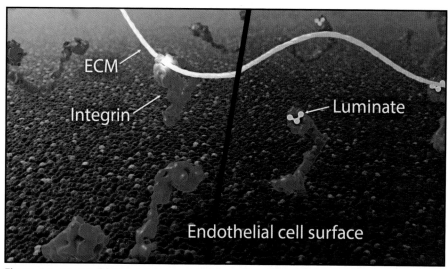

Figure 4-1. Integrin inhibition. Integrins regulate cell functions and interactions among cells and between cells and the extracellular matrix (ECM). As they bind or attach to the ECM, integrins activate intracellular signaling pathways and proteolytic changes that promote angiogenesis. Luminate inhibits the connection between the integrins and the ECM, preventing the downstream angiogenic effects. (Reprinted with permission from Allegro Ophthalmics.)

antagonist that blocks 3 different integrin receptor sites ($\alpha v\beta 3$, $\alpha v\beta 5$, and $\alpha 5\beta 1$) that mediate a number of angiogenic processes, including endothelial cell migration, proliferation, differentiation, and maturation (Figure 4-1).[54-56] Since Luminate inhibits all 3 of these receptors associated with angiogenesis, early clinical evidence suggests that it is effective in preventing the formation of new blood vessels as well as shrinking and stopping leakage from existing blood vessels.

In a phase I study, 15 patients with chronic DME received 3 injections of Luminate monthly after a 90-day washout period from any previous therapy.[54,57] The study participants were then observed for 3 months without additional treatment. Mean visual improvement was approximately 11 letters gained (2 lines of vision), with 8 individuals (53%) gaining at least 3 lines of vision. Importantly, no participants lost vision, even during the 3 months off treatment, and the safety during the study was excellent. These results also suggested that Luminate may be potent enough to work as monotherapy for DME. Many of the study patients improved on Luminate despite a previous history of 10 to 12 anti-VEGF injections prior to study enrollment.[54] Currently, the drug is in phase II clinical trials as potential monotherapy for DME compared to bevacizumab and focal laser.[58]

Luminate additionally carries a dual function in that it inhibits a fourth integrin receptor site ($\alpha 3\beta 1$) involved in vitreolysis, and is being separately investigated as a potential agent to pharmacologically induce a posterior vitreous detachment in patients with nonproliferative diabetic retinopathy, as well as those with vitreomacular adhesion or vitreomacular traction.[59,60]

Systemic Therapy

AKB-9778

AKB-9778 (Aerpio Therapeutics) is a small molecule that inhibits vascular endothelial protein tyrosine phosphatase (VE-PTP), which acts as a negative regulator of the Tie2 receptor. Under normal conditions, Tie2 activity is maintained by binding of the activating ligand, Angiopoietin-1 (Ang1), which stimulates phosphorylation and downstream signaling.[61,62] When phosphorylated, Tie2 promotes quiescence and unresponsiveness to stimuli that cause endothelial-cell proliferation and/or leakiness (ie, VEGF).[61,62] In diseased states, such as DME, the negative regulators of Tie2, Ang2, and VE-PTP become upregulated. Specifically, VE-PTP dephosphorylates Tie2, resulting in vascular destabilization and leakage.[63,64] By inhibiting VE-PTP, AKB-9778 promotes normal Tie2 signaling to be restored independent of Ang2 levels, and makes endothelial cells less responsive to VEGF and other pro-permeability/proangiogenic factors.[65]

Of particular interest is the means of drug administration. AKB-9778 is delivered via subcutaneous injection by the patients themselves. This may be perceived as a unique advantage, as insulin-dependent diabetics are already comfortable self-administering such injections within the confines of their home. This may in turn lead to reduced clinic visits. An additional benefit of this systemic route is the potential for broader stimulation of Tie2 and stabilization of vascular beds elsewhere in the body, particularly those of the kidney, which may be beneficial in diabetics. It additionally causes a small reduction in systolic blood pressure, which may be desirable with this demographic of patients.[65]

In a phase IIa study (TIME-2) of AKB-9778 in 144 patients with DME over a 3-month period, the combination of AKB-9778 (15 mg dosed twice daily) together with monthly 0.3 mg intravitreal ranibizumab injections provided a clinically significant benefit in anatomic reduction of fluid on OCT (mean reduction 164 μm) compared to ranibizumab alone (mean reduction 109 μm).[66] The investigators additionally observed a trend toward improved visual acuity in the combination arm (6.3 letters gained vs 5.7 letters gained in the ranibizumab monotherapy arm). AKB-9778 was well tolerated, with no treatment group differences in ocular or systemic adverse events observed. A phase III trial is currently underway.

X-82

X-82 (Tyrogenex) is an orally available tyrosine kinase dual inhibitor of all isoforms of VEGF and PDGF receptors, and is currently in development for the treatment of neovascular AMD and solid tumors. The results of an open-label, dose-escalation phase I study released in 2015 found that X-82 maintained or improved vision in all 35 neovascular AMD patients during the 6-month study period.[67,68] Six treatment regimens at 4 dose levels (ranging from 50 mg every other day to 300 mg daily) of X-82 were evaluated. The outcomes showed an overall trend toward higher visual acuity of 4.3 letters gained, and a trend toward decreased foveal thickness of approximately 48 μm at 24 weeks. X-82 was generally well tolerated with no dose-limiting toxicities reported. There were 25 of 35 patients who completed the full 24-week treatment period; of the 25 patients, 15 (60%) required no rescue ranibizumab injections and had a mean visual acuity improvement of 5.3 letters throughout the study. Eight participants—1 receiving 100 mg daily, 5 receiving

200 mg daily, and 2 receiving 300 mg daily—experienced significant reductions in fluid on OCT imaging within the first few weeks of initiating X-82.[69]

These encouraging phase I results of X-82 supported Tyrogenex progressing forward with the phase II APEX (neovascular AMD in previously treated Eylea patients with X-82) trial.[70] APEX is a randomized, double-masked, placebo-controlled, dose-finding study being conducted to evaluate the safety and efficacy of X-82 plus aflibercept as needed (Eylea, Regeneron Pharmaceuticals) compared to aflibercept monotherapy. The primary endpoints of this study are the mean change in visual acuity from day 1 to week 52 and the reduction in the number of injections needed for the study period.

Topical Therapy

Squalamine

Squalamine lactate (OHR-102, Ohr Pharmaceutical) is a small-molecule, antiangiogenic drug with an intracellular mechanism of action that inhibits endothelial cell proliferation. A cholesterol-like compound originally isolated from the liver of the dogfish shark, *Squalus acanthias*,[71,72] squalamine inhibits aberrant neovascularization through the blockade of numerous angiogenic factors, including basic fibroblast growth factor, PDGF, and VEGF.[73-75] It enters cells via an active process and, once inside, is able to sequester intracellular calmodulin,[76] preventing receptor activation and causing broad inhibition of multiple downstream factors. The greatest effect of squalamine appears to be on inactivation of new endothelial cell formation, with no appreciable effect on unstimulated endothelium.[75]

A topical formulation of this agent is capable of transscleral penetration, resulting in high levels of active drug delivered to the choroid and retina. In a randomized, multicenter, masked, placebo-controlled, phase II clinical trial (IMPACT) completed in 2015, 142 patients with neovascular AMD received an intravitreal injection of ranibizumab at day 0, and then were randomized 1:1 to receive either placebo eye drops or squalamine 0.2% solution administered twice daily. Study participants were then followed monthly and retreated with ranibizumab pro re nata (PRN) based on strict OCT-guided criteria.[77,78]

The primary endpoint of the study, number of retreatment injections required, was not met, as both groups ended up receiving a similar number of ranibizumab injections. However, the results demonstrated improved visual function in the squalamine and ranibizumab combination group vs ranibizumab monotherapy alone. Specifically, in patients with classic CNV, 44% of eyes receiving combination therapy achieved a 3 or more line visual acuity gain after 9 months vs 29% in the anti-VEGF monotherapy group. These eyes also achieved a mean gain in visual acuity of 11 letters in the combination arm, as compared to 5 letters gained with the anti-VEGF monotherapy group, a clinically meaningful benefit of 6 letters. Less of an advantage was seen in the overall population (classic containing and occult-only CNV lesions).[77,78] Phase III clinical development (MAKO) for the treatment of neovascular AMD is currently ongoing.[79]

Similarly, a separate phase II study evaluating squalamine in the treatment of macular edema secondary to branch and central retinal vein occlusion has suggested that combination therapy together with ranibizumab resulted in increased visual acuity compared to anti-VEGF monotherapy.[80] Following an initial 10-week combination therapy treatment period, patients who continued to receive a combination of squalamine drops twice daily plus ranibizumab PRN achieved greater visual acuity gains at week 38 (27.8 letters gained) than members of the control group who received ranibizumab PRN alone (23.3 letters gained), a clinically meaningful difference of 4.5 letters. Patients treated with squalamine required a mean of 2.0 ranibizumab injections between weeks 10 and 38, compared with a mean of 3.3 injections for the monotherapy group during the same time period. In both studies, no safety issues were encountered.

PAN-90806

PAN-90806 (PanOptica Inc) is a potent, selective, small-molecule VEGF inhibitor that has been shown to be effective when applied as a topical eye drop in mouse models of neovascular AMD and diabetic retinopathy.[81] Preliminary results reported from a phase I/II study revealed signals of anti-VEGF biological activity across all PAN-90806 monotherapy dose arms in patients with neovascular AMD, including at the lowest doses.[82] Reproducible pharmacokinetic findings demonstrated excellent target tissue distribution to the retina and choroid, with concentrations sustained at 17 hours post-dose. Full study results from the AMD trial were reported in late 2016, which enrolled 50 patients with treatment-naïve neovascular AMD, and confirmed positive biological response to topical PAN-90806 in 45-50% of treated individuals, including outcomes such as visual acuity, vascular leakage, and lesion morphology.[83] Based on these results, the company plans to initiate a phase I/II clinical trial of a next-generation formulation of topical PAN-90806 for the treatment of neovascular AMD in 2017. PanOptica has also initiated a phase I trial of PAN-90806 in patients with proliferative diabetic retinopathy.[84]

Regorafenib

Regorafenib (formerly BAY 73-4506, Bayer AG) is a multiple tyrosine kinase inhibitor that inhibits VEGFR-1, VEGFR-2, and VEGFR-3, Tie2, and other tyrosine kinase receptors.[85] An oral version of this drug is currently FDA-approved for the treatment of metastatic colorectal cancer and advanced gastrointestinal stromal tumors.

A topical formulation of regorafenib has been packaged into an oily suspension for improved intraocular delivery. Preclinical studies have shown that topical administration of regorafenib (1 mg/mL) was helpful in preventing alkali-induced corneal neovascularization in a rat model.[86] Phase I studies have shown that the solution was well tolerated in humans. Daily use of varying doses of regorafenib eye drops are currently being studied in a phase II clinical trial (DREAM) in patients with neovascular AMD to evaluate its efficacy, safety, and tolerability after 4 and 12 weeks of treatment.[87]

LHA510

LHA510 (Alcon) is a topically delivered molecule currently under investigation for maintenance therapy in neovascular AMD. A randomized, double-masked, vehicle-controlled study is ongoing to analyze the safety and efficacy of single and multiple dosing regimens of LHA510.[88] The purpose will be to determine if LHA510 is able to reduce the number of rescue intravitreal ranibizumab injections required for recurrent active CNV during the course of 84 days of successive topical drop therapy.

References

1. Comparison of Age-Related Macular Degeneration Treatments Trials (CATT) Research Group, Maguire MG, Martin DF, et al. Five-year outcomes with anti-vascular endothelial growth factor treatment of neovascular age-related macular degeneration: the Comparison of Age-Related Macular Degeneration Treatments Trials. *Ophthalmology.* 2016;123(8):1751-1761.

2. Pechan P, Rubin H, Lukason M, et al. Novel anti-VEGF chimeric molecules delivered by AAV vectors for inhibition of retinal neovascularization. *Gene Ther.* 2009;16(1):10-16.

3. Maclachlan TK, Lukason M, Collins M, et al. Preclinical safety evaluation of AAV2-sFLT01: a gene therapy for age-related macular degeneration. *Mol Ther.* 2011;19:326-334.

4. Heier JS. Preliminary results of phase 1 study with AAV2-sFLT01 as gene therapy for treatment of exudative AMD: one-year results of phase 1 clinical trial with rAAV.sFLT-1. Paper presented at: The Retina Society 2014 Annual Meeting; September 11-14, 2014; Philadelphia, PA.

5. Heier JS. Gene therapy for exudative AMD: one-year results of phase 1 clinical trial with rAAV. sFLT-1. Paper presented at: The American Society of Retinal Specialists (ASRS) 2014 Annual Meeting; August 9-13, 2014; San Diego, CA.

6. Avalanche Biotechnologies, Inc. announces positive top-line phase 2a results for AVA-101 in wet age-related macular degeneration. Adverum Biotechnologies Website. http://investors.avalanche-biotech.com/phoenix.zhtml?c=253634&p=irol-newsArticle&ID=2059444. Published June 15, 2015. Accessed May 17, 2016.

7. AVA-201. Adverum Biotechnologies Website. http://avalanchebiotech.com/science/ava-201/. Accessed May 17, 2016.

8. Balaggan KS, Binley K, Esapa M, et al. EIAV vector-mediated delivery of endostatin or angiostatin inhibits angiogenesis and vascular hyperpermeability in experimental CNV. *Gene Ther.* 2006;13(15):1153-1165.

9. Binkley K, Widdsowson PS, Kelleher M, et al. Safety and biodistribution of an equine infectious anemia virus-based gene therapy, Retinostat, for age-related macular degeneration. *Hum Gene Ther.* 2012;23(9):980-991.

10. Phase I dose escalation safety study of retinostat in advanced age-related macular degeneration (AMD) (GEM). ClinicalTrials.gov Website. https://clinicaltrials.gov/ct2/show/NCT01301443. Accessed May 17, 2016.

11. OXB-201 (RetinoStat). A novel gene-based treatment for neovascular "wet" age-related macular degeneration. OxfordBioMedica Website. http://www.oxfordbiomedica.co.uk/oxb-201-retinostat-r/. Accessed May 17, 2016.

12. Tietz J, Schmid G, Konrad J, et al. Affinity and potency of RTH258 (ESBA1008), a novel inhibitor of vascular endothelial growth factor a for the treatment of retinal disorders. *Invest Ophthalmol Vis Sci.* 2015;56(7):1501.

13. Gaudreault J, Gunde T, Floyd HS, et al. Preclinical pharmacology and safety of ESBA1008, a single-chain antibody fragment, investigated as potential treatment for age related macular degeneration. *Invest Ophthalmol Vis Sci.* 2012;53(14):3025.

14. Singerman LJ, Weichselberger A, Sallstig P. OSPREY trial: randomized, active-controlled, phase II study to evaluate safety and efficacy of RTH258, a humanized single-chain anti-VEGF antibody fragment, in patients with neovascular AMD. Paper presented at: The Association for Research in Vision and Ophthalmology (ARVO) 2015 Annual Meeting; May 3-7, 2015; Denver, CO.

15. Efficacy and safety of RTH258 versus aflibercept. ClinicalTrials.gov Website. https://clinicaltrials. gov/ct2/show/NCT02307682?term=rth258&rank=2. Accessed May 17, 2016.

16. Singh R. Safety and efficacy of RTH258 delivered via intravitreal injection or microvolume injection/infusion for neovascular age-related macular degeneration. Paper presented at: The American Society of Retina Specialists (ASRS) 2015 Annual Meeting; July 11-14, 2015; Vienna, Austria.

17. Souied EH, Devin F, Mauget-Faÿsse M, et al. Treatment of exudative age-related macular degeneration with a designed ankyrin repeat protein that binds vascular endothelial growth factor: a phase I/II study. *Am J Ophthalmol.* 2014;158(4):724-732.e2.

18. Stahl A, Stumpp MT, Schlegel A, et al. Highly potent VEGF-A-antagonistic DARPins as anti-angiogenic agents for topical and intravitreal applications. *Angiogenesis.* 2013;16(1):101-111.

19. Stage 3 phase 2 study of DARPin abicipar pegol (previously MP0112) supports progressing to phase III development program. http://www.molecularpartners.com/wp-content/uploads/2014/10/201407_positive_phase2_for_darpin_abicipar.pdf. Accessed May 17, 2016.

20. Safety and efficacy of abicipar pegol in patients with neovascular age-related macular degeneration. ClincialTrials.gov Website. https://clinicaltrials.gov/ct2/show/NCT02462486. Accessed May 17, 2016.

21. Lashkari K, Ma J, Teague GC, Arroyo J. Expression of VEGF-C, VEGF-D and their cognate receptors in experimental choroidal neovascularization and clinical AMD. Paper presented at: The Association for Research in Vision and Ophthalmology (ARVO) 2013 Annual Meeting; May 5-9, 2013; Seattle, WA.

22. Lashkari K, Ma J, Teague GC, Guo C, Baldwin ME. VEGF-C and VEGF-D blockade by VGX-300 inhibits choroidal neovascularization and leakage in a mouse model of wet AMD. Paper presented at: The Association for Research in Vision and Ophthalmology (ARVO) 2014 Annual Meeting; May 4-8, 2014; Orlando, FL.

23. Lashkari K, Ma J, Sun Y, Teague GC, Baldwin ME. VGX-300, a 'trap' for VEGF-C and VEGF-D, inhibits choroidal neovascularization and vascular leakage in a mouse model of wet AMD. Paper presented at: The Association for Research in Vision and Ophthalmology (ARVO) 2015 Annual Meeting; May 3-7, 2015; Denver, CO.

24. Study evaluating the safety, pharmacokinetics and pharmacodynamics of OPT-302 with or without Lucentis in patients with wet AMD. ClinicalTrials.gov Website. https://clinicaltrials.gov/ct2/show/NCT02543229. Accessed May 17, 2016.

25. Opthea phase 1 wet AMD clinical trial with OPT-302 meets primary safety objective. http://www.opthea.com/news.

26. US Food and Drug Administration. Information on biosimilars. http://www.fda.gov/Drugs/DevelopmentApprovalProcess/HowDrugsareDevelopedandApproved/ApprovalApplications/TherapeuticBiologicApplications/Biosimilars/.

27. Safety study of PF582 versus lucentis in patients with age related macular degeneration. https://clinicaltrials.gov/ct2/show/NCT02121353. Accessed May 17, 2016.

28. A Safety and Efficacy Study of DE-120 Injectable Solution for Age-related Macular Degeneration (VAPOR1). ClinicalTrials.gov Website. https://clinicaltrials.gov/ct2/show/NCT02401945. Accessed May 17, 2016.

29. Carmeliet P. Mechanisms of angiogenesis and arteriogenesis. *Nat Med.* 2000;6(4):389-395.

30. Benjamin LE, Hemo I, Keshet E. A plasticity window for blood vessel remodelling is defined by pericyte coverage of the preformed endothelial network and is regulated by PDGF-B and VEGF. *Development.* 1998;125(9):1591-1598.

31. Bergers G, Song S, Meyer-Morse N, Bergsland E, Hanahan D. Benefits of targeting both pericytes and endothelial cells in the tumor vasculature with kinase inhibitors. *J Clin Invest.* 2003;111(9):1287-1295.

32. Armulik A, Abramsson A, Betsholtz C. Endothelial/pericyte interactions. *Circ Res.* 2005;97(6):512-523.

33. Dugel PU. Developments in therapy for neovascular AMD. *Retina Today.* 2013;8:54-57.

34. Lindahl P, Johansson BR, Levéen P, Betsholtz C. Pericyte loss and microaneurysm formation in PDGF-B-deficient mice. *Science.* 1997;277(5323):242-245.

35. Furuhashi M, Sjöblom T, Abramsson A, et al. Platelet-derived growth factor production by B16 melanoma cells leads to increased pericyte abundance in tumors and an associated increase in tumor growth rate. *Cancer Res.* 2004;64(8):2725-2733.

36. Armulik A, Abramsson A, Betsholtz C. Endothelial/pericyte interactions. *Circ Res.* 2005;97(6):512-523.

37. Greenberg JI, Shields DJ, Barillas SG, et al. A role for VEGF as a negative regulator of pericyte function and vessel maturation. *Nature.* 2008;456(7223):809-813.

38. Jo N, Mailhos C, Ju M, et al. Inhibition of platelet-derived growth factor B signaling enhances the efficacy of anti-vascular endothelial growth factor therapy in multiple models of ocular neovascularization. *Am J Pathol.* 2006;168(6):2036-2053.

39. Dugel PU. Anti-PDGF combination therapy in neovascular age-related macular degeneration: results of a phase 2b study. *Retina Today.* 2013;65-71.

40. Dugel PU. Anti-platelet derived growth factor: where do we stand? Paper presented at: The American Academy of Ophthalmology (AAO) 2012 Annual Meeting; November 10, 2012; Chicago, IL.

41. A phase 3 safety and efficacy study of Fovista (E10030) intravitreous administration in combination with Lucentis compared to Lucentis monotherapy. ClinicalTrials.gov Website. https://clinicaltrials.gov/ct2/show/NCT01944839. Accessed May 17, 2016.

42. Heier JS. Combined anti-PDGF/anti-VEGF therapy in neovascular AMD. Paper presented at: The Angiogenesis, Exudation, and Degeneration 2015 Annual Meeting; February 7, 2015; Miami, FL.

43. Study of intravitreal REGN2176-3 in patients with neovascular ("wet") age-related macular degeneration (AMD) (CAPELLA). ClinicalTrials.gov Website. https://clinicaltrials.gov/ct2/show/NCT02418754. Accessed May 17, 2016.

44. Davis S, Aldrich TH, Jones PF, et al. Isolation of angiopoietin-1, a ligand for the TIE2 receptor, by secretion-trap expression cloning. *Cell.* 1996;87:1161-1169.

45. Maisonpierre PC, Suri C, Jones PF, et al. Angiopoietin-2, a natural antagonist for Tie2 that disrupts in vivo angiogenesis. *Science.* 1997;277:55-60.

46. Anti-angiOpoeitin 2 Plus Anti-vascular eNdothelial Growth Factor as a therapY for Neovascular Age Related Macular Degeneration: Evaluation of a fiXed Combination Intravitreal Injection (ONYX). https://clinicaltrials.gov/ct2/show/NCT02713204?term=nesvacumab&rank=4. Accessed May 17, 2016.

47. Anti-vasculaR Endothelial Growth Factor plUs Anti-angiopoietin 2 in Fixed comBination therapY: Evaluation for the Treatment of Diabetic Macular Edema (RUBY). ClinicalTrials.gov Website. https://clinicaltrials.gov/ct2/show/NCT02712008?term=nesvacumab&rank=5. Accessed May 17, 2016.

48. Chakravarthy U, Schwab D, Cech P, et al. The novel bispecific monoclonal anti-VEGF/anti-Ang2 antibody RG7716 shows promise in wet age-related macular degeneration patients with suboptimal response to prior anti-VEGF monotherapy. Abstract presented at: The Association for Research in Vision and Ophthalmology (ARVO) 2016 Annual Meeting; May 1-5, 2016; Seattle, WA. *Invest Ophthalmol Vis Sci.* 2016; 57.

49. Hu Z, Sun Y, Garen A. Targeting tumor vasculature endothelial cells and tumor cells for immunotherapy of human melanoma in a mouse xenograft model. *Proc Natl Acad Sci U S A.* 1999;96(14):8161-8166.

50. Cho Y, Cao X, Shen D, et al. Evidence for enhanced tissue factor expression in age-related macular degeneration. *Lab Invest.* 2011;91(4):519-526.

51. Cocco E, Hu Z, Richter CE, et al. HI-con1, a factor VII-IgGFc chimeric protein targeting tissue factor for immunotherapy of uterine serous papillary carcinoma. *Br J Cancer.* 2010;103(6):812-819.

52. Tezel TH, Bodek E, Sönmez K, et al. Targeting tissue factor for immunotherapy of choroidal neovascularization by intravitreal delivery of factor VII-Fc chimeric antibody. *Ocul Immunol Inflamm.* 2007;15(1):3-10.

53. Wells JA, Berger BB, Gonzales C, et al. Multicenter phase 1 clinical trial targeting tissue factor for the treatment of neovascular AMD. *Invest Ophthalmol Vis Sci.* 2012;53:E-Abstract 450.

54. Kuppermann BD. A dual-mechanism drug for vitreoretinal diseases. *Retina Today.* 2015;10:85-87.

55. Friedlander M, Theesfeld C, Sugita M, et al. Involvement of integrins alpha v beta 3 and alpha v beta 5 in ocular neovascular diseases. *Proc Natl Acad Sci U S A.* 1996;93:9764-9769.

56. Ramakrishnan V, Bhaskar V, Law DA, et al. Preclinical evaluation of an anti-alpha5beta1 integrin antibody as a novel anti-angiogenic agent. *J Exp Ther Oncol.* 2006;5:273-286.

57. Quiroz-Mercado H. Integrin peptide therapy as a next-generation class of treatment for vascular eye disease. Paper presented at: T he American Academy of Ophthalmology (AAO) 2011 Annual Meeting; October 22-25, 2011; Orlando, FL.

58. A phase 2 randomized, controlled, double-masked, multicenter clinical trial designed to evaluate the safety and exploratory efficacy of Luminate (ALG-1001) as compared to Avastin and focal laser photocoagulation in the treatment of diabetic macular edema. ClinicalTrials.gov Website. https://clinicaltrials.gov/ct2/show/NCT02348918. Accessed May 17, 2016.

59. Oliveira LB, Meyer CH, Kumar J, et al. RGD peptide-assisted vitrectomy to facilitate induction of a posterior vitreous detachment: a new principle in pharmacological vitreolysis. *Curr Eye Res.* 2002;25:333-340.

60. Kuppermann BD, Boyer DS, Kaiser PK, et al. Topline results from prospective, double-masked, placebo controlled phase 2 clinical study evaluating Luminate (ALG-1001) in patients with symptomatic focal vitreomacular adhesion. Paper presented at: The Association for Research in Vision and Ophthalmology (ARVO) 2016 Annual Meeting; May 1-5, 2016; Seattle, WA. *Invest Ophthalmol Vis Sci.* 2016;57.

61. Suri C, Jones PF, Patan S, et al. Requisite role of angiopoietin-1, a ligand for the TIE2 receptor, during embryonic angiogenesis. *Cell.* 1996;87:1171-1180.

62. Thurston G, Suri C, Smith K, et al. Leakage-resistant blood vessels in mice transgenically overexpressing angiopoietin-1. *Science.* 1999;286:2511-2514.

63. Yacyshyn OK, Lai PF, Forse K, et al. Tyrosine phosphatase beta regulates angiopoietin-Tie2 signaling in human endothelial cells. *Angiogenesis.* 2009;12:25-33.

64. Winderlich M, Keller L, Cagna G, et al. VE-PTP control blood vessel development by balancing Tie-2 activity. *J Cell Biol.* 2009;185(4):657-671.

65. Campochiaro PA, Sophie R, Tolentin M, et al. Treatment of diabetic macular edema with an inhibitor of vascular endothelial-protein tyrosine phosphatase that activates Tie-2. *Ophthalmology.* 2015;122:545-554.

66. Khanani A. The Tie2 activator AKB-9778, used in combination with ranibizumab, enhances reduction of diabetic macular edema compared to ranibizumab monotherapy. Abstract presented at: The Association for Research in Vision and Ophthalmology (ARVO) Annual Meeting; May 1-5, 2016; Seattle, WA. *Invest Ophthalmol Vis Sci.* 2016;57.

67. Jackson T. A phase 1 study of oral tyrosine kinase inhibitor (X-82) in previously treated wet age-related macular degeneration. Paper presented at: The 15th EURETINA Congress; September 17-20, 2015; Nice, France.

68. Chaudhry NA. Oral VEGF receptor/PDGR receptor inhibitor X-82. Paper presented at: The American Academy of Ophthalmology (AAO) Retina 2015 Annual Meeting; November 13-14, 2015; Las Vegas, NV.

69. Rosenfeld PJ, Slakter JS, Boyer DS, et al. A phase 1 safety study of an orally available tyrosine kinase inhibitor X-82 in previously treated wet AMD patients. Abstract presented at the Association for Research in Vision and Ophthalmology (ARVO) 2015 Annual Meeting; May 3-7, 2015; Denver, CO.

70. X-82 to treat age-related macular degeneration. ClinicalTrials.gov Website. https://clinicaltrials.gov/ct2/show/NCT02348359. Accessed May 17, 2016.

71. Rao MN, Shinnar AE, Noecker LA, et al. Aminosterols from the dogfish shark *Squalus acanthias. J Nat Prod.* 2000;63(5):631-635.

72. Cho J, Kim Y. Sharks: a potential source of antiangiogenic factors and tumor treatments. *Mar Biotechnol (NY).* 2002;4(6):521-525.

73. Genaidy M, Kazi AA, Peyman GA, et al. Effect of squalamine on iris neovascularization in monkeys. *Retina.* 2002;22:772-778.

74. Higgins RD, Yan Y, Geng Y, et al. Regression of retinopathy by squalamine in a mouse model. *Pediatr Res.* 2004;56:144-149.

75. Sills AK Jr, Williams JI, Tyler BM, et al. Squalamine inhibits angiogenesis and solid tumor growth in vivo and perturbs embryonic vasculature. *Cancer Res.* 1998;58(13):2784-2792.

76. Ciulla TA, Criswell MH, Danis RP, et al. Squalamine lactate reduces choroidal neovascularization in a laser-injury model in the rat. *Retina.* 2003;23:808-814.

77. Slakter JS, Ciulla TA, Elman MJ, et al. Final results from a phase 2 study of squalamine lactate ophthalmic solution 0.2% (OHR-102) in the treatment of neovascular age-related macular degeneration (AMD). Abstract presented at: The Association for Research in Vision and Ophthalmology (ARVO) 2015 Annual Meeting; May 3-7, 2015; Denver, CO.

78. Heier JS. Final results from a phase 2 study of squalamine lactate ophthalmic solution 0.2% (OHR-102) in neovascular age-related macular degeneration (AMD). Paper presented at: The American Society of Retina Specialists (ASRS) 2015 Annual Meeting; July 11-14, 2015; Vienna, Austria.

79. Efficacy and safety study of squalamine ophthalmic solution in subjects with neovascular AMD (MAKO). ClinicalTrials.gov Website. https://clinicaltrials.gov/ct2/show/NCT02727881. Accessed May 17, 2016.

80. Wroblewski J. Squalamine lactate ophthalmic solution for the treatment of macular edema secondary to branch and central retinal vein occlusion: final data analysis. Paper presented at: The American Society of Retina Specialists (ASRS) 2015 Annual Meeting; July 11-14, 2015; Vienna, Austria.

81. Wax MB. PanOptica 90806: a novel topical agent for the treatment of wet age-related macular degeneration. Paper presented at: The Retina Society 2011 Annual Meeting; September 21-25, 2011; Rome, Italy.

82. Chaney PG. Phase 1/2 dose-ranging study of PAN-90806 in treatment-naïve patients with wet AMD. Paper presented at: The American Academy of Ophthalmology (AAO) Ophthalmology Innovation Summit. November 12, 2015; Las Vegas, NV.

83. Cousins SW. PAN-90806 - a novel topical treatment for neovascular AMD. Paper presented at: The American Academy of Ophthalmology (AAO) 2016 Annual Meeting; October 14-15, 2016; Chicago, IL.

84. Study of topical ocular PAN-90806 in PDR. ClinicalTrials.gov Website. https://clinicaltrials.gov/ct2/show/NCT02475109.

85. Eisen T, Joensuu H, Nathan PD, et al. Regorafenib for patients with previously untreated metastatic or unresectable renal-cell carcinoma: a single-group phase 2 trial. *Lancet Oncol.* 2012;13(10):1055-1062.

86. Onder HI, Erdurmus M, Bucak YY, Simavli H, Oktay M, Kukner AS. Inhibitory effects of regorafenib, a multiple tyrosine kinase inhibitor, on corneal neovascularization. *Int J Ophthalmol.* 2014;7(2):220-225.

87. Regorafenib eye drops: investigation of efficacy and safety in neovascular age related macular degeneration (DREAM). ClinicalTrials.gov Website. https://www.clinicaltrials.gov/ct2/show/NCT02222207. Accessed May 17, 2016.

88. LHA510 proof-of-concept study as a maintenance therapy for patients with wet age-related macular degeneration. ClinicalTrials.gov Website. https://clinicaltrials.gov/ct2/show/NCT02355028. Accessed May 17, 2016.

5

Intravitreal Delivery

Nora Muakkassa, MD; Kendra Klein, MD; and
Elias Reichel, MD

Intravitreal injection of medication was first described in 1947 with the use of penicillin for late postoperative endophthalmitis.[1] Antiviral agents were first injected intravitreally for the treatment of cytomegalovirus retinitis in the late 1980s.[2] Intravitreal injection of corticosteroids for diabetic macular edema was first described in 2002 and became commonplace for the treatment of retinal vein occlusion and diabetic macular edema.[3-5]

In 2004, pegaptanib became the first anti-vascular endothelial growth factor (VEGF) agent the United States (US) Food and Drug Administration (FDA) approved for intravitreal injection for the treatment of neovascular age-related macular degeneration (AMD). Since then, additional anti-VEGF agents have become available and include bevacizumab, ranibizumab, and aflibercept. Currently, ranibizumab and aflibercept are FDA approved for the treatment of neovascular AMD, macular edema due to retinal vein occlusion, diabetic macular edema, and diabetic retinopathy. Large, randomized, controlled trials to assess injection technique are lacking; however, there have been many large studies to help establish general guidelines.[6]

Preexisting Conditions

Guidelines based on roundtable deliberations conducted after a review of published studies of intravitreal injections from 2004 to 2014 addressed several issues related to the injection process, including preexisting ocular conditions. The authors suggest that there are no absolute contraindications to intravitreal injection, but there are several clinical scenarios that warrant special consideration.[6]

Patients with preexisting ocular hypertension or glaucoma should be managed by the treating physician according to the standard of care or preferred practice pattern.

Duker JS, Liang MC, eds.
Anti-VEGF Use in
Ophthalmology (pp. 47-56).
© 2017 Taylor & Francis Group.

Intravitreal injection should not be withheld secondary to ocular hypertension or glaucoma if treatment is necessary for preservation of vision. In these patients, the injecting physician should consider monitoring intraocular pressure after injection, but routine anterior chamber paracentesis is not recommended. It may be beneficial, however, in those with highly elevated intraocular pressure due to neovascular glaucoma.

In addition, previous ocular surgery does not preclude a patient from receiving an intravitreal injection, although the physician should avoid the site of prior incisional glaucoma surgery. Anticoagulation does not need to be withheld prior to injection. Patients with active external infection, including severe blepharitis, hordeolum, or cellulitis, should have the injection postponed until the infection has been adequately treated and cleared.[6] In reviewing our cases of endophthalmitis after intravitreal injection, we found approximately one-third had an underlying systemic infection. Therefore, we recommend deferring injection, if possible, until after the infection has been adequately treated.

There are no data in the literature discussing the safety of intravitreal injections of anti-VEGF agents in the setting of active uveitis. If possible, we recommend controlling intraocular inflammation prior to injection.

Anesthesia

Many patients who receive intravitreal injections of anti-VEGF agents require frequent injections on a regular basis, and in some, the fear of pain and discomfort may lead to considerable anxiety. A pain-free injection is paramount in maintaining comfort and ensuring compliance to a treatment regimen. An ideal anesthetic provides maximum pain reduction without inflicting additional discomfort or increasing the risk of side effects. Other considerations include the ease of anesthetic application, the time required to administer the anesthetic, and cost.[7]

There has been no consensus as to which mode of anesthesia is optimal for pain control in intravitreal injections. Commonly used methods of topical anesthesia include topical drops (0.5% proparacaine, 0.5% tetracaine, 2% aqueous lidocaine), topical 2% lidocaine jelly, topical 3.5% lidocaine gel, or subconjunctival 2% lidocaine. In the 2008 American Society of Retina Specialists (ASRS) Preferences and Trends (PAT) survey, 36% of practitioners used a pledget or cotton-tip applicator soaked with anesthetic, 24% used subconjunctival lidocaine, 21% used topical anesthetic drops, and 18% used a viscous anesthetic.[8]

In a prospective, masked, randomized study, Blaha et al[7] compared the effectiveness of 4 different anesthetic methods for intravitreal injection: 0.5% proparacaine, 0.5% tetracaine, a pledget of 4% lidocaine, or subconjunctival injection of 2% lidocaine. There was no statistically significant difference between the subjective patient pain scores.[7] Furthermore, the use of subconjunctival lidocaine is associated with chemosis and subconjunctival hemorrhage.[7,9] In another randomized study, there was no significant difference in patient pain scales in patients receiving 0.5% tetracaine hydrochloride drops and a 4% lidocaine pledget, 0.5% tetracaine hydrochloride drops alone, or 4% cocaine drops alone.[10]

Viscous anesthetics have been shown to provide adequate anesthesia for cataract surgery and are frequently used as an anesthetic for intravitreal injection.[11,12] They are reported to be equally efficacious as subconjunctival injections in providing anesthesia with less patient discomfort and fewer side effects.[9,13] Lidocaine jelly (2%), formulated for urogenital use, has been used off-label as an ocular anesthetic. The viscous nature of lidocaine jelly is beneficial in maintaining prolonged anesthetic contact with the ocular surface. Concerns have been raised over the jelly anesthetic forming a physical barrier over the conjunctiva, thus preventing povidone-iodine from contacting the conjunctival surface. In laboratory experiments, culture plates showed increased numbers of colony-forming units on plates treated with povidone-iodine after application of lidocaine jelly in comparison to application of povidone-iodine alone.[14] However, there is no clinical evidence suggesting higher rates of endophthalmitis with the use of lidocaine jelly.[15,16] In 2008, preservative-free lidocaine gel 3.5% (Akten, Akorn) was FDA approved for ocular use. It is 50% less viscous than lidocaine jelly, potentially lowering the risk of bacterial entrapment and allowing better penetration of povidone-iodine.[12]

Allergy to topical anesthetics is rare, with an incidence of less than 1% of the general population. Allergic episodes attributed to topical anesthetics are typically adverse reactions rather than true hypersensitivities, but documented cases of contact dermatitis to anesthetics have been reported. Alternatives include a trial of anesthetic from another class (ie, amides such as lidocaine vs benzoic acid esters such as proparacaine or tetracaine), skin patch testing to verify true allergy, or trial of a preservative-free formula if allergy to preservative is suspected. Ice in a sterile glove has also been reported as an effective anesthetic for intravitreal injection in a patient with a severe lidocaine allergy.[17]

Setting

There is a large variability in practice patterns regarding sterility of injections, ranging from an operating room setting under sterile conditions to office-based injections without the use of lid speculums, gloves, or masks (Figure 5-1). According to the 2013 ASRS PAT survey, 98.2% of retina specialists in the US perform their injections in the office while only 47.3% of their international colleagues do the same. The large remainder of injections performed internationally are given in a surgery center (33.2%) or a hospital (16.4%).[18]

In 2014, Brynskov et al[19] reported a 0.00% incidence of endophthalmitis in 20,293 injections performed in a positive-pressure ventilated operating room under sterile conditions. The authors compared results of major studies of rates of endophthalmitis after intravitreal injection. In 5 studies in which intravitreal injections were performed in the operating room, the rate of endophthalmitis was 0.014% and in 11 studies with an office setting, the rate was 0.038%.[19] Another study reported no difference in the rate of endophthalmitis between injections performed in the operating room vs the office.[20]

Masks

There is concern for oropharyngeal droplet transmission during intravitreal injection potentially increasing the risk of endophthalmitis. This is supported by data from a meta-analysis in which *Streptococcus* species were 3 times more commonly isolated after intravitreal injection as compared to postoperative endophthalmitis.[21] Speaking while not wearing a face mask, by either the patient or physician, has been shown to increase bacterial dispersal in a setting simulating an intravitreal injection.[22] There is significantly less bacterial dispersal either when a face mask is worn or when talking is

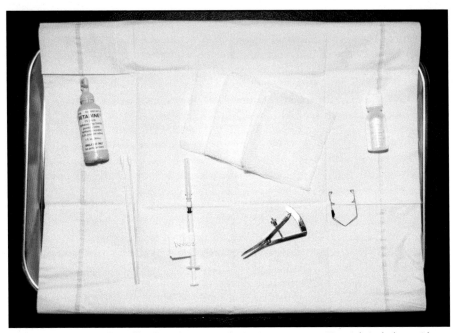

Figure 5-1. Example of an office-based intravitreal injection tray setup. Materials include povidone-iodine 5%, sterile lid speculum, sterile calipers, anti-vascular endothelial growth factor agent in a 1 cc syringe with a 30-gauge needle attached, sterile cotton-tipped applicators, balanced salt solution, and gauze.

avoided.[22,23] Given the evidence above, published guidelines recommend either using a surgical mask or minimizing speaking during preparation and injection.[6,24] According to the 2013 ASRS PAT survey, 78% of US members follow these guidelines.[18]

Gloves

In a survey of US retina specialists, 58% reported using gloves, and of those, 58% use sterile gloves.[25] However, there is no evidence to support the use of gloves to prevent endophthalmitis. In general, the use of nonsterile or sterile gloves is recommended as part of routine infection control in the office setting.[6]

Sterile Drapes

There is no evidence in the literature to suggest the use of sterile drapes decreases the risk of endophthalmitis.[6] In one retrospective study that did not use sterile gloves or drapes, the rate of endophthalmitis was 0.057%, comparable with the overall rates reported in the literature.[26] A 2011 survey found that only 12% of retina specialists in the US use a sterile drape for intravitreal injections.[25]

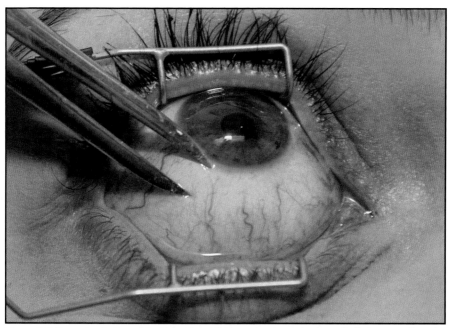

Figure 5-2. Preparing for intravitreal injection. A lid speculum is used to keep the lashes away from the injection site. A sterile caliper is used to mark the injection site, 4 mm posterior to the limbus.

Lid Speculum

In 2011, 90% to 92% of retina specialists reported routinely using a lid speculum for intravitreal injections.[25,27] There is no evidence to suggest that there is a lower rate of endophthalmitis with lid speculum use.[28,29] Care should be taken to avoid the needle contacting the lashes or any other nonsterile objects.[6] The most common way to perform this is with a lid speculum (Figure 5-2), although other techniques have been described.[29,30]

Povidone-Iodine

Endophthalmitis is the most feared complication of intravitreal injection. The rate of endophthalmitis after intravitreal injection reported in the literature ranges from 0.0053% to 0.2%.[31-39] The rate is most likely around 0.05%.[21,40,41] The most commonly isolated organisms are coagulase-negative *Staphylococcus* and *Streptococcus* species.[40]

Povidone-iodine is the only antimicrobial agent that has been proven to decrease the rate of postsurgical endophthalmitis; however, there have been no randomized, controlled trials to determine its efficacy in preventing endophthalmitis after intravitreal injection.[42] Its use has been universally accepted as an important way to decrease rates of endophthalmitis.

While many patients report having allergies to povidone-iodine, true allergy is rare, and no cases of anaphylaxis after ocular application have been reported in the literature.

A skin patch test can be performed to verify an allergy; however, redness does not necessarily equate to allergy and therefore may lead to a false-positive result.[6] Aqueous chlorhexidine has been demonstrated to be effective and safe for ophthalmic use in animal models, but human studies are lacking.[43] Topical antibiotic use immediately preceding intravitreal injection likely does not allow sufficient time to kill many species of bacteria.[44] When used for 3 days prior to injection, topical gatifloxacin decreases rates of positive conjunctival bacterial cultures compared to controls. However, when used in conjunction with povidone-iodine, there was no additional benefit over povidone-iodine use alone.[45]

Topical Antibiotics

The use of periprocedural topical antibiotics with intravitreal injection has been somewhat controversial over the past 10 years. In the 2009 ASRS PAT survey, 82.5% of members used topical antibiotics after intravitreal injection, while in 2015, only 39% of international members and 3.2% of US members did the same.[46,47]

The use of topical antibiotics as an adjunct to povidone-iodine does not decrease bacterial growth on the conjunctiva when compared to povidone-iodine alone.[45] Furthermore, the repeated use of topical antibiotics after intravitreal injections increases the rates of drug-resistant bacteria on the ocular surface.[48] Topical moxifloxacin or gatifloxacin use results in vitreous concentrations lower than the minimum inhibitory concentration for the bacterial species most likely to cause endophthalmitis and therefore are unlikely to be of benefit.[49]

These reports have been substantiated by clinical studies showing no added benefit of periprocedural antibiotics in lowering the rate of endophthalmitis.[31,32,38,39,50,51] Only 2.1% of retina specialists in the US continue to prescribe antibiotics before and after intravitreal injection.[47] Given the evidence, in 2014, an expert panel advised against the routine use of periprocedural topical antibiotics and stressed the importance of povidone-iodine use.[6]

Needle Gauge and Length

Thirty-gauge needles measuring one-half to five-eighths inches in length are the most commonly used needles for injection of anti-VEGF agents. One may also use 31-gauge and 32-gauge needles.[6]

Injection Site

Injections should be performed approximately 3.5 mm or 4 mm posterior to the limbus in pseudophakic and phakic eyes, respectively, with the goal of injecting through the pars plana and toward the center of the globe. Calipers may be used to mark the site of injection (Figure 5-2). There are no formal recommendations advising in which quadrant to perform an injection. Some physicians prefer to use the inferotemporal quadrant for better exposure and for ease of injection in the case of lid squeezing and resultant Bell's reflex. Others prefer to use the superior quadrants to theoretically decrease risk of endophthalmitis as the glaucoma literature has shown higher rates of endophthalmitis with inferior blebs.[52] However, studies have shown no difference in the rate of endophthalmitis between superior and inferior hemisphere injection sites.[28]

Reflux

Reflux often occurs after intravitreal injection and typically presents as a subconjunctival bleb. The contents and significance of this reflux is unknown. Some theorize it is liquefied vitreous, while others believe it may be aqueous or the drug itself.[53-55] Advantages of reflux include allowing the intraocular pressure to equilibrate. Disadvantages include possible loss of drug and a theoretical passageway for bacteria to enter the globe. Studies show less reflux and higher intraocular pressure with increasing needle gauge and with tunneled injections.[56-58] Clinically, there has been no proven benefit with a tunneled approach so a perpendicular injection is typically used.[6]

Reflux can be avoided by occluding the injection site with a sterile cotton-tipped swab immediately after injection. Conjunctival displacement, while allowing reflux, theoretically provides a less direct pathway for bacteria to enter the globe; however, this has not been shown to decrease the rate of postinjection endophthalmitis.[28] We advocate allowing reflux to occur to equilibrate intraocular pressure.

Bilateral Injections

Simultaneous, bilateral intravitreal injections in the office have been shown to be well tolerated by patients, and if offered, patients should be counseled on the risk of having a bilateral complication.[59] Expert panel guidelines advise using caution when performing bilateral injections and recommend that the injecting physician treat each eye as a separate procedure with separate instruments. Furthermore, if a compounded medication is used, the authors recommend using a medication with a different lot number for each eye.[6]

Postoperative Care

Postinjection antibiotics are not recommended as they can contribute to bacterial resistance and have not been shown to decrease the risk of postinjection endophthalmitis, as discussed previously. Patients should be instructed to avoid eye rubbing and use artificial tears as needed. Physicians may consider overnight patching of patients who are especially sensitive to povidone-iodine. Physicians should review the signs and symptoms of endophthalmitis with all patients and provide 24-hour emergency contact information.[6]

Complications

Complications of intravitreal injection include infectious endophthalmitis, noninfectious endophthalmitis, ocular hypertension, subconjunctival or intraocular hemorrhage, lens injury, and retinal detachment.[24] Infectious endophthalmitis is the most feared complication of intravitreal injection. Sterile intraocular inflammation may also occur and can mimic infectious endophthalmitis. The absence of pain is not a reliable marker of sterile inflammation, and administration of intravitreal antibiotics should be strongly considered.[28,60] Retinal detachment after intravitreal injection is rare,[33,61] but likely occurs either because of induction of a posterior vitreous detachment or incorrect injection technique.[60] Transient, and, rarely, sustained, elevation in intraocular pressure may occur following intravitreal injection.[57,62-64] If the intraocular pressure is greater than the central retinal artery perfusion pressure, occlusion of the central retinal artery may occur. Gross visual acuity assessment should be performed to ensure the retina is perfused prior to discharging the patient from the office.[6]

References

1. Schneider J, Frankel S. Treatment of late postoperative intraocular infections with intraocular injection of penicillin. *Arch Ophthalmol.* 1947;37:304-307.

2. Cantrill HL, Henry K, Melroe NH, Knobloch WH, Ramsay RC, Balfour HH. Treatment of cytomegalovirus retinitis with intravitreal ganciclovir. *Ophthalmology.* 1989;96(3):367-374.

3. Martidis A, Duker JS, Greenberg PB, et al. Intravitreal triamcinolone for refractory diabetic macular edema. *Ophthalmology.* 2002;109(5):920-927.

4. Ip MS, Scott IU, VanVeldhuisen PC, et al. A randomized trial comparing the efficacy and safety of intravitreal triamcinolone with observation to treat vision loss associated with macular edema secondary to central retinal vein occlusion: the standard care vs corticosteroid for retinal vein occlusion (SCORE) study report 5. *Arch Ophthalmol.* 2009;127(9):1101-1114.

5. Diabetic Retinopathy Clinical Research Network. A randomized trial comparing intravitreal triamcinolone acetonide and focal/grid photocoagulation for diabetic macular edema. *Ophthalmology.* 2008;115(9):1447-1449, 1449.e1-e10.

6. Avery RL, Bakri SJ, Blumenkranz MS, et al. Intravitreal injection technique and monitoring: updated guidelines of an expert panel. *Retina.* 2014;34(Suppl 1):S1-S18.

7. Blaha GR, Tilton EP, Barouch FC, Marx JL. Randomized trial of anesthetic methods for intravitreal injections. *Retina.* 2011;31(3):535-539.

8. Mittra R, Pollack J. American Society of Retina Specialists Preferences and Trends Membership Survey. Chicago; 2008.

9. Kozak I, Cheng L, Freeman WR. Lidocaine gel anesthesia for intravitreal drug administration. *Retina.* 2005;25(8):994-998.

10. Yau GL, Jackman CS, Hooper PL, Sheidow TG. Intravitreal injection anesthesia—comparison of different topical agents: a prospective randomized controlled trial. *Am J Ophthalmol.* 2011;151(2):333-337.e2.

11. Assia EI, Pras E, Yehezkel M, Rotenstreich Y, Jager-Roshu S. Topical anesthesia using lidocaine gel for cataract surgery. *J Cataract Refract Surg.* 1999;25(5):635-639.

12. Shah HR, Reichel E, Busbee BG. A novel lidocaine hydrochloride ophthalmic gel for topical ocular anesthesia. *Local Reg Anesth.* 2010;3(1):57-63.

13. Friedman SM, Margo CE. Topical gel vs subconjunctival lidocaine for intravitreous injection: a randomized clinical trial. *Am J Ophthalmol.* 2006;142(5):887-888.

14. Boden JH, Myers ML, Lee T, Bushley DM, Torres MF. Effect of lidocaine gel on povidone-iodine antisepsis and microbial survival. *J Cataract Refract Surg.* 2008;34(10):1773-1775.

15. Lad EM, Maltenfort MG, Leng T. Effect of lidocaine gel anesthesia on endophthalmitis rates following intravitreal injection. *Ophthalmic Surg Lasers Imaging.* 2012;43(2):115-120.

16. Inman ZD, Anderson NG. Incidence of endophthalmitis after intravitreal injection of antivascular endothelial growth factor medications using topical lidocaine gel anesthesia. *Retina.* 2011;31(4):669-672.

17. Lindsell LB, Miller DM, Brown JL. Use of topical ice for local anesthesia for intravitreal injections. *JAMA Ophthalmol.* 2014;132(8):1010-1011.

18. Stone T, Mittra R, Raef S. American Society of Retina Specialists 2013 Preferences and Trends: Membership Survey. Chicago; 2013.

19. Brynskov T, Kemp H, Sørensen TL. No cases of endophthalmitis after 20,293 injections in an operating room setting. *Retina*. 2014;34(5):951-957.

20. Tabandeh H, Boscia F, Sborgia A, et al. Endophthalmitis associated with intravitreal injections: office-based setting and operating room setting. *Retina*. 2014;34(1):18-23.

21. McCannel CA. Meta-analysis of endophthalmitis after intravitreal injection of anti-vascular endothelial growth factor agents: causative organisms and possible prevention strategies. *Retina*. 2011;31(4):654-661.

22. Wen JC, McCannel CA, Mochon B, Garner OB. Bacterial dispersal associated with speech in the setting of intravitreous injections. *Arch Ophthalmol*. 2011;129(12):1551-1554.

23. Doshi RR, Leng T, Fung AE. Reducing oral flora contamination of intravitreal injections with face mask or silence. *Retina*. 2012;32(3):473-476.

24. Doshi RR, Bakri SJ, Fung AE. Intravitreal injection technique. *Semin Ophthalmol*. 2011;26(3):104-113.

25. Green-Simms AE, Ekdawi NS, Bakri SJ. Survey of intravitreal injection techniques among retinal specialists in the United States. *Am J Ophthalmol*. 2011;151(2):329-332.

26. Cheung CS, Wong AW, Lui A, Kertes PJ, Devenyi RG, Lam WC. Incidence of endophthalmitis and use of antibiotic prophylaxis after intravitreal injections. *Ophthalmology*. 2012;119(8):1609-1614.

27. Mittra RA, Jumper JM. American Society of Retina Specialists 2010 Preferences and Trends: Membership Survey. Chicago, IL; 2010.

28. Shah CP, Garg SJ, Vander JF, Brown GC, Kaiser RS, Haller JA. Outcomes and risk factors associated with endophthalmitis after intravitreal injection of anti-vascular endothelial growth factor agents. *Ophthalmology*. 2011;118(10):2028-2034.

29. Fineman MS, Hsu J, Spirn MJ, Kaiser RS. Bimanual assisted eyelid retraction technique for intravitreal injections. *Retina*. 2013;33(9):1968-1970.

30. Shrier E. Cotton-tip applicator lid retraction technique for controlled intravitreal injection. *Retina*. 2014;34(6):1244-1246.

31. Bhatt SS, Stepien KE, Joshi K. Prophylactic antibiotic use after intravitreal injection: effect on endophthalmitis rate. *Retina*. 2011;31(10):2032-2036.

32. Bhavsar AR, Stockdale CR, Ferris FL III, Brucker AJ, Bressler NM, Glassman AR. Update on risk of endophthalmitis after intravitreal drug injections and potential impact of elimination of topical antibiotics. *Arch Ophthalmol*. 2012;130(6):809-810.

33. Bhavsar AR, Sandler DR. Eliminating antibiotic prophylaxis for intravitreal injections: a consecutive series of 18,839 injections by a single surgeon. *Retina*. 2015;35(4):783-788.

34. Moshfeghi AA, Rosenfeld PJ, Flynn HW, et al. Endophthalmitis after intravitreal vascular [corrected] endothelial growth factor antagonists: a six-year experience at a university referral center. *Retina*. 2011;31(4):662-668.

35. Dossarps D, Bron AM, Koehrer P, Aho-Glélé LS, Creuzot-Garcher C, FRCR net (FRenCh Retina specialists net). Endophthalmitis after intravitreal injections: incidence, presentation, management, and visual outcome. *Am J Ophthalmol*. 2015;160(1):17-25.e1.

36. Falavarjani KG, Modarres M, Hashemi M, et al. Incidence of acute endophthalmitis after intravitreal bevacizumab injection in a single clinical center. *Retina*. 2013;33:971-974.

37. Gregori NZ, Flynn HW Jr, Schwartz SG, et al. Current infectious endophthalmitis rates after intravitreal injections of anti-vascular endothelial growth factor agents and outcomes of treatment. *Ophthalmic Surg Lasers Imaging Retina*. 2015;46(6):643-648.

38. Meredith TA, McCannel CA, Barr C, et al. Postinjection endophthalmitis in the Comparison of Age-Related Macular Degeneration Treatments Trials (CATT). *Ophthalmology*. 2015;122(4):817-821.

39. Storey P, Dollin M, Pitcher J, et al. The role of topical antibiotic prophylaxis to prevent endophthalmitis after intravitreal injection. *Ophthalmology*. 2014;121(1):283-289.

40. Fileta JB, Scott IU, Flynn HW Jr. Meta-analysis of infectious endophthalmitis after intravitreal injection of anti-vascular endothelial growth factor agents. *Ophthalmic Surg Lasers Imaging Retina*. 2014;45(2):143-149.

41. Sigford DK, Reddy S, Mollineaux C, Schaal S. Global reported endophthalmitis risk following intravitreal injections of anti-VEGF: a literature review and analysis. *Clin Ophthalmol*. 2015;9:773-781.

42. Ciulla TA, Starr MB, Masket S. Bacterial endophthalmitis prophylaxis for cataract surgery: an evidence-based update. *Ophthalmology*. 2002;109(1):13-24.

43. Fagan XJ, Al-Qureshi S. Intravitreal injections: a review of the evidence for best practice. *Clin Exp Ophthalmol*. 2013;41(5):500-507.

44. Callegan MC, Novosad BD, Ramadan RT, Wiskur B, Moyer AL. Rate of bacterial eradication by ophthalmic solutions of fourth-generation fluoroquinolones. *Adv Ther*. 2009;26(4):447-454.

45. Moss JM, Sanislo SR, Ta CN. A prospective randomized evaluation of topical gatifloxacin on conjunctival flora in patients undergoing intravitreal injections. *Ophthalmology*. 2009;116(8):1498-1501.

46. Mittra R, Pollack J. American Society of Retina Specialists Preferences and Trends Membership Survey. Chicago, IL; 2009.

47. Stone T, Raef S. American Society of Retina Specialists 2015 Preferences and Trends: Membership Survey. Chicago, IL; 2015.

48. Dave SB, Toma HS, Kim SJ. Ophthalmic antibiotic use and multidrug-resistant Staphylococcus epidermidis: a controlled, longitudinal study. *Ophthalmology*. 2011;118(10):2035-2040.

49. Costello P, Bakri SJ, Beer PM, et al. Vitreous penetration of topical moxifloxacin and gatifloxacin in humans. *Retina*. 2006;26(2):191-195.

50. Schwartz SG, Grzybowski A, Flynn HW Jr. Antibiotic prophylaxis: different practice patterns within and outside the United States. *Clin Ophthalmol*. 2016;10:251-256.

51. Yu CQ, Ta CN. Prevention and treatment of injection-related endophthalmitis. *Graefes Arch Clin Exp Ophthalmol*. 2014;252(7):1027-1031.

52. Mac I, Soltau J. Glaucoma-filtering bleb infections. *Curr Opin Ophthalmol*. 2003;14(2):91-94.

53. Brodie FL, Ruggiero J, Ghodasra DH, Hui JZ, VanderBeek BL, Brucker AJ. Volume and composition of reflux after intravitreal injection. *Retina*. 2014;34(7):1473-1476.

54. Boon CJF, Crama N, Klevering BJ, van Kuijk FJ, Hoyng CB. Reflux after intravitreal injection of bevacizumab. *Ophthalmology*. 2008;115(7):1270.

55. Christoforidis JB, Williams MM, Epitropoulos FM, Knopp MV. Subconjunctival bleb that forms at the injection site after intravitreal injection is drug, not vitreous. *Clin Exp Ophthalmol*. 2013;41(6):614-615.

56. De Stefano VS, Abechain JJ, de Almeida LF, et al. Experimental investigation of needles, syringes and techniques for intravitreal injections. *Clin Exp Ophthalmol*. 2011;39(3):236-242.

57. Höhn F, Mirshahi A. Impact of injection techniques on intraocular pressure (IOP) increase after intravitreal ranibizumab application. *Graefes Arch Clin Exp Ophthalmol*. 2010;248(10):1371-1375.

58. Pang CE, Mrejen S, Hoang QV, Sorenson JA, Freund KB. Association between needle size, postinjection reflux, and intraocular pressure spikes after intravitreal injections. *Retina*. 2015;35(7):1401-1406.

59. Bakri SJ, Risco M, Edwards AO, Pulido JS. Bilateral simultaneous intravitreal injections in the office setting. *Am J Ophthalmol*. 2009;148(1):66-69.e1.

60. Falavarjani KG, Nguyen QD. Adverse events and complications associated with intravitreal injection of anti-VEGF agents: a review of literature. *Eye (Lond)*. 2013;27(7):787-794.

61. Sampat KM, Garg SJ. Complications of intravitreal injections. *Curr Opin Ophthalmol*. 2010;21(3):178-183.

62. Falkenstein IA, Cheng L, Freeman WR. Changes of intraocular pressure after intravitreal injection of bevacizumab (Avastin). *Retina*. 2007;27(8):1044-1047.

63. Bakri SJ, McCannel CA, Edwards AO, Moshfeghi DM. Persistent ocular hypertension following intravitreal ranibizumab. *Graefes Arch Clin Exp Ophthalmol*. 2008;246(7):955-958.

64. Adelman RA, Zheng Q, Mayer HR. Persistent ocular hypertension following intravitreal bevacizumab and ranibizumab injections. *J Ocul Pharmacol Ther*. 2010;26(1):105-110.

6

SUSTAINED DELIVERY OPTIONS UNDER STUDY

Michael N. Cohen, MD; Chirag P. Shah, MD, MPH; and
Jeffrey S. Heier, MD

Few therapeutic interventions have been as revolutionary or impactful as the advent of intravitreal anti-vascular endothelial growth factor (anti-VEGF) therapy.[1-4] Currently, the standard ophthalmologic route of administration is by direct injection into the vitreous cavity, providing a high, initial drug concentration that decreases over time. The rate of diffusion of the drug through the vitreous is determined by several factors including molecular weight, hydrophilicity, lipophilicity, and ionic charge.[5] Subsequent elimination is likely controlled anteriorly by aqueous flow dynamics and posteriorly by both retrochoroidal flow and transcellular transport, mediated by proteins in the retinal pigment epithelial cells.[6] Along with the half-life of the drug, these diffusion and elimination pharmacokinetics ultimately limit its durability, with studies demonstrating that VEGF suppression ranges from 26 to 69 days after intravitreal injection.[7] To combat this, patients require frequent injections, and vitreoretinal specialists attempt to individualize each treatment schedule to minimize the patient's total injection burden but still maximize their visual recovery.[8-10] Despite an overall favorable safety profile, intravitreal injections carry a risk of endophthalmitis, cataract, retinal tear or detachment, intraocular hemorrhage, and increased intraocular pressure. Patients face these risks with each injection, and, because of the frequency, can experience an economic and/or even emotional burden over time.[11] Perhaps the bigger problem is varying degrees of postinjection discomfort, either the result of the injection itself, or the use of topical betadine for infection prophylaxis. By developing a method, or device, capable of sustained medication delivery into the vitreous cavity and leading to a reduction, or even elimination of intravitreal injections, the landscape of intravitreal drug administration would change dramatically.

As the scope of intravitreal medications continues to intensify and expand, research efforts dedicated toward sustained delivery models continue to emerge. The most promising technologies for sustained anti-VEGF delivery will be discussed herein.

Duker JS, Liang MC, eds.
Anti-VEGF Use in
Ophthalmology (pp. 57-64).
© 2017 Taylor & Francis Group.

Refillable Reservoir Implants

Surgically implantable devices hold promise as vehicles to release the drug directly into the vitreous cavity; they can be equipped with a refillable reservoir capable of minimally invasive refills. Similar to a glaucoma drainage implant, these devices are surgically implanted, rest on bare sclera, and would remain in place as long as therapy is required, or until the device is no longer able to deliver the drug. Two different systems are being developed simultaneously: the Posterior MicroPump Drug Delivery System (Replenish Inc), which delivers nanoliter doses through a wireless, programmable dosing schedule, and the Port Delivery System (Genentech/Roche), which is designed to provide a continuous release of ranibizumab into the vitreous cavity.[12,13]

The MicroPump system relies on microelectrochemical system technology, consists of titanium, parylene, and silicone, and is implanted underneath conjunctiva and Tenon's capsule. It is composed of carefully sealed electronics responsible for powering the device and controlling the drug delivery mechanism, a drug reservoir chamber, a one-way, pressure-dependent valve, a refill port that can be accessed with a 31-gauge needle using a transconjunctival approach, and a cannula implanted directly into the pars plana.[14] Drug delivery is based on the low-power process of electrolysis, which electrochemically induces water to change phase to oxygen and hydrogen gas, generating pressure in the drug reservoir and forcing the drug out through the cannula. The length of time required to deliver a specific drug dose is determined by the speed and magnitude of the applied current. Interestingly, the device should be compatible with any available medication intended for intravitreal injection.

After demonstrating the device was biocompatible and safe in animal models, it was subsequently implanted in human participants.[12,14] Researchers conducted a single-center, single-arm, open-label study involving 11 patients with diabetic macular edema, and implanted the Posterior MicroPump Drug Delivery System for the purpose of delivering ranibizumab therapy over a course of 90 days. All 11 surgical implantations were completed without complication, and no serious adverse events occurred during the follow-up period. Four of 11 patients did not receive the full dose of ranibizumab, highlighting several different causes of suboptimal dosing, which will likely be addressed in future models. As the primary goal of this study was to demonstrate safety and tolerability of the device, no comparisons were made between bolus injections of ranibizumab and the microdose infusions via the MicroPump. Of note, there was no statistical difference in the visual acuity and central foveal thickness between baseline and the final visit. Clinical trials for United States Food and Drug Administration (FDA) approval are under design.

The Ranibizumab Port Delivery System is surgically placed in the pars plana with a 3.2 mm sutureless incision and is covered by conjunctiva. After completion of surgical fixation, the proximal end of the device is subconjunctival but external to the sclera, while the body of the implant extends into the vitreous cavity. Designed to work exclusively with ranibizumab, the device's 500 µg reservoir comes preloaded with the drug. The implant controls the rate and duration of ranibizumab delivery, providing a continuous release of drug into the vitreous cavity between each refill procedure. Reservoir refills are carried out in the office with a custom refill needle.[15]

Results of the phase I, proof-of-concept study were released in 2012 and discussed during the 2012 American Academy of Ophthalmology Retina Subspecialty Day.[13] Twenty treatment-naïve patients, newly diagnosed with neovascular age-related macular degeneration (AMD), were selected for implantation of the Port Delivery System. Surgical implantation of the device was complicated by 4 potentially sight-threatening adverse events (20%): 1 case of endophthalmitis, 2 cases of persistent vitreous hemorrhage, and 1 traumatic cataract. At the end of the study, only 1 patient with persistent vitreous hemorrhage had a poor visual outcome, and the other 3 had improved visual acuity from baseline. At the 1 year primary endpoint of the study, most patients attained significant visual acuity improvement from baseline, gaining an average of 12 letters, and demonstrated a corresponding anatomical improvement in central retinal thickness. Interestingly, patients required a mean of 4.2 refills during the 1 year period. After 1 year, the study protocol called for the explanation of the device in 6 patients and the continued observation of all others for an additional 24 months. There were no other adverse events reported, and patients tolerated the refilling and explantation procedures well.

As this was a proof-of-concept study only, it was not powered to sufficiently demonstrate efficacy as a primary outcome measure. A phase II trial (LADDER) is currently underway and estimated to be completed in October 2017. This is a multicenter, randomized, double-blinded, active-treatment controlled study to evaluate the safety and efficacy of different doses of ranibizumab delivered via the Port Delivery System to help find the optimum drug concentration for sustained delivery.[16] Low, medium, and high doses of ranibizumab delivered through the Port Delivery System will be compared to monthly intravitreal ranibizumab injections. In an effort to address safety concerns from device implantation during the phase I study, a surgical training program will aim to help minimize risks of the procedure. There is hope that completion of the phase II study will allow clinicians and researchers to achieve a better understanding of true sustained delivery anti-VEGF performance.

Injectable Particulate Systems

Advances in nanotechnology allow for the potential use of nanoparticles for enhanced drug penetration and/or targeting and sustained release. Specific classes of nanoparticles that have potential in the future of anti-VEGF delivery are liposomes and microspheres/nanospheres. Verisomes and hydrogels are 2 additional injectable particulate technologies of particular interest.

Liposomes are small, closed-lipid vesicles that are made of a modifiable phospholipid bilayer. Their size, exact lipid composition, and electric charge can be customized, allowing them to be excellent drug carriers.[17] Additionally, they have almost no toxicity, an extremely low antigenicity, and can be biodegradable. Early research in animal models suggests that intravitreal injection of liposomes containing a drug may allow for controlled and sustained release, an increase in half-life of the drug, and a decrease in potential toxicity.[18-20] In one animal study, aqueous and vitreous concentrations of bevacizumab were compared after either liposomal bevacizumab injection or standard bevacizumab injection. Those that received liposomal bevacizumab showed concentrations that were five-fold higher on day 42 when compared to eyes that received free bevacizumab injections.[21] Still in the preclinical stage, there are several limitations including the potential for blurred vision after injection, low drug load, poor stability when a water-soluble drug is encapsulated, and limited storage conditions.[16]

Although similar to liposomes in both shape and size, microspheres have greater stability and drug-carrying capacity.[22] Microspheres are spherical preparations whose particles have diameters ranging from 1 μm to 1000 μm; preparations whose particles have smaller diameters (nanomicrons) are called nanospheres. The drugs are encapsulated in natural and/or synthetic polymers, allowing them to target certain tissues and achieve a state of sustained, continuous release. Frequently used polymers include polylactic acid, polyglycolic acid, and poly (lactic-co-glycolic acid) (PLGA). Research has demonstrated that polylactic acid and PLGA can be inserted without any evidence of histologic or functional toxicity to the retina.[23] For comparison, the sustained-release dexamethasone intravitreal implant, Ozurdex (Allergan Inc), is a biodegradable PLGA device. Polylactic acid, polyglycolic acid, and PLGA are also all used as suture material, vascular grafts, and bone screws and all are FDA-approved for drug delivery.[24]

More than a decade ago, a microsphere system was used in an animal model to provide a continuous release of pegaptanib over several weeks.[25] These particles demonstrated promising in vitro results of sustained anti-VEGF release; however, there are no active clinical trials at this time.[11,26]

Verisome (Icon Bioscience Inc) is a proprietary technology designed for sustained and controlled delivery of small molecules, proteins, or antibodies for up to one year.[27] The Verisome-based drug is injected into the vitreous cavity with a 30-gauge needle and forms a single spherule that settles inferiorly. The system is biodegradable, and its subsequent reduction in size reflects the degradation of both the delivery system and release of active drug.[11] Positive results have been demonstrated in a phase I trial using a single intravitreal injection of IBI-20089 (a proprietary drug formulated with the steroid triamcinolone acetonide) to treat patients with macular edema due to retinal vein occlusion.[26] Combination therapy with IBI-20089 and ranibizumab for patients with neovascular AMD is currently in phase II clinical trials.[11] A Verisome system formulated with an anti-VEGF drug is still in preclinical stages.

Similar to Verisome technology, hydrogels can also be injected in a liquid form, via a small-gauge needle, into the vitreous. Hydrogels are polymeric networks that permit the alteration of diffusion and permeation characteristics, allowing for the creation of an optimal drug delivery system.[28] These hydrogels lack hydrophobic interactions that normally denature biomolecules, and are therefore excellent for encapsulating biomacromolecules. Although these natural polymers provide increased biodegradability, increased biocompatibility, and biologically recognizable moieties, they still might provoke inflammatory responses within the body.[29]

Ocular Therapeutix is in the preclinical stages of developing a polyethylene glycol hydrogel that contains anti-VEGF drug particles. The bioresorbable hydrogel creates a tight meshwork that permits complete embedding of the drug molecules, allowing for controlled release of drug and stability over time. As the hydrogel degrades with hydrolysis, the anti-VEGF molecules dissolve from the surrounding particles and diffuse through the hydrogel and into the surrounding tissue. They have pioneered a coiling process that, because of its "coiled" configuration, allows a larger amount of drug to be deposited than would have been possible without the conformational change (Figure 6-1). Animal studies have been promising thus far, demonstrating a favorable safety profile over a 2-month period, and a very favorable pharmacokinetic profile of its sustained release formulation over a 28-day period.[30,31] The technology remains in the preclinical stages of development, with the goal of drug efficacy set at 4 to 6 months for each injection.

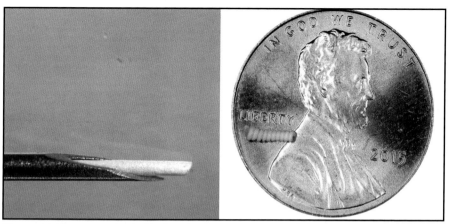

Figure 6-1. Illustration of coiled hydrogel insertion through a small-gauge needle (the preformed dried hydrogel fiber hydrates in situ to form a cell) and its size compared to a penny. (Reprinted with permission from Ocular Therapeutix.)

Encapsulated Cell Technology

In an effort to circumvent the injection or implantation of a finite amount of drug product, encapsulated cell technology (Neurotech Pharmaceuticals), uses genetically transformed cells to produce and secrete a continuous amount of target drug in vivo. The essential tool behind this sustained delivery platform is a malleable and resilient cell line (proprietary to Neurotech), which is derived from human retinal pigment epithelial cells. Reportedly able to survive in conditions low in both oxygen concentration and nutrients, these cells are amenable to genetic engineering by plasmid transfection, allowing them to secrete various therapeutic proteins including growth factors, fusion proteins, and antibodies.[11,32] The implant, which has been placed in more than 400 individuals over the last 5 years (using different cells), consists of a semipermeable external membrane that is capped by a titanium loop and sutured to the sclera. The cells rest in an internal scaffolding, in an environment specifically targeted for their growth and development. The semipermeability of the external casing not only acts to protect the internal contents from an immune response from the body, but also allows oxygen and nutrients to diffuse in and permits the therapeutic proteins created by the cells to diffuse out into the vitreous cavity.

Although several therapeutic products are in development, the NT 503 cell line is of particular interest, as it is genetically modified to continuously create and secrete a VEGF antagonist that was tested to possess the potency, affinity, and inhibitory abilities similar, or better to, that of aflibercept.[33] The sustained therapeutic effect comes from the maintained, steady-state intravitreal concentration, which exceeds the concentration of maintenance-dose monthly bevacizumab injections.[34] Early reports supported safety of the device[35] but a subsequent phase II clinical trial was recently stopped because of poor efficacy. Although there were no safety concerns, efficacy and delivery of the medication will need to be addressed for future efforts.[36]

Figure 6-2. A noninvasive, sustained delivery system using the process of iontophoresis. The probe is placed directly over the pars plana allowing for transmission of drug into the vitreous cavity. (Reprinted with permission from Visulex.)

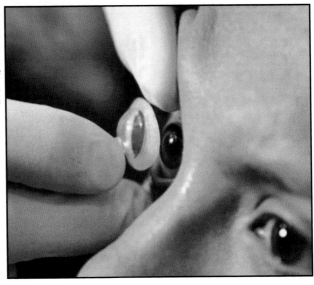

Iontophoresis

In the process of iontophoresis, an electric current is used to drive molecules across the sclera and into the vitreous cavity.[37] Higher current densities should lead to a higher ocular drug concentration. This noninvasive technique is currently under development by several companies (Eyegate II, Eyegate Pharma, Visulex, Aciont). In order to allow precise drug delivery, a plastic probe is placed directly over the pars plana (Figure 6-2), eliminating the need to physically traverse through the anterior segment structures (cornea, iris, lens).[27] This system remains intriguing because of its noninvasive nature; without entering the eye, many of the risks associated with intravitreal injection are eliminated. Although there have been successful proof-of-concept studies with animal models demonstrating that iontophoresis provides appropriate concentrations of triamcinolone acetonide and ranibizumab into ocular tissues of rabbits, there are currently no human trials evaluating anti-VEGF therapy through iontophoresis planned or in development.[38-40]

Conclusions

The promise of sustained delivery therapy for patients requiring repeated anti-VEGF medications seems to be on the near horizon. Although some technologies are further along in development than others, there will likely be several systems for physicians to choose from in the future. It is essential to remain informed and educated on the benefits, risks, and differences between each option.

References

1. Rosenfeld PJ, Brown DM, Heier JS, et al. Ranibizumab for neovascular age-related macular degeneration. *N Engl J Med.* 2006;355(14):1419-1431.

2. Brown DM, Michels M, Kaiser PK, et al. Ranibizumab versus verteporfin photodynamic therapy for neovascular age-related macular degeneration: two-year results of the ANCHOR study. *Ophthalmology.* 2009;116(1):57-65.e5.

3. CATT Research Group, Martin DF, Maguire MG, et al. Ranibizumab and bevacizumab for neovascular age-related macular degeneration. *N Engl J Med.* 2011;364(20):1897-1908.

4. Heier JS, Brown DM, Chong V, et al. Intravitreal aflibercept (VEGF Trap-eye) in wet age-related macular degeneration. *Ophthalmology.* 2012;119(12):2537-2548.

5. Durairaj C, Shah JC, Senapati S, Kompella UB. Prediction of vitreal half-life based on drug physicochemical properties: quantitative structure-pharmacokinetic relationships (QSPKR). *Pharm Res.* 2009;26(5):1236-1260.

6. Kim SH, Lutz RJ, Wang NS, Robinson MR. Transport barriers in transscleral drug delivery for retinal diseases. *Ophthalmic Res.* 2007;39:244-254.

7. Krohne TU, Muether PS, Stratmann NK, et al. Influence of ocular volume and lens status on pharmacokinetics and duration of action of intravitreal vascular endothelial growth factor inhibitors. *Retina.* 2014;35(1):69-74.

8. Gupta OP, Shienbaum G, Patel AH, Fecarotta C, Kaiser RS, Regillo CD. A treat and extend regimen using ranibizumab for neovascular age-related macular degeneration clinical and economic impact. *Ophthalmology.* 2010;117(11):2134-2140.

9. Oubraham H, Cohen SY, Samimi S, et al. Inject and extend dosing versus dosing as needed: a comparative retrospective study of ranibizumab in exudative age-related macular degeneration. *Retina.* 2011;31(1):26-30.

10. Toalster N, Russell M, Ng P. A 12-month prospective trial of inject and extend regimen for ranibizumab treatment of age-related macular degeneration. *Retina.* 2013;33:1351-1358.

11. Bansal P, Garg S, Sharma Y, Venkatesh P. Posterior segment drug delivery devices: current and novel therapies in development. *J Ocul Pharmacol Ther.* 2016;32(3):135-144.

12. Gutiérrez-Hernández JC, Caffey S, Abdallah W, et al. One-year feasibility study of Replenish MicroPump for intravitreal drug delivery: a pilot study. *Transl Vis Sci Technol.* 2014;3(4):8.

13. Loewenstein A, Laganovska G. First-in-human results of a refillable drug delivery implant providing release of ranibizumab in patients with neovascular AMD. Paper presented at: The American Academy of Ophthalmology Retina Subspecialty Day; November 9, 2012; Chicago, IL.

14. Humayun M, Santos A, Altamirano JC, et al. Implantable MicroPump for drug delivery in patients with diabetic macular edema. *Transl Vis Sci Technol.* 2014;3(6):5.

15. Englander M, Shah CP, Heier JS. Extended release of ranibizumab with the Port Delivery System. *Retina Times.* 2015;33(2):20-21.

16. Genentech, Inc. Study of the efficacy and safety of the ranibizumab port delivery system for sustained delivery of ranibizumab in participants with subfoveal neovascular age-related macular degeneration (LADDER). ClinicalTrials.gov. https://clinicaltrials.gov/ct2/show/NCT02510794. Published July 17, 2015. Accessed May 8, 2016.

17. Honda M, Asai T, Oku N, Araki Y, Tanaka M, Ebihara N. Liposomes and nanotechnology in drug development: focus on ocular targets. *Int J Nanomedicine.* 2013;8:495-504.

18. Tremblay C, Barza M, Szoka F, Lahav M, Baum J. Reduced toxicity of liposome-associated amphotericin B injected intravitreally in rabbits. *Invest Ophthalmol Vis Sci.* 1985;26(5):711-718.

19. Fishman PH, Peyman GA, Lesar T. Intravitreal liposome-encapsulated gentamicin in a rabbit model. Prolonged therapeutic levels. *Invest Ophthalmol Vis Sci.* 1986;27(7):1103-1106.

20. Peyman GA, Khoobehi B, Tawakol M, et al. Intravitreal injection of liposome-encapsulated ganciclovir in a rabbit model. *Retina.* 1987;7(4):227-229.

21. Abrishami M, Zarei-Ghanavati S, Soroush D, Rouhbakhsh M, Jaafari MR, Malaekeh-Nikouei B. Preparation, characterization, and in vivo evaluation of nanoliposomes-encapsulated bevacizumab (Avastin) for intravitreal administration. *Retina.* 2009;29(5):699-703.

22. Wang J, Jiang A, Joshi M, Christoforidis J. Drug delivery implants in the treatment of vitreous inflammation. *Mediators Inflamm.* 2013;2013:780634.

23. Jain R, Shah NH, Malick AW, Rhodes CT. Controlled drug delivery by biodegradable poly(ester) devices: different preparative approaches. *Drug Dev Ind Pharm.* 1998;24(8):703-727.

24. Yeh, S, Albini TA, Moshfeghi AA. A peek down the pipeline: emerging drug-delivery options for retinal diseases. *Adv Ocul Care.* 2015;32-37.

25. Carrasquillo KG, Ricker JA, Rigas IK, Miller JW, Gragoudas ES, Adamis AP. Controlled delivery of the anti-VEGF aptamer EYE001 with poly(lactic-co-glycolic) acid microspheres. *Invest Ophthalmol Vis Sci.* 2003;44(1):290-299.

26. Osswald CR, Kang-Mieler JJ. Controlled and extended in vitro release of bioactive anti-vascular endothelial growth factors from a microsphere-hydrogel drug delivery system. *Curr Eye Res.* 2016;41(9):1216-1222.

27. Lim JI, Fung AE, Wieland M, Hung D, Wong V. Sustained-release intravitreal liquid drug delivery using triamcinolone acetonide for cystoid macular edema in retinal vein occlusion. *Ophthalmology.* 2011;118(7):1416-1422.

28. Shah SS, Denham LV, Elison JR, et al. Drug delivery to the posterior segment of the eye for pharmacologic therapy. *Expert Rev Ophthalmol.* 2010;5(1):75-93.

29. Lin CC, Metters AT. Hydrogels in controlled release formulations: network design and mathematical modeling. *Adv Drug Del Rev.* 2006;58:1379-1408.

30. Jarrett PK, Elhayek RF, Guedez S, Rosales C, Jarrett TS, Sawhney A. Tolerability of intravitreal hydrogel depots for anti-VEGF sustained release in a rabbit model. *Invest Ophthalmol Vis Sci.* 2015;56(7):1496.

31. Elhayek RF, Jarrett PK, Sawhney A, et al. Pharmacokinetics of bevacizumab sustained release from intravitreal hydrogel depots in a rabbit model compared to a single Avastin dose. *Invest Ophthalmol Vis Sci.* 2015;56(7):1522.

32. Neurotech. Platform & Pipeline. http://www.neurotechusa.com/ect-platform.html. Accessed April 7, 2016.

33. Rivera M, Nystuen A, Kauper K, et al. Analysis of binding affinity and inhibitory capacity of NT-503 produced VEGF antagonist compared to Aflibercept. *Invest Ophthalmol Vis Sci.* 2015;56(7):228.

34. Rivera M, Lelis A, Bouchard B, et al. Pharmacokinetics of a VEGF antagonist delivered by an intraocular encapsulated cell technology implant. *Invest Ophthalmol Vis Sci.* 2012;53(14):474.

35. Guerrero-Naranjo JL, Quiroz-Mercado H, Sanchez-Bermudez G, et al. Safety of implantation of the NT-503 device in patients with choroidal neovascularization secondary to age-related macular degeneration. *Invest Ophthalmol Vis Sci.* 2013;54(15):3298.

36. Neurotech. Platform & Pipeline. http://www.neurotechusa.com/phone/nc-503-ect.html Accessed May 26, 2016.

37. Sarraf D, Lee DA. The role of iontophoresis in ocular drug delivery. *J Ocul Pharmacol.* 1994;10(1):69-81.

38. Singh RP, Mathews ME, Kaufman M, Riga A. Transcleral delivery of triamcinolone acetonide and ranibizumab to retinal tissues using macroesis. *Br J Ophthalmol.* 2010;94(2):170-173.

39. Higuchi W, Tuitupou AL, Kochambilli RP, et al. Delivery of sustained release formulation of triamcinolone acetonide to the rabbit eye using the VisulexTM Ocular Iontophoresis Device. *Invest Ophthalmol Vis Sci.* 2006;47(13):5108.

40. Molokhia SA, Papangkorn K, Mix D, et al. Transscleral iontophoretic delivery of Avastin in vivo: drug distribution and safety aspects. *Invest Ophthalmol Vis Sci.* 2012;53(14):491.

Section II

Use of Anti-Vascular Endothelial Growth Factor Agents in Clinical Practice

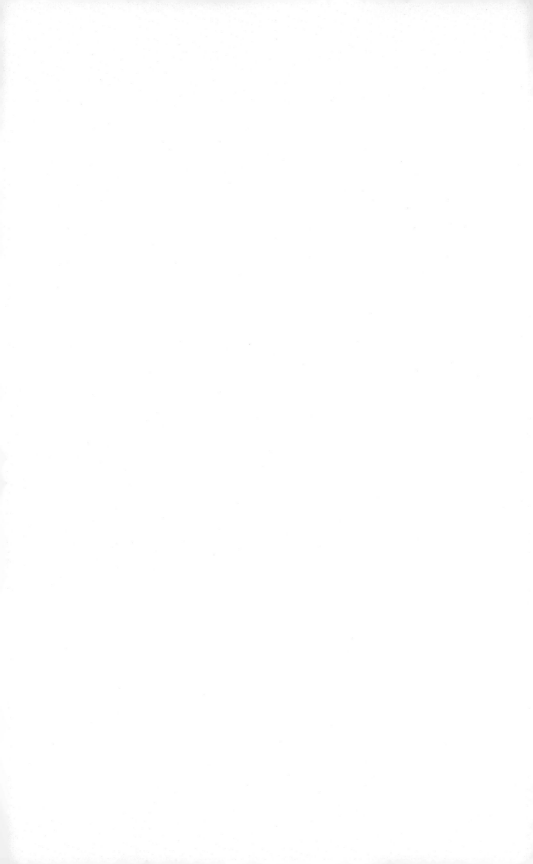

7

Neovascular Age-Related Macular Degeneration

Michael D. Lewen, MD and
Andre J. Witkin, MD

Age-related macular degeneration (AMD) is a leading cause of vision loss among adults worldwide, and advances in its management represent one of the most successful recent achievements in medicine. AMD can cause severe central vision loss in advanced disease, which is marked by geographic atrophy in the non-neovascular or "dry" form and by the growth of abnormal choroidal neovascular membranes (CNV) in neovascular or "wet" disease. The targeted inhibition of vascular endothelial growth factor (VEGF) has revolutionized the treatment of neovascular AMD, and these medications are currently among the most frequently used in all of medicine.[1]

Epidemiology

Population-based studies in the United States (US), Australia, and Europe estimate the prevalence of neovascular AMD to range between 0.41% and 1.55% in adults older than 40 years of age, with higher prevalence in Caucasian compared to African American individuals.[2] The incidence in predominantly Caucasian populations over a 15-year period is estimated at 2.0% to 4.4%.[3,4] Both the prevalence and incidence of neovascular AMD increase dramatically with age, particularly after the age of 70.[2-4] Although the neovascular form represents a small percentage of AMD overall, it accounts for the overwhelming degree of severe vision loss due to AMD.[5]

Significant risk factors associated with development of AMD include tobacco use, hypertension, increased body mass index, hyperopia, and certain genetic markers.[6,7] Clinical features of nonexudative AMD, including soft, indistinct drusen and pigmentary abnormalities, are considered high-risk features for the development of neovascularization. In addition, the presence of CNV in one eye increases the risk of development in the fellow eye,[8] the incidence of which was approximately 33% at 2 years in recent landmark studies of neovascular AMD.[9,10] Over 7 years of follow-up, these patients demonstrated bilateral neovascular disease in 51% of the cohort.[11]

Duker JS, Liang MC, eds.
*Anti-VEGF Use in
Ophthalmology (pp. 67-79).*
© 2017 Taylor & Francis Group.

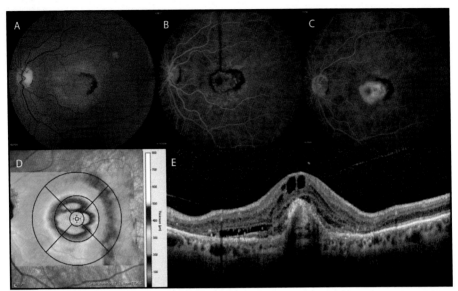

Figure 7-1. A patient with neovascular age-related macular degeneration and type 2, or "classic," choroidal neovascularization (CNV). (A) Color fundus photograph and (B) early- and (C) late-phase fluorescein angiography show subretinal hemorrhage with early leakage of a well-defined CNV that hyperfluoresces with less-distinct margins in the late frame. (D) Retinal thickness map and (E) foveal horizontal optical coherence tomography B-scan reveal a hyper-reflective CNV complex with increased central retinal thickness and associated intra- and subretinal fluid.

Pathophysiology and Clinical Features

The etiology and pathogenesis of AMD is multifactorial and has not been completely elucidated, though progression includes degeneration of Bruch's membrane and the retinal pigment epithelium (RPE). This can lead to formation of abnormal capillary-like vessels that emanate from the choriocapillaris and invade into the sub-RPE space (type 1) or subneurosensory retinal space (type 2); these abnormal fibrovascular complexes are termed *choroidal neovascular membranes* (CNV).[12,13] Less commonly, CNV may originate from abnormal vessels within the retinal circulation and grow to invade the sub-RPE space, categorized as retinal angiomatous proliferation (type 3).[14] CNV are prone to leaking serous fluid, lipid, or hemorrhage that can be observed clinically as exudation or intra- or subretinal hemorrhage (Figures 7-1A and 7-2).

Depending on the anatomical location and severity of neovascularization, patients may experience abrupt changes in vision ranging from distortion of straight lines, known as metamorphopsia, to profoundly decreased central vision. Clinical examination typically demonstrates a decrease in visual acuity, and if left untreated, this visual loss can be rapidly progressive. Although fundus findings are often suggestive of neovascular AMD, subtle cases may be difficult to diagnose on examination alone. Therefore, ancillary testing is crucial in confirming the diagnosis of neovascular AMD.

Fluorescein angiography (FA) has long been considered the gold standard in diagnosis of neovascular AMD. FA classically shows leakage of dye at the site of the CNV, as the blood vessel endothelium in CNV has improperly formed tight junctions allowing for

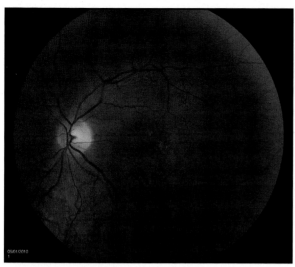

Figure 7-2. Color fundus photograph demonstrates exudate surrounding an area of hemorrhage and a lesion suspicious for choroidal neovascularization, as well as mottling of the retinal pigment epithelium inferiorly.

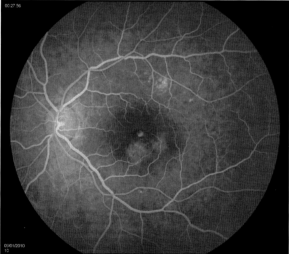

Figure 7-3. Fluorescein angiography corresponding to the fundus image in Figure 7-2 confirms the presence of neovascularization as a well-defined hyperfluorescent focus in the fovea. The adjacent ill-defined areas of hyperfluorescence inferiorly correspond to the retinal pigment epithelium mottling seen in Figure 7-2 and are suggestive of proliferation of the choroidal neovascularization in the subretinal pigment epithelium space as a type 1, or "occult," choroidal neovascularization.

extravasation of fluorescein dye over time. The appearance of CNV can vary depending on its location. Type 2 CNV, termed *classic* on FA, appears early as well-defined hyperfluorescent lesions that leak in mid- to late-frames (Figure 7-1). Type 1 CNV, termed *occult* on FA, is ill defined, and leakage often appears only in later frames (Figures 7-2 and 7-3). In type 3 CNV, a focal "hot spot" is often visualized at the point of anastomosis between retinal and choroidal circulations. Indocyanine green angiography is another technique to image CNV and can be particularly useful in differentiating neovascularization associated with AMD from other known variants such as polypoidal choroidal vasculopathy.

Optical coherence tomography (OCT) has become the most commonly used imaging modality in managing neovascular AMD, as it allows for precise, rapid, and noninvasive cross-sectional and volumetric analysis of the retinal architecture. Intra- or subretinal

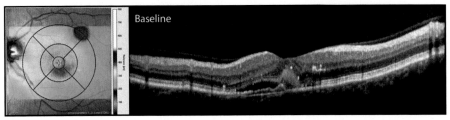

Figure 7-4. Retinal thickness map and foveal horizontal optical coherence tomography B-scan corresponding to Figures 7-2 and 7-3 show a subfoveal hyper-reflective lesion, consistent with choroidal neovascularization. There is an adjacent shallow retinal pigment epithelial detachment with overlying subretinal fluid, and intraretinal exudate is scattered throughout the retinal layers.

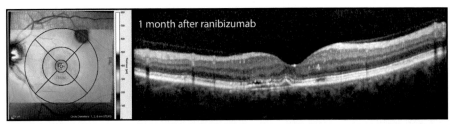

Figure 7-5. Retinal thickness map and optical coherence tomography B-scan corresponding to Figure 7-4 one month following intravitreal ranibizumab therapy. The subfoveal hyper-reflective lesion is no longer visible and there is interval improvement of the subretinal fluid with return of the foveal contour.

fluid, signs of neovascular disease, can be detected in untreated eyes with CNV and also serve as signs of persistent disease activity once therapy has been initiated. These subtle anatomic changes might otherwise be clinically undetectable but can easily be visualized with OCT (Figures 7-1, 7-4, and 7-5).

The natural history of neovascular AMD is rapid progression to severe loss of visual acuity. In a meta-analysis of more than 4000 treatment-naïve patients with neovascular AMD, the mean change in visual acuity worsened from 1 line lost at 3 months to 2.7 lines lost at 12 months and 4 lines lost at 24 months. At 3 years, more than 40% of untreated patients experienced severe vision loss (defined as a decrease of more than 6 lines) and more than 75% of patients had visual acuity worse than 20/200.[15] End-stage disease is characterized by atrophy of the neurosensory retina and RPE or fibrovascular scar tissue formation, often termed a *disciform scar*.

Evolution of Treatment

Prior to anti-VEGF therapy, the treatment for neovascular AMD consisted of thermal laser photocoagulation and photodynamic therapy (PDT) with verteporfin (Visudyne). A small percentage of eyes with extrafoveal CNV had improvements in visual acuity from direct laser photocoagulation;[16] however, laser photocoagulation for subfoveal CNV resulted in poor visual outcomes, and its use was largely abandoned after the development of PDT. The Treatment of Age-Related Macular Degeneration with PDT (TAP) study demonstrated benefit from PDT for subfoveal CNV lesions that were "predominantly classic," with greater than 50% of the CNV lesion being classic.[17] Treatment success, however, was largely defined in terms of slowing or limiting visual loss, not visual improvement.

The discovery of VEGF and its major role in neovascular AMD dramatically changed the treatment paradigm, and PDT and thermal laser have largely become historical treatments for this disease. VEGF is a glycoprotein that is instrumental in angiogenesis, endothelial cell growth, and increased vascular permeability.[18] Of the multiple VEGF genes, VEGF-A is the predominant form. There are several isoforms of VEGF-A based on the size of the protein products; $VEGF_{165}$ is the principal isoform in humans.[19] The larger isoforms can be further modified by enzymes resulting in smaller proteins that have different biologic activities or properties such as the capacity to easily diffuse through retinal tissue.[20]

Shortly after VEGF was isolated and sequenced, increased intraocular levels of VEGF were demonstrated in the setting of retinal ischemia and neovascularization.[21,22] Mouse models were shown to develop CNV in the setting of VEGF overexpression,[23] and engineered antibodies against VEGF demonstrated efficacy in decreasing leakage from and formation of CNV in animal studies,[24] thus ushering in the era of anti-VEGF treatment for neovascular AMD. The following 4 anti-VEGF medications have been used for treatment of neovascular AMD (Table 7-1):

1. Pegaptanib sodium
2. Ranibizumab
3. Bevacizumab
4. Aflibercept

Although pegaptanib sodium was the first anti-VEGF medication on the market for treatment of neovascular AMD, its use quickly declined as more effective treatments became available, and its use for treatment of neovascular AMD is now largely of historical significance.

Bevacizumab and Ranibizumab

Bevacizumab (Avastin) is a full-length recombinant humanized antibody that binds to all isoforms of VEGF[19,25] and was US Food and Drug Administration (FDA) approved in 2004 for the treatment of colon cancer in combination with chemotherapy. It was initially thought the size of bevacizumab as a full-length antibody would preclude efficient diffusion through the retina to reach its site of action within the choroid, so a similar but truncated molecule was developed, ranibizumab, specifically formulated for intravitreal injection.[19,26] Ranibizumab (Lucentis) is a recombinant humanized antibody fragment that also binds to and blocks all active forms of VEGF.

Prior to the FDA approval of ranibizumab, a small pilot study of 9 patients with neovascular AMD were treated with intravenous, systemic bevacizumab. The results were encouraging, with a mean improvement of vision and positive anatomical outcomes as evidenced by decreased central retinal thickness and reduction or complete absence of leakage of the CNV.[27] Soon after, another pilot study demonstrated that off-label use of bevacizumab for intravitreal injection was well tolerated and very effective,[28] and despite early concerns that bevacizumab would be a poor candidate for intravitreal use because of its large molecular structure, its intravitreal use became widespread.

Table 7-1. Landmark Trials of Anti-Vascular Endothelial Growth Factor Agents for Treatment of Macular Degeneration With Best-Corrected Visual Acuity Results:
One-Year Data

Trial (Year)	Total n	Study Groups	Mean Change in Best-Corrected Visual Acuity[a] (Letters)
VISION[b] (2004)	1186	• Pegaptanib 0.3 mg every 6 weeks • Pegaptanib 1.0 mg every 6 weeks • Pegaptanib 3.0 mg every 6 weeks • Sham injection every 6 weeks	−8 −7 −10 −15
ANCHOR (2006)	423	• Ranibizumab 0.3 mg monthly + sham Photodynamic therapy • Ranibizumab 0.5 mg monthly + sham Photodynamic therapy • Sham injection monthly + active PDT	+8.5 +11.3 −9.5
MARINA (2006)	716	• Ranibizumab 0.3 mg monthly • Ranibizumab 0.5 mg monthly • Sham injection monthly	+5.9 +7.2 −10.4
CATT (2011)	1208	• Ranibizumab 0.5 mg monthly • Ranibizumab 0.5 mg pro re nata • Bevacizumab 1.25 mg monthly • Bevacizumab 1.25 mg pro re nata	+8.5 +6.8 +8.0 +5.9
VIEW 1+2 (2012)	2419	• Aflibercept 0.5 mg monthly • Aflibercept 2.0 mg monthly • Aflibercept 2.0 mg every 2 months • Ranibizumab 0.5 mg monthly	+8.3 +9.3 +8.4 +8.7
HARBOR (2013)	1098	• Ranibizumab 0.5 mg monthly • Ranibizumab 0.5 mg pro re nata • Ranibizumab 2.0 mg monthly • Ranibizumab 2.0 mg pro re nata	+10.1 +8.2 +9.2 +8.6

[a]Compared with baseline vision at the start of the trial.
[b]Data are approximate values.

Subsequent large clinical studies involving ranibizumab proved to be a monumental paradigm shift in the management of neovascular AMD. In 2006, 2 phase III studies (ANCHOR and MARINA) demonstrated that ranibizumab dramatically improved visual outcomes for all forms of CNV in AMD and led to its FDA approval. This was in stark contrast to the previous standard of slowing or minimizing vision loss. In both studies, more than 90% of the treatment arms met the primary endpoint of less than 15 letters of vision lost at 1 year, compared to approximately 60% in the control arms.[29,30] More than 25% of treated patients had improvement in vision of 15 letters or more, with a mean gain of visual acuity across all treatment groups. In the 0.5 mg dose groups at 1 year, patients demonstrated a mean improvement of 11.3 letters in ANCHOR and 7.2 letters in MARINA.[29,30] The control groups in both studies lost vision compared with baseline.

Severe vision loss was exceedingly rare in the treated groups and visual improvement was maintained throughout the 2-year study period.

Bevacizumab remained a compelling alternative to ranibizumab, however, in large part because aliquots of bevacizumab made for intravitreal administration by compounding pharmacies allowed for significant cost savings with a seemingly comparable therapeutic effect. The equivalency of intravitreal bevacizumab to ranibizumab was unproven until 2 large, randomized clinical trials in the US (Comparison of Age-Related Macular Degeneration Treatments Trials [CATT]) and the United Kingdom (IVAN) published data in 2011 and 2012. The results of the 2-year studies confirmed that bevacizumab was noninferior to ranibizumab in safety and efficacy.[31,32] Furthermore, the average cost of 1 year of monthly ranibizumab was $23,400 compared with $595 for 1 year of monthly bevacizumab.[31] For this reason, many physicians use intravitreal bevacizumab as first-line therapy for the treatment of neovascular AMD.

Aflibercept

Aflibercept is the highest-affinity VEGF inhibitor to date.[33] It is a decoy receptor that binds all isoforms of VEGF-A, VEGF-B, and placental growth factor, and is composed of the binding regions of VEGF receptors 1 and 2 combined with the fragment crystallizable, or constant region, of human immunoglobulin G1.[33,34] Two phase III trials (VIEW 1 and 2) compared aflibercept given monthly and every 2 months with monthly ranibizumab. After one year, all of the aflibercept groups were determined to be noninferior to monthly ranibizumab based on visual acuity and anatomical outcomes.[35] Noninferiority compared with monthly ranibizumab was again demonstrated at the 2-year mark, with the every 2-month aflibercept group requiring 5 fewer injections on average.[36] The results of these studies led to FDA approval of aflibercept in 2011.

Alternative Dosing Regimens

CATT and IVAN not only compared bevacizumab with ranibizumab, but also evaluated fixed, monthly injections vs as-needed treatment (pro re nata, PRN) in order to potentially decrease the frequency and total number of injections required.[31,32] OCT was essential for these studies, as a primary criterion for PRN treatment was evidence of activity on OCT. This technique was previously evaluated in a smaller study (PrONTO).[37] At 24 months, mean treatments were 12.6 ranibizumab injections and 14.1 bevacizumab injections in the PRN arms. When comparing the 2 treatment regimens, there was a small but statistically significant loss of efficacy in the PRN compared to monthly treatment (–2.23 letters) group, although both had significant visual acuity gains over the course of the study.[32] In the HARBOR study, the mean number of ranibizumab injections was 13.3 over 24 months, with 5.6 given during the second year. The average treatment interval was 9.9 weeks.[38] However, similar to CATT and IVAN, the PRN dosing group did not meet the noninferiority endpoint in comparison to monthly treatment, again suggesting a small loss of efficacy when using PRN treatment in comparison to monthly injections.

An alternative dosing regimen is termed *treat-and-extend*. In this regimen, treatment is individualized so as to minimize not only the number of injections but also patient visits, which are typically monthly in the PRN treatment arms. Treat-and-extend involves administering initial monthly anti-VEGF injections until stability is achieved, at which point the follow-up visit is scheduled 1 or 2 weeks longer than the previous visit. At this subsequent exam, if there is no disease activity, an injection is still administered and the follow-up interval is again extended; if there is disease activity, an injection is given and follow-up is scheduled at the previous time interval. This pattern is repeated until an individualized treatment schedule is determined.[39] Studies of the treat-and-extend regimen with ranibizumab and bevacizumab report positive visual outcomes consistent with the fixed, monthly dosing studies, with patients requiring an average of 8.36 and 7.94 injections during the first year, with the mean longest period of extension of 79.9 and 92.4 days, respectively.[40,41]

Both PRN treatment with monthly monitoring or a treat-and-extend approach can provide significant therapeutic benefits while helping to decrease the financial and practical burden associated with frequent exams and injections. These regimens have therefore become the most commonly used by retina physicians in everyday practice. However, monthly anti-VEGF injection with ranibizumab remains the gold standard based on the clinical trials, and at this point is the regimen to which other treatments for neovascular AMD are compared.

Approaches to Treatment Resistance

Despite the efficacy of ranibizumab and bevacizumab in the majority of patients, the anticipated treatment response is clearly not achieved in all individuals. A small but not insignificant percentage of patients suffer moderate to severe vision loss despite treatment. In the MARINA and ANCHOR trials, 10% of patients in the monthly ranibizumab arms lost 15 letters or more at 2 years.[29,30] CATT demonstrated persistent retinal fluid on OCT in 51.5% and 67.4% of patients who received monthly ranibizumab and bevacizumab for 2 years, respectively.[31]

Such patients, who for unknown reasons respond incompletely to treatment with ranibizumab or bevacizumab, may demonstrate additional improvement with aflibercept (Figure 7-6). In recent studies, patients who received more than 30 prior injections of ranibizumab or bevacizumab demonstrated a statistically significant improvement in central retinal thickness following treatment with aflibercept.[42,43] While some of these patients demonstrated improved visual acuity, the positive anatomical outcome did not necessarily correlate with improved vision.

Another strategy for patients with inadequate treatment response includes increased frequency or dosage.[44,45] Although increased dosage is currently off-label, some have suggested using a quadruple dose of ranibizumab (2.0 mg) in non-responders.[46] Alternatively, biweekly alternating ranibizumab and bevacizumab may limit costs and the possibility of tachyphylaxis.[47]

Finally, combination therapy with anti-VEGF and thermal laser or PDT may be considered for select patients. Although thermal laser is rarely used, it may be helpful in select cases of extrafoveal CNV. PDT may be used alone or in combination with anti-VEGF therapy, as well as in combination with corticosteroids, otherwise known as *triple therapy*.[48–51]

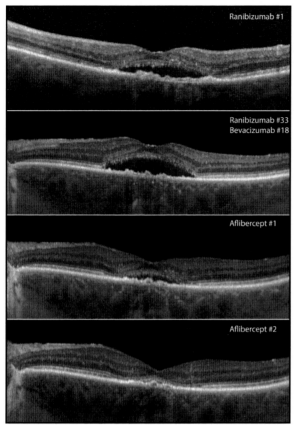

Figure 7-6. Optical coherence tomography B-scans of a patient with neovascular age-related macular degeneration showing limited response to repeated doses of intravitreal ranibizumab and bevacizumab (top 2 panels) and rapid response to intravitreal aflibercept (bottom two panels). (Reprinted with permission from Allen Ho, MD.)

Prognosis

Historically, the diagnosis of neovascular AMD meant a likely prognosis of blindness. Anti-VEGF therapeutics have dramatically improved outcomes. A population-based study in Denmark demonstrated a 50% reduction in the incidence of blindness (visual acuity 20/200 or worse) from AMD coinciding with the advent of intravitreal ranibizumab and bevacizumab.[52] With treatment, fewer patients suffer legal blindness due to neovascular AMD despite the increasing prevalence of this disease.[53-55]

Notwithstanding these advancements, much has yet to be learned about the prognosis of neovascular AMD with long-term anti-VEGF treatment. It is not altogether uncommon for patients to require ongoing treatment for several years, which can add up to many injections. The HORIZON trial reported data on patients who were followed and treated for 2 additional years after completion of the early ranibizumab trials ANCHOR, MARINA, and FOCUS. Four years of treatment with ranibizumab was well tolerated in these patients.[56]

The SEVEN-UP trial was an observational study published in 2013 in which 65 patients who were originally administered intensive ranibizumab therapy in ANCHOR, MARINA, and HORIZON were recruited to evaluate the long-term course of neovascular

AMD. These patients were not actively enrolled in a treatment protocol and were not necessarily maintained on an aggressive regimen at the time of examination for SEVEN-UP, therefore many of these patients had poor visual outcomes. Among the cohort, an average of approximately 2 anti-VEGF injections/year were administered following the conclusion of the HORIZON study, although 41% of patients had received no treatment during this interval.[11] At a mean overall treatment time of 7.3 years, about one-third of study eyes had visual acuity of 20/70 or better and one-third of the cohort was 20/200 or worse. Twenty-three percent of patients had visual acuity of 20/40 or better, and almost half of the patient cohort was stable or improved compared with their baseline acuity at the start of the original ranibizumab trials. There was an overall mean decline in vision of 8.6 letters; however, the subset of patients who had been treated more aggressively had a mean gain of 3.9 letters since the conclusion of HORIZON.[11]

Also of note, CATT showed that patients who were treated most aggressively with monthly injections were more likely to develop geographic atrophy,[31] suggesting that frequent anti-VEGF therapy may promote formation of geographic atrophy. Conversely, 98.2% of patients in SEVEN-UP had evidence of macular atrophy on fundus autofluorescence, a study in which patients were under-treated with anti-VEGF therapy, indicating this may partially be due to the natural history of the disease.[11]

Conclusion

Even in the anti-VEGF era, neovascular AMD remains a chronic and progressive disease. The positive effects of treatment are often temporary and maintenance of visual acuity necessitates regular, ongoing intervention. Some anatomical changes, which may occur as a result of neovascularization, cannot be improved with anti-VEGF treatment and can result in permanent visual loss despite treatment. Nevertheless, relentless progression of vision loss is no longer the standard outcome in patients with neovascular AMD, as anti-VEGF therapies usually are able to maintain vision and often allow for the distinct possibility of visual recovery. This profound advancement has improved the quality of life for countless individuals, and forthcoming therapeutics as well as individualized treatment approaches offer hope for continued improvement in the management of neovascular AMD.

References

1. Medicare Part B: Expenditures for new drugs concentrated among a few drugs, and most were costly for beneficiaries. U.S Government Accountability Office. http://www.gao.gov/products/GAO-16-12. Published October 23, 2015. Accessed March 1, 2016.

2. Friedman DS, O'Colmain BJ, Muñoz B, et al. Prevalence of age-related macular degeneration in the United States. *Arch Ophthalmol.* 2004;122(4):564-572.

3. Klein R, Klein BE, Knudtson MD, Meuer SM, Swift M, Gangnon RE. Fifteen-year cumulative incidence of age-related macular degeneration: the Beaver Dam Eye Study. *Ophthalmology.* 2007;114(2):253-262.

4. Joachim N, Mitchell P, Burlutsky G, Kifley A, Wang JJ. The incidence and progression of age-related macular degeneration over 15 years: the Blue Mountains Eye Study. *Ophthalmology.* 2015;122(12):2482-2489.

5. Ferris FL 3rd, Fine SL, Hyman L. Age-related macular degeneration and blindness due to neovascular maculopathy. *Arch Ophthalmol.* 1984;102(11):1640-1642.

6. Age-Related Eye Disease Study Research Group. Risk factors associated with age-related macular degeneration. A case-control study in the age-related eye disease study: Age-Related Eye Disease Study Report Number 3. *Ophthalmology*. 2000;107(12):2224-2232.

7. Buitendijk GH, Rochtchina E, Myers C, et al. Prediction of age-related macular degeneration in the general population: the Three Continent AMD Consortium. *Ophthalmology*. 2013;120(12):2644-2655.

8. Age-Related Eye Disease Study Research Group. The age-related eye disease study severity scale for age-related macular degeneration: Age-Related Eye Disease Study Report Number 17. *Arch Ophthalmol*. 2005;123(11):1484-1498.

9. Maguire MG, Daniel E, Shah AR, et al. Incidence of choroidal neovascularization in the fellow eye in the comparison of age-related macular degeneration treatment trials. *Ophthalmology*. 2013;120(10):2035-2041.

10. Barbazetto IA, Saroj N, Shapiro H, Wong P, Ho AC, Freund KB. Incidence of new choroidal neovascularization in fellow eyes of patients treated in the MARINA and ANCHOR trials. *Am J Ophthalmol*. 2010;149(6):939-946.

11. Rofagha S, Bhisitkul RB, Boyer DS, Sadda SR, Zhang K. Seven-year outcomes in ranibizumab-treated patients in ANCHOR, MARINA, and HORIZON: a multicenter cohort study (SEVEN-UP). *Ophthalmology*. 2013;120(11):2292-2299.

12. Green WR, Enger C. Age-related macular degeneration histopathologic studies: the 1992 Lorenz E. Zimmerman Lecture. *Ophthalmology*. 1993;100(10):1519-1535.

13. Sarks SH. New vessels formation beneath the retinal pigment epithelium in senile eyes. *Br J Ophthalmol*. 1973;57(12):951-965.

14. Freund KB, Ho IV, Barbazetto IA, et al. Type 3 neovascularization: the expanded spectrum of retinal angiomatous proliferation. *Retina*. 2008;28(2):201-211.

15. Wong TY, Chakravarthy U, Klein R, et al. The natural history and prognosis of neovascular age-related macular degeneration: a systemic review of the literature and meta-analysis. *Ophthalmology*. 2008;115(1):116-126.

16. Macular Photocoagulation Study Group. Argon laser photocoagulation for neovascular maculopathy: three-year results from randomized clinical trials. *Arch Ophthalmol*. 1986;104(5):694-701.

17. Bressler NM, Treatment of Age-Related Macular Degeneration with Photodynamic Therapy (TAP) Study Group. Photodynamic therapy of subfoveal choroidal neovascularization in age-related macular degeneration with verteporfin: two-year results of 2 randomized clinical trials—TAP report 2. *Arch Ophthalmol*. 2001;119(2):198-207.

18. Keck PJ, Hauser SD, Krivi G, et al. Vascular permeability factor, an endothelial mitogen related to PDGF. *Science*. 1989;246(4935):1309-1312.

19. Ferrara N, Damico L, Shams N, Lowman H, Kim R. Development of ranibizumab, an anti-vascular endothelial growth factor antigen binding fragment, as therapy for neovascular age-related macular degeneration. *Retina*. 2006;26(8):859-870.

20. Adamis AP, Shima DT. The role of vascular endothelial growth factor in ocular health and disease. *Retina*. 2005;25(2):111-118.

21. Miller JW, Adamis AP, Shima DT, et al. Vascular endothelial growth factor/vascular permeability factor is temporally and spatially correlated with ocular angiogenesis in a primate model. *Am J Pathol*. 1994;145(3):574-584.

22. Aiello LP, Avery RL, Arrigg PG, et al. Vascular endothelial growth factor in ocular fluid of patients with diabetic retinopathy and other retinal disorders. *N Engl J Med*. 1994;331(22):1480-1487.

23. Schwesinger C, Yee C, Rohan RM, et al. Intrachoroidal neovascularization in transgenic mice overexpressing vascular endothelial growth factor in the retinal pigment epithelium. *Am J Pathol*. 2001;158(3):1161-1172.

24. Krzystolik MG, Afshari MA, Adamis AP, et al. Prevention of experimental choroidal neovascularization with intravitreal anti-vascular endothelial growth factor antibody fragment. *Arch Ophthalmol*. 2002;120(3):338-346.

25. Gordon MS, Margolin K, Talpaz M, et al. Phase I safety and pharmacokinetic study of recombinant human anti-vascular endothelial growth factor in patients with advanced cancer. *J Clin Oncol.* 2001;19(3):843-850.

26. Mordenti J, Cuthbertson RA, Ferrara N, et al. Comparisons of the intraocular tissue distribution, pharmacokinetics, and safety of 125I-labeled full-length and Fab antibodies in rhesus monkeys following intravitreal administration. *Toxicol Pathol.* 1999;27(5):536-544.

27. Michels S, Rosenfeld PJ, Puliafito CA, Marcus EN, Venkatraman AS. Systemic bevacizumab (Avastin) therapy for neovascular age-related macular degeneration twelve-week results of an uncontrolled open-label clinical study. *Ophthalmology.* 2005;112(6):1035-1047.

28. Rosenfeld PJ, Moshfeghi AA, Puliafito CA. Optical coherence tomography findings after an intravitreal injection of bevacizumab (Avastin) for neovascular age-related macular degeneration. *Ophthalmic Surg Lasers Imaging.* 2005;36(4):331-335.

29. Brown DM, Michels M, Kaiser PK, Heier JS, Sy JP, Ianchulev T. Ranibizumab versus verteporfin photodynamic therapy for neovascular age-related macular degeneration: two-year results of the ANCHOR study. *Ophthalmology.* 2009;116(1):57-65.

30. Rosenfeld PJ, Brown DM, Heier JS, et al. Ranibizumab for neovascular age-related macular degeneration. *N Engl J Med.* 2006;355(14):1419-1431.

31. Comparison of Age-related Macular Degeneration Treatments Trials (CATT) Research Group, Martin DF, Maguire MG, et al. Ranibizumab and bevacizumab for treatment of neovascular age-related macular degeneration: two-year results. *Ophthalmology.* 2012;119(7):1388-1398.

32. Chakravarthy U, Harding SP, Rogers CA, et al. Alternative treatments to inhibit VEGF in age-related choroidal neovascularisation: 2-year findings of the IVAN randomised controlled trial. *Lancet.* 2013;382(9900):1258-1267.

33. Papadopoulos N, Martin J, Ruan Q, et al. Binding and neutralization of vascular endothelial growth factor (VEGF) and related ligands by VEGF Trap, ranibizumab and bevacizumab. *Angiogenesis.* 2012;15(2):171-185.

34. Holash J, Davis S, Papadopoulos N, et al. VEGF-Trap: a VEGF blocker with potent antitumor effects. *Proc Natl Acad Sci U S A.* 2002;99(17):11393-11398.

35. Heier JS, Brown DM, Chong V, et al. Intravitreal aflibercept (VEGF trap-eye) in wet age-related macular degeneration. *Ophthalmology.* 2012;119(12):2537-2548.

36. Schmidt-Erfurth U, Kaiser PK, Korobelnik JF, et al. Intravitreal aflibercept injection for neovascular age-related macular degeneration: ninety-six-week results of the VIEW studies. *Ophthalmology.* 2014;121(1):193-201.

37. Lalwani GA, Rosenfeld PJ, Fung AE, et al. A variable-dosing regimen with intravitreal ranibizumab for neovascular age-related macular degeneration: year 2 of the PrONTO Study. *Am J Ophthalmol.* 2009;148(1):43-58.

38. Ho AC, Busbee BG, Regillo CD, et al. Twenty-four-month efficacy and safety of 0.5 mg or 2.0 mg ranibizumab in patients with subfoveal neovascular age-related macular degeneration. *Ophthalmology.* 2014;121(11):2181-2192.

39. Spaide R. Ranibizumab according to need: a treatment for age-related macular degeneration. *Am J Ophthalmol.* 2007;143(4):679-680.

40. Gupta OP, Shienbaum G, Patel AH, Fecarotta C, Kaiser RS, Regillo CD. A treat and extend regimen using ranibizumab for neovascular age-related macular degeneration: clinical and economic impact. *Ophthalmology.* 2010;117(11):2134-2140.

41. Shienbaum G, Gupta OP, Fecarotta C, Patel AH, Kaiser RS, Regillo CD. Bevacizumab for neovascular age-related macular degeneration using a treat-and-extend regimen: clinical and economic impact. *Am J Ophthalmol.* 2012;153(3):468-473.

42. Wykoff CC, Brown DM, Maldonado ME, Croft DE. Aflibercept treatment for patients with exudative age-related macular degeneration who were incomplete responders to multiple ranibizumab injections (TURF trial). *Br J Ophthalmol.* 2014;98(7):951-955.

43. Chang AA, Li H, Broadhead GK, et al. Intravitreal aflibercept for treatment-resistant neovascular age-related macular degeneration. *Ophthalmology.* 2014;121(1):188-192.

44. Brown DM, Chen E, Mariani A, Major JC Jr. Super-dose anti-VEGF (SAVE) trial: 2.0 mg intra-vitreal ranibizumab for recalcitrant neovascular macular degeneration-primary end point. *Ophthalmology*. 2013;120(2):349-354.

45. Stewart MW, Rosenfeld PJ, Penha FM, et al. Pharmacokinetic rationale for dosing every 2 weeks versus 4 weeks with intravitreal ranibizumab, bevacizumab, and aflibercept (vascular endothelial factor Trap-eye). *Retina*. 2012;32(3):434-457.

46. Fung AT, Kumar N, Vance SK, et al. Pilot study to evaluate the role of high-dose ranibizumab 2.0 mg in the management of neovascular age-related macular degeneration in patients with persis-tent/recurrent macular fluid <30 days following treatment with intravitreal anti-VEGF therapy (the LAST Study). *Eye (Lond)*. 2012;26:1181-1187.

47. Witkin AJ, Rayess N, Garg SJ, et al. Alternating bi-weekly intravitreal ranibizumab and beva-cizumab for refractory neovascular age-related macular degeneration with pigment epithelial detachment. *Semin Ophthalmol*. 2015;4:1-7.

48. Kaiser PK, Boyer DS, Cruess AF, Slakter JS, Pilz S, Weisberger A. Verteporfin plus ranibizumab for choroidal neovascularization in age-related macular degeneration: twelve-month results of the DENALI study. *Ophthalmology*. 2012;119(5):1001-1010.

49. Larsen M, Schmidt-Erfurth U, Lanzetta P, et al. Verteporfin plus ranibizumab for choroidal neo-vascularization in age-related macular degeneration: twelve-month MONT BLANC study results. *Ophthalmology*. 2012;119(5):992-1000.

50. Kovacs KD, Quirk MT, Kinoshita T, et al. A retrospective analysis of triple combination therapy with intravitreal bevacizumab, posterior sub-Tenon's triamcinolone acetonide, and low-fluence verteporfin photodynamic therapy in patients with neovascular age-related macular degeneration. *Retina*. 2011;31(3):446-452.

51. Forte R, Bonavolonta P, Benayoun Y, Adenis JP, Robert PY. Intravitreal ranibizumab and beva-cizumab in combination with full-fluence verteporfin therapy and dexamethasone for exudative age-related macular degeneration. *Ophthalmic Res*. 2011;45(3):129-134.

52. Bloch SB, Larsen M, Munch IC. Incidence of legal blindness from age-related macular degenera-tion in Denmark: year 2000 to 2010. *Am J Ophthalmol*. 2012;153(2):209-213.

53. Bressler NM, Doan QV, Varma R, et al. Estimated cases of legal blindness and visual impairment avoided using ranibizumab for choroidal neovascularization: non-hispanic white population in the United States with age-related macular degeneration. *Arch Ophthalmol*. 2011;129(6):709-717.

54. Campbell JP, Bressler SB, Bressler NM. Impact of availability of anti-vascular endothelial growth factor therapy on visual impairment and blindness due to neovascular age-related macular degen-eration. *Arch Opthalmol*. 2012;130(6):794-795.

55. Mitchell P, Bressler N, Doan QV, et al. Estimated cases of blindness and visual impairment from neovascular age-related macular degeneration avoided in Australia by ranibizumab treatment. *PLoS One*. 2014;9(6):e101072.

56. Singer MA, Awh CC, Sadda S, et al. HORIZON: an open-label extension trial of ranibizumab for choroidal neovascularization secondary to age-related macular degeneration. *Ophthalmology*. 2012;119(6):1175-1183.

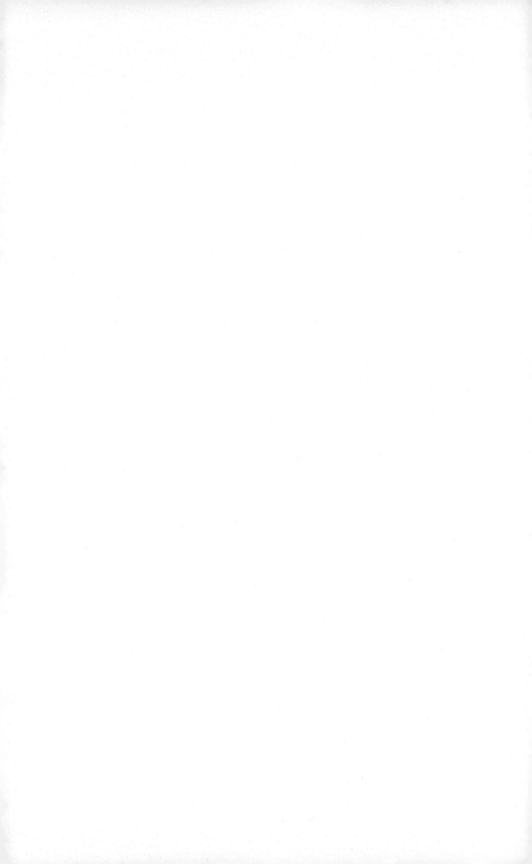

8

Choroidal Neovascularization, Not Age-Related Macular Degeneration

Darin R. Goldman, MD

Choroidal neovascularization (CNV) may result from various pathological entities. The end result is an abnormal vascular complex that breaks through Bruch's membrane into the subretinal space with consequent leakage of serous and hemorrhagic contents. When this occurs in proximity to the fovea, there may be significant deleterious effects to central visual acuity. Neovascular age-related macular degeneration (AMD) is the most common cause for CNV. However, there are numerous "other" pathological conditions that may result in CNV or CNV-like entities. These include pathological myopia, angioid streaks, traumatic sequela (ie, choroidal rupture), ocular histoplasmosis, polypoidal choroidal vasculopathy (PCV), central serous chorioretinopathy, hereditary macular dystrophies, inflammatory retinochoroidopathies, optic nerve drusen, and choroidal tumors.[1] Idiopathic CNV can also occur. Although these other causes for CNV have a much lower incidence than neovascular AMD, they tend to occur in younger patients, in whom their potential lifetime impact may be much greater.

Historically, various treatments have been employed to treat CNV with causes other than neovascular AMD. These include thermal laser photocoagulation,[2] verteporfin photodynamic therapy (PDT),[3-6] submacular CNV extraction,[7] and intravitreal steroids.[8,9] With these treatment modalities, rates of vision loss could be slowed under the best of circumstances. None of these therapies resulted in an overall improvement in vision on average.

Vascular endothelial growth factor (VEGF) is integral to normal angiogenesis for a multitude of physiological processes.[10] However, abnormally increased levels of VEGF can result in devastating pathological consequences. One of the major common denominators among all disease entities that cause CNV is abnormally high levels of VEGF. VEGF levels are highest in AMD, followed by myopic CNV, and then PCV.[11] Neovascular AMD is the most common cause of CNV and results in an enormous burden to society from a public health standpoint.[12] Over the last decade, anti-VEGF therapy has been revolutionary in the treatment of neovascular AMD. Anti-VEGF therapy

Duker JS, Liang MC, eds.
Anti-VEGF Use in Ophthalmology (pp. 81-100).
© 2017 Taylor & Francis Group.

with ranibizumab elevated treatment from historical benchmarks of decreasing the rate of vision loss to providing visual stabilization in the majority and visual improvement in a significant portion of eyes.[13,14]

Many non-AMD causes of CNV have experienced a similar revolution regarding treatment benefit due to the development of anti-VEGF agents.[15] However, the lower prevalence of these other causes for CNV, in comparison to neovascular AMD, creates a significant barrier to the development of disease-specific treatment. As such, there remains no on-label anti-VEGF therapy for any of the non-AMD causes for CNV other than due to high myopia in the United States (US), even though they are used routinely in an off-label manner. This off-label approach to anti-VEGF treatment for these conditions began by extrapolating from the extensive scientific record pertaining to neovascular AMD. The body of literature devoted to non-AMD causes for CNV continues to grow but still does not compare in its rigor to those for AMD. Myopic CNV is the most frequently encountered non-AMD cause of CNV. Other entities that will be discussed in this chapter include PCV, angioid streaks, central serous chrioretinopathy, and presumed ocular histoplasmosis syndrome (POHS).

Myopic Choroidal Neovascularization

High myopia (> 6.0 diopters) along with its intrinsic axial elongation (> 25 mm to 26 mm) results in degenerative changes in various layers of the globe including Bruch's membrane and the retinal pigment epithelium (RPE). CNV is the most common sight-threatening pathology associated with high myopia, present in more than 10% of highly myopic eyes[16] and bilaterally in 15% of eyes.[17] CNV develops spontaneously as an abnormal vascular complex that traverses through a weak area in Bruch's membrane (lacquer crack). The CNV complex generally occurs in proximity to and underneath the fovea with resultant fluid, hemorrhage, and/or fibrosis that leads to vision loss or metamorphopsia. VEGF levels are significantly elevated in the presence of myopic CNV, although less so than in AMD.[11] These high VEGF levels are effectively suppressed with anti-VEGF therapy.[18]

The typical appearance of myopic CNV is that of a subfoveal grayish membrane. Associated exudation is usually minimal and, if present, hemorrhage is also typically minimal (Figure 8-1[A]). Fluorescein angiographic (FA) appearance is usually that of a classic, or type 2, CNV leakage pattern (Figure 8-1[B]). Optical coherence tomography (OCT) shows a CNV complex present between the neurosensory retina and the RPE, which is typically highly reflective, well-circumscribed and dome shaped, with minimal associated sub- or intraretinal fluid (Figure 8-2). The diagnosis of myopic CNV is made with the combination of clinical examination, FA, and OCT.

The natural history of CNV due to myopia is more favorable than that of neovascular AMD. Large disciform scarring is less common and the disease is not bilateral as often as AMD. However, overall the prognosis is still poor with 43% of eyes losing 2 or more lines of vision and 60% of eyes having final visual acuity of 20/200 or worse.[19] The loss of vision in eyes with CNV from myopia is progressive over time[20] and contributes significantly as a cause for vision loss and blindness throughout the world.[17] Specifically, the natural history of CNV in pathological myopia is significantly worse in patients older than 50 compared to those younger than 50.[21] In a 3-year natural history study, 43% of patients younger than 40 maintained 20/40 or better visual acuity and only 11% had

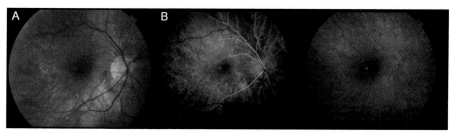

Figure 8-1. (A) Color photograph and (B) fluorescein angiography in myopic choroidal neovascular membrane. There is increased hyperfluorescence centrally corresponding to the choroidal neovascular membrane.

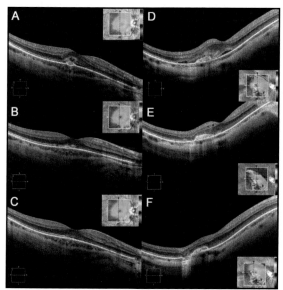

Figure 8-2. Optical coherence tomography of myopic choroidal neovascular membrane at (A, D) baseline, (B, E) 1 and (C, F) 2 months following treatment with anti-vascular endothelial growth factor therapy. There is resolution of the overlying fluid as well as reduction in the size of the subretinal membrane visible on optical coherence tomography.

visual acuity worse than 20/200.[22] In contrast, more than 50% of those aged over 40 had visual acuity worse than 20/200. Because of the more favorable natural history in younger patients, consideration should be given to a more conservative treatment approach in this demographic. Other factors that may play a role in the ultimate visual prognosis include presenting visual acuity, location of CNV, and degree of myopia. High myopia is increasing in prevalence with an estimated one billion people to be affected worldwide by 2050.[23] High myopia is more common in Asian countries, thought to be due to environmental factors such as decreased time spent outdoors and increased near work activities.[24]

Until recently, the only Food and Drug Administration-approved treatment for myopic CNV in the US was PDT with Visudyne (Novartis AG), which is associated with less significant vision loss compared to sham at 2 years.[4] However, this result was not statistically significant, with 64% of the PDT group avoiding loss of more than or equal to 8 lines of vision compared to 49% in the sham group. PDT has also been combined with intravitreal steroid, which allowed for fewer PDT treatment sessions, however, without any visual advantage and with the added risks of cataract and glaucoma.[8,25] Anti-VEGF therapy has emerged more recently as an effective off-label treatment for myopic CNV; available agents include bevacizumab, ranibizumab, and aflibercept. Intravitreal ranibizumab was approved for this indication in early 2017 and is currently the only FDA-approved treatment for myopic CNV in the US.

Intravitreal bevacizumab[26-30] and ranibizumab[31-34] have been studied for the treatment of myopic CNV in a number of retrospective and prospective uncontrolled case series (Table 8-1). For bevacizumab, the percentage of eyes gaining 15 or more letters of vision ranged from 30% to 70%, the mean improvements in logMAR visual acuity averaged 0.24, and the mean number of injections ranged from 1.8 to 3.6 over one year. The best visual gains were noted in a study that had a high portion of treatment-naïve eyes in comparison to the other studies, with only 10% of eyes receiving prior PDT.[27] Although other studies found worse visual acuity outcomes with anti-VEGF therapy after PDT, a 2009 retrospective study did not find any differences in visual acuity outcomes whether PDT treatment was previously received or not.[30]

For ranibizumab, the percentage of eyes gaining 15 or more letters of vision ranged from 25% to 40.3%, the mean gain in Early Treatment Diabetic Retinopathy Study (ETDRS) letters was 10, and the mean number of injections ranged from 2.3 to 4.1 over one year. The majority of visual gains were achieved after the first injection.[31] Positive predictors of visual outcome included better baseline best-corrected visual acuity (BCVA) and extra-foveal CNV location. With continued treatment, BCVA continued to improve over time with 25%, 30%, and 35% of eyes experiencing BCVA gains of 3 or more lines of vision at 1, 2, and 3 years, respectively.[32] In this study, a mean of 4.1, 2.4, and 1.1 injections were performed over the first, second, and third years, respectively, showing a trend toward less treatment being required over time. The REPAIR study showed that 14.4% of eyes improved from the worse-seeing eye to the better-seeing eye of the patient, and the greatest improvement in visual acuity occurred after the first month.[33]

Furthermore, mean central foveal thickness (CFT) was consistently reduced with both bevacizumab and ranibizumab. Overall, patients younger than 50 years of age experienced better vision outcomes[27,29,30,32] and required fewer injections.[30] The percentage of eyes gaining 3 or more lines of vision (bevacizumab 30% to 70%, ranibizumab 25% to 40.3%) were superior when compared to 6% in the PDT-treatment group and 3% in the placebo-treatment group of the Verteporfin In Photodynamic Therapy Trial.[3] Another study showed that more than 50% of eyes achieved final visual acuity of 20/40 or better and only 2% of eyes had final visual acuity worse than 20/200.[28] Six-line or better visual acuity gains were achieved in 13% of eyes compared to 0% in the Verteporfin In Photodynamic Therapy Trial.[28]

Regarding treatment regimen, anti-VEGF dosing with 3 consecutive monthly injections at initiation of treatment has not been shown to be more effective compared to 1 initiation dose followed by an as-needed treatment approach (1-pro re nata [prn]).[34] One study retrospectively evaluated 46 treatment-naïve eyes with subfoveal myopic CNV treated with 0.5 mg intravitreal ranibizumab.[34] At 12 months, the mean number of injections given to the 1 initial injection group was 2.32 and to the 3 initial injections group was 3.57. No differences in visual outcome were found between the 2 groups. When 1-prn dosing is followed, required retreatment over the first year can range from 0.8 to 3.1 injections.[28,30,32-34]

Aflibercept has also been evaluated for the treatment of myopic CNV and shown to be superior to sham treatment. In the MYRROR study, 122 patients with myopic CNV[35] were treated with either 2 mg intravitreal aflibercept at baseline and then as needed up to 44 weeks or sham treatment up to week 20 and rescue aflibercept treatment if needed

Table 8-1. Anti-VEGF Treatment of Myopic CNVM

	Study Design	Dose (1-prn or 3 loading)	# Eyes	% Gaining ≥ 3 Lines VA[a]	Mean Change VA (logMAR)[a]	Mean Change VA (ETDRS)[a]	Mean # Injections
Bevacizumab							
Chan 2009	Retrospective	3 loading	29	[b]	0.24		3.6
Ruiz-Moreno 2009	Retrospective	3 loading	29	[b]	0.17		[b]
Gharbiya 2010	Prospective	3 loading	20	70.0%	0.36		[b]
Ikuno 2009	Retrospective	1-prn	63	40.0%	0.24		2.4
Ruiz-Moreno 2010	Retrospective	1-prn	107	30.0%	0.19		1.8
Ranibizumab							
Calvo-Gonzales 2011	Prospective	3 loading	67	40.3%		11.9	3.9
Franqueira 2012	Retrospective	1-prn	40	25.0%		4.3	4.1
Tufail 2013	Prospective	1-prn	65	36.9%		13.8	3.6
Kung 2014	Retrospective	1-prn (*n* = 25)	46	[b]	0.35		2.32
		3 loading (*n* =21)	N/A	[b]	0.33		3.57

VEGF = vascular endothelial growth factor; CNVM = choroidal neovascular membrane; 1-prn = one injection followed by as-needed treatment; 3 loading = 3 serial monthly loading injections followed by as needed treatment; VA = visual acuity; ETDRS = Early Treatment Diabetic Retinopathy Study; N/A = not applicable.
[a]At 12 months.
[b]Not reported.

at week 24 and beyond. The mean number of aflibercept injections in the treatment arm was 4.2 and in the sham arm was 3.0 at 48 weeks. At week 24, the intravitreal aflibercept group gained a mean of 12.1 letters of vision compared to 2 letters lost in the sham group, and 38.9% of eyes in the aflibercept group gained 3 lines or more compared to 9.7% in the sham group. Anatomical outcomes similarly favored the aflibercept treatment arm. At week 48 (crossover allowed in sham group at week 24), the aflibercept group gained 13.5 letters compared to 3.9 in the sham/aflibercept crossover group. These findings were all statistically significant. Another retrospective study showed that only 1 aflibercept injection was required to obtain CNV resolution in 55% of eyes and the mean number of injections over an 18-month study period was only 2.1, similar when compared to bevacizumab and ranibizumab. They also found that the mean number of aflibercept injections in patients younger than 50 years of age was 1.5 compared to 2.7 in patients 50 years or older at 18 months.[36]

Other agents have been compared to anti-VEGF in their effectiveness for the treatment of myopic CNV. In a study retrospectively evaluating 53 eyes with myopic CNV treated with either 20 mg sub-Tenon triamcinolone or 1 mg intravitreal bevacizumab,[37] the mean number of treatments over 12 months was 1.3 in the triamcinolone group and 2.1 in the bevacizumab group. Visual acuity outcomes were superior in the bevacizumab group with 32% gaining more than 3 lines compared to 15% in the triamcinolone group. Mean BCVA changes at 12 months were 1.9 letters gained in the bevacizumab group compared to 0.3 letters lost in the triamcinolone group. These results support the superior efficacy of bevacizumab over sub-Tenon triamcinolone.

Two other studies compared patients treated with 0.5 mg ranibizumab to 1.25 mg bevacizumab at baseline and then as needed.[38,39] No statistically significant visual or anatomic difference was found between the 2 groups and the mean number of injections was also similar between the groups in both studies. BCVA improved significantly in all treatment arms, but there was a trend favoring more significant reduction of CFT in the ranibizumab group.[39]

A prospective, multicenter study of 55 eyes compared PDT to intravitreal bevacizumab at 2 years.[40] Group 1 was treated with PDT at baseline and then every 3 months as needed. Group 2 was treated with 3 serial intravitreal bevacizumab injections for the first 3 months followed by as-needed treatment. At 2 years, there was a statistically significant improvement in BCVA in the bevacizumab group only. The mean number of PDT treatments was 1.8 over the first year and 0.2 over the second year. The mean number of intravitreal bevacizumab injections was 3.6 over the first year and 0.6 over the second year. This study supported the superiority of bevacizumab to PDT. Similar findings were reported for ranibizumab in RADIANCE, a 1-year randomized, controlled trial that enrolled 277 patients at 76 centers worldwide.[41] Patients were randomized into 3 groups: group 1 received 0.5 mg ranibizumab on day 1, month 1, and then as needed; group 2 received 0.5 mg ranibizumab on day 1 and then as needed; group 3 received PDT on day 1 and then PDT and/or ranibizumab from month 3 at the discretion of the investigator. Both group 1 (+10.5 letters) and group 2 (+10.6 letters) achieved significantly better visual outcomes compared to group 3 (+2.2 letters) at 3 months, prior to ranibizumab rescue being allowed in group 3. Group 1 and group 2 achieved significantly better gains of 15 or more ETDRS letters compared to group 3 at three months (group 1 = 38.1%; group 2 = 43.1%; group 3 = 14.5%), and at one year, 53.3% of eyes in group 1 and 51.7% in group 2 gained 15 or more ETDRS letters, while only 32.7% of eyes in group 3 achieved the same improvement, even allowing for ranibizumab rescue beyond 3 months. The mean number of ranibizumab injections was 4.6, 3.5, and 2.4 in groups 1, 2, and 3, respectively. This study was the first randomized, controlled trial to demonstrate the superiority of ranibizumab over PDT for the treatment of myopic CNV and data from this study ultimately led to the FDA approval for ranibizumab in myopic CNV. Furthermore, even with rescue ranibizumab treatment after month 3, the visual outcomes in group 3 never caught up to group 1 or group 2, supporting the notion that early initiation of anti-VEGF treatment is consistent with best visual acuity outcomes.

The combination of PDT with anti-VEGF therapy has also been investigated to evaluate if there is a synergistic benefit to improve visual acuity outcomes and/or reduce treatment burden. Neither of these 2 outcomes has been definitively demonstrated. One retrospective study compared 3 groups of patients with myopic CNV totaling 79 eyes that were treated with either PDT, anti-VEGF (ranibizumab or bevacizumab), or a combination of PDT and anti-VEGF.[42] Treatment protocol was induction of treatment by each method followed by as-needed treatment. They concluded the combination group was the only group to achieve a statistically significant BCVA improvement although this was likely flawed by a type 2 error. The visual acuity outcomes were quite similar between the anti-VEGF monotherapy group (0.16 logMAR gain) and combination therapy group (0.22 logMAR gain), both of which showed a trend toward improvement, whereas the PDT monotherapy group (0.09 logMAR gain) showed a trend toward stability. They did show, however, that the combination of PDT and anti-VEGF treatment may reduce the required anti-VEGF treatment burden.

However, combination PDT and anti-VEGF therapy did not appear to have an advantage over anti-VEGF monotherapy in other studies.[43] One report of 34 eyes treated with either combination PDT and intravitreal bevacizumab or bevacizumab monotherapy[43] showed both groups had a significant improvement in mean BCVA at one year and there were no statistically significant differences between groups regarding visual outcomes. The mean number of treatments required was significantly lower in the combination group, although this difference was easily accounted for by the required 3 monthly loading doses in the monotherapy group. Overall, it is not clear that PDT offers any benefit in reducing the required anti-VEGF treatment burden.

In summary, anti-VEGF therapy for myopic CNV has supplanted any previous treatment modality because of its superior efficacy. Both ranibizumab and aflibercept have gained on-label approval for myopic CNV in numerous countries around the world; ranibizumab was only recently FDA-approved and is the only on-label treatment available for the treatment of myopic CNV in the US.

Despite this, treatment of myopic CNV with anti-VEGF therapy has evolved into the standard of care.[44] Intravitreal anti-VEGF therapy for myopic CNV results in moderate visual acuity gains of 3 or more ETDRS lines at 1 year in 30% to 38.9% of eyes,[30,32,33,35] similar findings to those seen following anti-VEGF therapy for neovascular AMD (34% in ANCHOR,[14] 40% in MARINA[13]). Level-one evidence exists for the effectiveness of both ranibizumab[41] and aflibercept[35] for the treatment of myopic CNV, but there has not been an adequately powered study to sufficiently determine if one anti-VEGF agent is superior (or inferior) to the others. Other studies have shown anti-VEGF monotherapy superior to PDT monotherapy and there does not appear to be any added benefit of additional or combination PDT for treating myopic CNV. In addition, there is no clear benefit of 3 serial monthly loading doses followed by as-needed treatment compared to 1 initial dose followed by as-needed treatment, although the latter strategy does have the advantage of a reduced treatment burden.[45] Overall, earlier initiation of anti-VEGF therapy is

Figure 8-3. (Top) Color and (middle) red-free photograph with fluorescein angiography (bottom) in polypoidal choroidal vasculopathy. Exudates and hemorrhage are visible superotemporal to the optic disc with additional exudation in the inferotemporal macula and nasal to the optic disc. There is hyperfluorescence in the same area superotemporal to the disc on fluorescein angiography. (Reprinted with permission from Jay S. Duker, MD.)

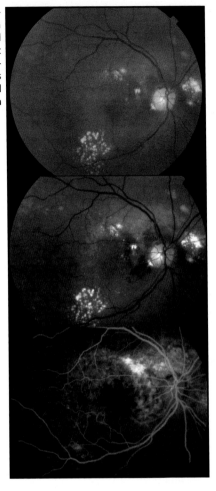

associated with better long-term visual outcomes. We recommend prompt initiation of anti-VEGF therapy at the first sign of myopic CNV, followed by monthly initial follow-up and an as-needed treatment approach following the first injection. In patients older than 50 to 55 year, more aggressive therapy should be considered, as their visual prognosis is generally worse than younger patients.

Polypoidal Choroidal Vasculopathy

PCV is widely considered a subtype of neovascular AMD but it is more accurately described as a distinct choroidal vascular abnormality that can resemble neovascular AMD. The primary pathology lies in the choroidal vasculature, underneath the RPE, where abnormal polypoid and branching vascular complexes can be visualized on angiography. VEGF levels have been shown to be elevated in the aqueous of PCV eyes.[11] Patients typically have pronounced RPE detachments with prominent hemorrhage and exudate (Figure 8-3). In patients with presumed neovascular AMD in whom a suboptimal

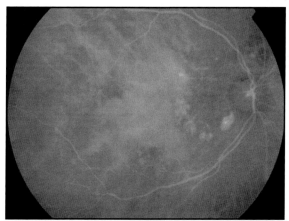

Figure 8-4. Indocyanine green angiography in polypoidal choroidal vasculopathy shows many clusters of polyps around the nerve and in the nasal macula. (Reprinted with permission from Jay S. Duker, MD.)

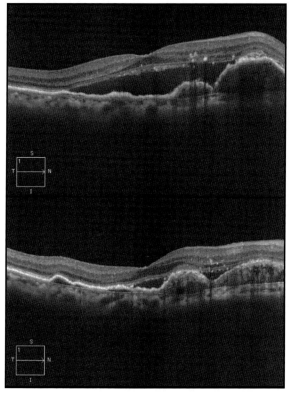

Figure 8-5. Optical coherence tomography in polypoidal choroidal vasculopathy. There are multiple retinal pigment epithelial detachments with overlying subretinal fluid. Treatment response after anti-vascular endothelial growth factor therapy is demonstrated in the lower panel. (Reprinted with permission from Jay S. Duker, MD.)

treatment response is seen following anti-VEGF therapy, PCV should be considered as the underlying diagnosis.[46] Identifying PCV can be challenging, requires a high level of suspicion, and often necessitates specialized diagnostic testing such as indocyanine green angiography (Figure 8-4). OCT is useful to monitor response after treatment (Figure 8-5) and can also aid in the initial diagnosis. PCV can cause severe vision impairment without treatment due to exudation and hemorrhage from leaking or ruptured polyps. It most commonly occurs in adults during the sixth decade and is more common in Asian and African American populations.[47] The natural history seems to be divergent with a large portion experiencing spontaneous improvement. However, more than half of eyes will develop progressive vision loss worse than 20/200 without treatment.[48] Various treatment agents have been used in PCV with a more recent emphasis on anti-VEGF therapy.

Bevacizumab, ranibizumab, and aflibercept have demonstrated efficacy for treating PCV. A retrospective study of 35 eyes evaluated symptomatic macular PCV treated with 2.5 mg intravitreal bevacizumab at baseline and then as needed for one year.[49] Mean BCVA and CFT both improved from baseline to one year. Another smaller, prospective study evaluated 12 eyes with PCV treated monthly with intravitreal ranibizumab.[50] They found vision to be stabilized with 6 monthly injections, with a mean improvement of 6.6 ETDRS letters.

As monotherapy, ranibizumab has demonstrated superior visual outcomes compared to PDT. LAPTOP, a prospective, randomized trial, compared ranibizumab to PDT for PCV.[51] Significantly more patients in the ranibizumab group gained vision at 12 months (30.4% vs 17.0%) although there was no significant difference in CFT reduction between the 2 arms. After 3 initial monthly ranibizumab treatments, the mean number of retreatments was 1.5 in the ranibizumab arm. After one initial PDT treatment, the mean number of retreatments was 0.8 in the PDT arm. Other studies have shown the benefit of aflibercept, with polyp resolution in 66% of eyes at 3 months[52] and similar improvements in mean visual acuity at 12 months with either every 2-month or as-needed treatment after a 3-month loading dose.[53]

Given a less robust treatment response to anti-VEGF therapy for PCV compared to AMD, there has been a greater interest in combination therapy with PDT. The EVEREST study randomized 59 treatment-naïve patients with symptomatic macular PCV[54] to PDT and ranibizumab, PDT monotherapy, or ranibizumab monotherapy. The results showed that PDT monotherapy, or in combination with ranibizumab, achieved a significantly greater degree of complete polyp regression compared to ranibizumab monotherapy at 6 months (77.8%, 71.4% vs 28.6%). However, this did not translate into any significant differences in visual acuity outcomes, although there was a trend favoring both ranibizumab groups. Visual acuity gains of 15 or more letters were greatest in the ranibizumab monotherapy group (33.3%) compared to the PDT/ranibizumab combination group (21%) and the PDT monotherapy group (19%). This study provides evidence that PDT may address the unique underlying pathology in PCV distinct from anti-VEGF therapy, whereby regression of polyps is induced. This may provide a longer-acting treatment effect and less reliance on continued anti-VEGF therapy, although there is no clear, long-term visual benefit.

When combined with bevacizumab, whether PDT is performed initially or delayed 3 months does not appear to affect outcomes. In a prospective study of 60 eyes with PCV, all patients received intravitreal ranibizumab for 3 consecutive months and then as needed, but 1 group was randomized to receive PDT at baseline and the other group at 3 months.[55] Mean visual acuity improved significantly in both groups at 12 months with no significant difference between the 2 groups. Both groups had similar amounts of eyes experiencing 15 or more ETDRS letter gains at 12 months (44.8%, initial PDT; 48.4%, delayed PDT). Similarly, CFT decreased significantly in both groups with no difference between the 2 groups. Of note, when combination PDT and anti-VEGF therapy is performed, half-fluence PDT should be considered if there is only a single polyp to reduce the risk of potential choroidal ischemia.[56]

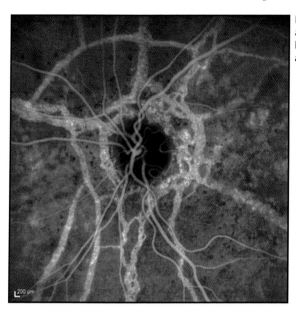

Figure 8-6. Indocyanine green angiography in angioid streaks, highlighting streaks radiating from and around the optic nerve.

In some cases of PCV recalcitrant to either bevacizumab or ranibizumab, aflibercept appears to be effective. A retrospective study of 43 eyes with PCV administered intravitreal aflibercept to patients who previously proved refractory to treatment with ranibizumab.[57] After switching to aflibercept, mean visual acuity (20/48 to 20/43) and CFT (245 μm to 131 μm) improved significantly at 3 months. Complete regression of polypoidal lesions was also achieved in 50% of eyes. In treatment-naïve patients, aflibercept has not clearly demonstrated a benefit over other anti-VEGF agents, although this has not been evaluated in a randomized, controlled fashion. A retrospective evaluation of 98 treatment-naïve eyes with PCV treated with either intravitreal aflibercept or ranibizumab[58] showed no significant differences in functional or anatomic outcomes between the 2 groups at 12 months, although complete polyp regression was higher in the aflibercept group (39.5% vs 21.6%).

In summary, functional outcomes with PDT and anti-VEGF therapies are similar to monotherapy for PCV with a tendency toward better visual outcomes with anti-VEGF monotherapy but higher rates of polyp regression with PDT. As a primary treatment modality, both PDT and anti-VEGF can be considered first line. A combination approach using both modalities has the potential for a synergistic effect and reduced overall treatment burden. In cases recalcitrant to bevacizumab or ranibizumab, aflibercept may have additional benefit.

Angioid Streaks

Angioid streaks are curvilinear breaks in a pathologically weakened/abnormally calcified Bruch's membrane that typically emanate from the optic nerve head out toward the peripheral retina (Figure 8-6). These may occur as an isolated entity or be associated with systemic diseases such as pseudoxanthoma elasticum. Secondary CNV is a common complication of angioid streaks, occurring in the majority of eyes, and may cause

Figure 8-7. (A) Color photograph, (B) fluorescein angiography, (C) optical coherence tomography, and (D) red free photograph of choroidal neovascularization (CNV) due to angioid streaks. Color photograph shows the CNV with hemorrhage, fluorescein angiography demonstrates a typical classic CNV appearance, and optical coherence tomography shows a subretinal CNV with associated subretinal fluid.

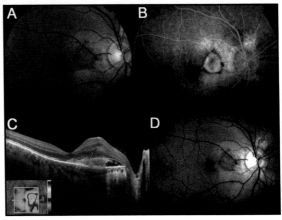

devastating visual consequences. CNV due to angioid streaks are considerably less common than those due to myopia and, as such, the body of evidence pertaining to treatment of this specific CNV subtype is limited. The required treatment burden for this subtype of CNV tends to be more than for myopic CNV due to a higher rate of recurrence, but less than that for CNV due to neovascular AMD. On FA, CNV due to angioid streaks typically exhibit a classic leakage pattern (Figure 8-7).

Both bevacizumab and ranibizumab have been evaluated for the treatment of CNV secondary to angioid streaks in case series, where they have shown efficacy that exceeds PDT. When CNV due to angioid streaks is treated with PDT, vision is generally stabilized or lost over time, whereas mean visual acuity gains have been shown consistently with both bevacizumab[59-61] and ranibizumab[62,63] at 12 months and beyond (Table 8-2). Studies have shown that 72.7% of patients had improved vision at 12 months when treated with bevacizumab[59] and vision was stabilized or improved in 85.7% of eyes when treated with ranibizumab.[62] In studies with an as-needed treatment protocol, the mean number of injections per 12-month period was 2.5. Overall, visual improvement with anti-VEGF averages 0.21 logMAR units, which compares favorably to PDT, where eyes lost 3 letters of visual acuity at 12 months.[64] It remains unclear how frequently treatment is needed, with a mean interval of 4.1 months[59] but may be more frequent.[60]

Anti-VEGF therapy appears to be effective in stabilizing and/or improving visual acuity in the majority of eyes with CNV due to angioid streaks in the short term and is superior to any previously used options such as PDT and thermal laser photocoagulation. The treatment burden appears to be more than with other non-AMD causes of CNV. Unlike for neovascular AMD, the evidence for efficacy of anti-VEGF therapy relies mostly on retrospective and nonstandardized clinical studies.[65] Longer-term and larger studies are needed to make more definitive conclusions regarding treatment frequency and superiority of one anti-VEGF agent over another.

Central Serous Chorioretinopathy

Central serous chorioretinopathy (CSR) is a mysterious condition affecting the macula whereby subretinal fluid accumulates, causing perturbations in vision. The underlying pathophysiology remains poorly understood, although both a hyperpermeable choroid

Table 8-2. Anti-VEGF Treatment of CNVM Secondary to Angioid Streaks

	Study Design	# Eyes	% Gaining ≥ 3 Lines VA	Mean Change VA (logMAR)	Mean Change VA (ETDRS)	Mean # Injections	Mean Follow-Up (Months)
Bevacizumab							
Neri 2009	Prospective	11		0.34		3.5	23.8
Sawa 2009	Retrospective	15		0.11		3.8	19
Wiegand 2009	Retrospective	9	44.4%			4.4	19
Ranibizumab							
Mimoun 2010	Retrospective	35	11.4%	0.12		5.7	24.1
Finger 2011	Prospective	7		0.29	12	12	12

VEGF = vascular endothelial growth factor; CNVM = choroidal neovascular membrane; VA = visual acuity; ETDRS = Early Treatment Diabetic Retinopathy Study.

and dysfunctional RPE are thought to be pivotal.[66] CSR is a common maculopathy that can adversely affect central visual function and is 6-fold more common in males than females.[67] Affected patients are typically between 30 and 50 years of age. Many putative risk factors exist for the development of CSR, the most conclusive being any form of exogenous corticosteroid use. Other risk factors include pregnancy, "Type A" personality, gastroesophageal reflux disease, and possibly sleep disturbances.[68] Acute CSR is usually a self-limited disease and resolves spontaneously within a few months. If subretinal fluid persists beyond 3 months, this is considered chronic CSR and treatment is generally

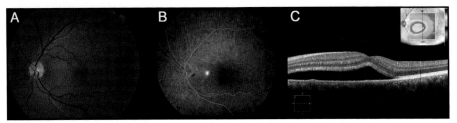

Figure 8-8. (A) Color photograph, (B) fluorescein angiography, and (C) optical coherence tomography in central serous chorioretinopathy. There is a nasal area of leakage on the fluorescein angiogram with associated subretinal fluid visible on optical coherence tomography.

considered as prolonged subretinal fluid can result in irreversible vision loss. This is particularly true in individuals over age 50, in whom secondary occult CNV is more common.[69] The classic appearance of CSR is that of a circular serous detachment of the neurosensory macula, typically overlying a pigment epithelial detachment (Figure 8-8[A]). FA shows a classic leakage pattern (Figure 8-8[B]) and gravitational tracks may be seen on FA or fundus autofluorescence. A thickened choroid is another universal finding on OCT (Figure 8-8[C]).

Given its wide acceptance for other neovascular conditions affecting the macula, anti-VEGF therapy has been used in chronic CSR despite evidence that VEGF levels are not elevated in CSR.[70] In a prospective study of chronic CSR comparing treatment with 2.5 mg intravitreal bevacizumab to observation, there was a statistically significant improvement in both BCVA and CFT in the treatment group at 6 months.[71] In contrast, a meta-analysis of 112 eyes with chronic CSR found no statistically significant difference in either functional or anatomic outcomes at 6 months.[71-73] Intravitreal ranibizumab, however, may shorten the mean time to resolution of subretinal fluid in patients with acute CSR compared to observation.[74]

Other studies have evaluated anti-VEGF therapy in comparison to PDT. In a study of low-fluence PDT compared to intravitreal ranibizumab for chronic CSR,[75] 88.9% of eyes in the PDT group had complete resolution of fluid while only 31.3% did in the ranibizumab group. Greater reductions in CFT were found in the PDT group up to 5 months. The mean change in BCVA was significantly greater in the PDT group compared to the ranibizumab group at 3 months but this difference was not retained at 12 months. Overall, treatment outcomes were superior in the PDT group compared to ranibizumab. In addition, injections of 2 mg intravitreal aflibercept were not shown to improve BCVA over 6 months.[76] These studies taken together do not demonstrate a clear benefit of anti-VEGF therapy for CSR.

In summary, the quality of evidence in support of anti-VEGF therapy for chronic CSR is poor and thus it is not generally recommended as monotherapy. Uncontrolled studies tend to report favorable results; however, randomized, controlled trials do not show any clear benefit.[72,75] However, anti-VEGF therapy should be considered in those cases of secondary CNV in CSR.[66] Photodynamic therapy has been shown to be superior to ranibizumab and remains the most effective treatment modality for chronic CSR without CNV.

Figure 8-9. (A, C) Color photograph, (B) fluorescein angiography, and (C) optical coherence tomography of choroidal neovascularization (CNV) due to presumed ocular histoplasmosis syndrome. The posterior pole shows peripapillary atrophy and multiple focal areas of atrophy in addition to the central CNV. There are additional focal areas of atrophy in the inferior periphery. Optical coherence tomography demonstrates a subfoveal CNV with associated fluid.

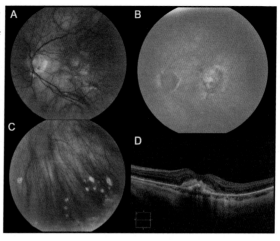

Presumed Ocular Histoplasmosis Syndrome

POHS is associated with infection with *Histoplasma capsulatum* and causes peripheral punched out lesions, peripapillary pigment, and CNV (Figure 8-9). POHS is endemic to certain regions, most notable the Ohio and Mississippi river valleys. The natural history of subfoveal CNV associated with POHS is devastating, with 77% of eyes retaining 20/100 visual acuity or worse after a median of 36.5 months.[77] Treatment of CNV secondary to POHS has been studied to a limited degree. Bevacizumab, ranibizumab, and aflibercept have shown efficacy in case series (Table 8-3); at 12 months, vision stabilized or improved in 84% to 85% of eyes.[78,79] The average number of required treatments was 3.75 over 12 months with as-needed treatment protocols. Anti-VEGF agents are the most effective treatment strategy for CNV due to POHS.

Various studies have grouped CNV due to non-AM D causes together to generate larger numbers of patients in attempt to make more statistically meaningful conclusions. However, these studies are difficult to interpret in a manner to make generalizations. These studies reaffirm the overall effectiveness of anti-VEGF therapy to treat all forms of non-AMD CNV.[45,80,81]

Conclusion

Myopic CNV is the most prevalent and important non-AMD cause of CNV worldwide with a significant potential for vision loss. Anti-VEGF therapy with bevacizumab, ranibizumab, and aflibercept has proven more effective than any prior class of therapy for myopic CNV, and ranibizumab was recently approved for use to treat myopic CNV in the US. Similarly, anti-VEGF therapy has proven effective in the treatment of CNV caused by PCV, angioid streaks, and POHS. Although anti-VEGF therapy has not clearly shown efficacy in treating primary central serous chorioretinopathy, it can be effective in the setting of secondary CNV. The overall frequency requirements of anti-VEGF treatment in non-AMD causes of CNV are less than that for AMD, but further studies are necessary

Table 8-3. Anti-VEGF Treatment of CNVM Secondary to
Presumed Ocular Histoplasmosis Syndrome

	Anti-VEGF Agent	# Eyes	% Gaining ≥ 3 Lines VA[a]	Mean Change VA (logMAR)[a]	Mean Change VA (ETDRS)	Mean # Injections/ 12 Months	Mean Follow-Up (Months)
Schadlu 2008	Bevacizumab	28		0.22			5.5
Cionni 2011	Bevacizumab	104	37.9%	0.24		3.1	21.1
Nielsen 2012	Bevacizumab/ Ranibizumab	54		0.30		4.4	26.8
Walia 2016	Aflibercept	5			12.4		12

VEGF = vascular endothelial growth factor; CNVM = choroidal neovascular membrane; VA = visual acuity; ETDRS = Early Treatment Diabetic Retinopathy Study.
[a] At 12 months.

to identify any differences between individual anti-VEGF agents and to clarify the best treatment frequency.

References

1. Spaide RF. Choroidal neovascularization in younger patients. *Curr Opin Ophthalmol.* 1999;10(3):177-181.

2. Krypton laser photocoagulation for neovascular lesions of ocular histoplasmosis. Results of a randomized clinical trial. Macular Photocoagulation Study Group. *Arch Ophthalmol.* 1987;105(11):1499-1507.

3. Verteporfin in Photodynamic Therapy Study Group. Photodynamic therapy of subfoveal choroidal neovascularization in pathologic myopia with verteporfin. 1-year results of a randomized clinical trial—VIP report no. 1. *Ophthalmology.* 2001;108(5):841-852.

4. Blinder KJ, Blumenkranz MS, Bressler NM, et al. Verteporfin therapy of subfoveal choroidal neovascularization in pathologic myopia: 2-year results of a randomized clinical trial—VIP report no. 3. *Ophthalmology.* 2003;110(4):667-673.

5. Rosenfeld PJ, Saperstein DA, Bressler NM, et al. Photodynamic therapy with verteporfin in ocular histoplasmosis: uncontrolled, open-label 2-year study. *Ophthalmology.* 2004;111(9):1725-1733.

6. Montero JA, Ruiz-Moreno JM. Verteporfin photodynamic therapy in highly myopic subfoveal choroidal neovascularisation. *Br J Ophthalmol.* 2003;87(2):173-176.

7. Hawkins BS, Bressler NM, Bressler SB, et al. Surgical removal vs observation for subfoveal choroidal neovascularization, either associated with the ocular histoplasmosis syndrome or idiopathic: I. Ophthalmic findings from a randomized clinical trial: Submacular Surgery Trials (SST) Group H Trial: SST Report No. 9. *Arch Ophthalmol.* 2004;122(11):1597-1611.

8. Montero JA, Ruiz-Moreno JM. Combined photodynamic therapy and intravitreal triamcinolone injection for the treatment of choroidal neovascularisation secondary to pathological myopia: a pilot study. *Br J Ophthalmol.* 2007;91(2):131-133.

9. Lee YA, Ho TC, Chen MS, Yang CH, Yang CM. Photodynamic therapy combined with posterior subtenon triamcinolone acetonide injection in the treatment of choroidal neovascularization. *Eye (Lond).* 2009;23(3):645-651.

10. Ferrara N, Gerber HP, LeCouter J. The biology of VEGF and its receptors. *Nat Med.* 2003;9(6):669-676.

11. Tong JP, Chan WM, Liu DT, et al. Aqueous humor levels of vascular endothelial growth factor and pigment epithelium-derived factor in polypoidal choroidal vasculopathy and choroidal neovascularization. *Am J Ophthalmol.* 2006;141(3):456-462.

12. Brown GC, Brown MM, Sharma S, et al. The burden of age-related macular degeneration: a value-based medicine analysis. *Trans Am Ophthalmol Soc.* 2005;103:173-184; discussion 184-186.

13. Brown DM, Kaiser PK, Michels M, et al. Ranibizumab versus verteporfin for neovascular age-related macular degeneration. *N Engl J Med.* 2006;355(14):1432-1444.

14. Rosenfeld PJ, Brown DM, Heier JS, et al. Ranibizumab for neovascular age-related macular degeneration. *N Engl J Med.* 2006;355(14):1419-1431.

15. Troutbeck R, Bunting R, van Heerdon A, Cain M, Guymer R. Ranibizumab therapy for choroidal neovascularization secondary to non-age-related macular degeneration causes. *Clin Experiment Ophthalmol.* 2012;40(1):67-72.

16. Grossniklaus HE, Green WR. Pathologic findings in pathologic myopia. *Retina.* 1992;12(2):127-133.

17. Wong TY, Ferreira A, Hughes R, Carter G, Mitchell P. Epidemiology and disease burden of pathologic myopia and myopic choroidal neovascularization: an evidence-based systematic review. *Am J Ophthalmol.* 2014;157(1):9-25.e12.

18. Chan WM, Lai TY, Chan KP, et al. Changes in aqueous vascular endothelial growth factor and pigment epithelial-derived factor levels following intravitreal bevacizumab injections for choroidal neovascularization secondary to age-related macular degeneration or pathologic myopia. *Retina.* 2008;28(9):1308-1313.

19. Hampton GR, Kohen D, Bird AC. Visual prognosis of disciform degeneration in myopia. *Ophthalmology*. 1983;90(8):923-926.

20. Yoshida T, Ohno-Matsui K, Yasuzumi K, et al. Myopic choroidal neovascularization: a 10-year follow-up. *Ophthalmology*. 2003;110(7):1297-1305.

21. Tabandeh H, Flynn HW Jr, Scott IU, et al. Visual acuity outcomes of patients 50 years of age and older with high myopia and untreated choroidal neovascularization. *Ophthalmology*. 1999;106(11):2063-2067.

22. Yoshida T, Ohno-Matsui K, Ohtake Y, et al. Long-term visual prognosis of choroidal neovascularization in high myopia: a comparison between age groups. *Ophthalmology*. 2002;109(4):712-719.

23. Holden BA, Fricke TR, Wilson DA, et al. Global prevalence of myopia and high myopia and temporal trends from 2000 through 2050. *Ophthalmology*. 2016;123(5):1036-1042.

24. Rose KA, Morgan IG, Smith W, Burlutsky G, Mitchell P, Saw SM. Myopia, lifestyle, and schooling in students of Chinese ethnicity in Singapore and Sydney. *Arch Ophthalmol*. 2008;126(4):527-530.

25. Chan WM, Lai TY, Wong AL, Liu DT, Lam DS. Combined photodynamic therapy and intravitreal triamcinolone injection for the treatment of choroidal neovascularisation secondary to pathological myopia: a pilot study. *Br J Ophthalmol*. 2007;91(2):174-179.

26. Chan WM, Lai TY, Liu DT, Lam DS. Intravitreal bevacizumab (Avastin) for myopic choroidal neovascularisation: 1-year results of a prospective pilot study. *Br J Ophthalmol*. 2009;93(2):150-154.

27. Gharbiya M, Allievi F, Mazzeo L, Gabrieli CB. Intravitreal bevacizumab treatment for choroidal neovascularization in pathologic myopia: 12-month results. *Am J Ophthalmol*. 2009;147(1):84-93. e81.

28. Ikuno Y, Sayanagi K, Soga K, et al. Intravitreal bevacizumab for choroidal neovascularization attributable to pathological myopia: one-year results. *Am J Ophthalmol*. 2009;147(1):94-100.e101.

29. Ruiz-Moreno JM, Montero JA, Gomez-Ulla F, Ares S. Intravitreal bevacizumab to treat subfoveal choroidal neovascularisation in highly myopic eyes: 1-year outcome. *Br J Ophthalmol*. 2009;93(4):448-451.

30. Ruiz-Moreno JM, Montero JA, Arias L, et al. Twelve-month outcome after one intravitreal injection of bevacizumab to treat myopic choroidal neovascularization. *Retina*. 2010;30(10):1609-1615.

31. Calvo-Gonzalez C, Reche-Frutos J, Donate J, Fernandez-Perez C, Garcia-Feijoo J. Intravitreal ranibizumab for myopic choroidal neovascularization: factors predictive of visual outcome and need for retreatment. *Am J Ophthalmol*. 2011;151(3):529-534.

32. Franqueira N, Cachulo ML, Pires I, et al. Long-term follow-up of myopic choroidal neovascularization treated with ranibizumab. *Ophthalmologica*. 2012;227(1):39-44.

33. Tufail A, Narendran N, Patel PJ, et al. Ranibizumab in myopic choroidal neovascularization: the 12-month results from the REPAIR study. *Ophthalmology*. 2013;120(9):1944-1945.e1941.

34. Kung YH, Wu TT, Huang YH. One-year outcome of two different initial dosing regimens of intravitreal ranibizumab for myopic choroidal neovascularization. *Acta Ophthalmol*. 2014;92(8):e615-e620.

35. Ikuno Y, Ohno-Matsui K, Wong TY, et al. Intravitreal aflibercept injection in patients with myopic choroidal neovascularization: the MYRROR study. *Ophthalmology*. 2015;122(6):1220-1227.

36. Brue C, Pazzaglia A, Mariotti C, Reibaldi M, Giovannini A. Aflibercept as primary treatment for myopic choroidal neovascularisation: a retrospective study. *Eye (Lond)*. 2016;30(1):139-145.

37. Wakabayashi T, Ikuno Y, Gomi F, Hamasaki T, Tano Y. Intravitreal bevacizumab vs sub-tenon triamcinolone acetonide for choroidal neovascularization attributable to pathologic myopia. *Am J Ophthalmol*. 2009;148(4):591-596.e591.

38. Gharbiya M, Giustolisi R, Allievi F, et al. Choroidal neovascularization in pathologic myopia: intravitreal ranibizumab versus bevacizumab—a randomized controlled trial. *Am J Ophthalmol*. 2010;149(3):458-464.e451.

39. Cha DM, Kim TW, Heo JW, et al. Comparison of 1-year therapeutic effect of ranibizumab and bevacizumab for myopic choroidal neovascularization: a retrospective, multicenter, comparative study. *BMC Ophthalmol*. 2014;14:69.

40. Ruiz-Moreno JM, Lopez-Galvez MI, Montero Moreno JA, Pastor Jimeno JC. Intravitreal bevacizumab in myopic neovascular membranes: 24-month results. *Ophthalmology*. 2013;120(7):1510-1511.e1511.

41. Wolf S, Balciuniene VJ, Laganovska G, et al. RADIANCE: a randomized controlled study of ranibizumab in patients with choroidal neovascularization secondary to pathologic myopia. *Ophthalmology.* 2014;121(3):682-692.e682.

42. Rishi P, Rishi E, Bhende M, et al. Comparison of photodynamic therapy, ranibizumab/bevacizumab or combination in the treatment of myopic choroidal neovascularisation: a 9-year-study from a single centre. *Br J Ophthalmol.* 2016;100(10):1337-1340.

43. Saviano S, Piermarocchi R, Leon PE, et al. Combined therapy with bevacizumab and photodynamic therapy for myopic choroidal neovascularization: A one-year follow-up controlled study. *Int J Ophthalmol.* 2014;7(2):335-339.

44. Adatia FA, Luong M, Munro M, Tufail A. The other CNVM: a review of myopic choroidal neovascularization treatment in the age of anti-vascular endothelial growth factor agents. *Surv Ophthalmol.* 2015;60(3):204-215.

45. Heier JS, Brown D, Ciulla T, et al. Ranibizumab for choroidal neovascularization secondary to causes other than age-related macular degeneration: a phase I clinical trial. *Ophthalmology.* 2011;118(1):111-118.

46. Broadhead GK, Hong T, Chang AA. Treating the untreatable patient: current options for the management of treatment-resistant neovascular age-related macular degeneration. *Acta Ophthalmol.* 2014;92(8):713-723.

47. Ciardella AP, Donsoff IM, Yannuzzi LA. Polypoidal choroidal vasculopathy. *Ophthalmol Clin North Am.* 2002;15(4):537-554.

48. Cheung CM, Yang E, Lee WK, et al. The natural history of polypoidal choroidal vasculopathy: a multi-center series of untreated Asian patients. *Graefes Arch Clin Exp Ophthalmol.* 2015;253(12):2075-2085.

49. Cheng CK, Peng CH, Chang CK, Hu CC, Chen LJ. One-year outcomes of intravitreal bevacizumab (Avastin) therapy for polypoidal choroidal vasculopathy. *Retina.* 2011;31(5):846-856.

50. Kokame GT, Yeung L, Lai JC. Continuous anti-VEGF treatment with ranibizumab for polypoidal choroidal vasculopathy: 6-month results. *Br J Ophthalmol.* 2010;94(3):297-301.

51. Oishi A, Kojima H, Mandai M, et al. Comparison of the effect of ranibizumab and verteporfin for polypoidal choroidal vasculopathy: 12-month LAPTOP study results. *Am J Ophthalmol.* 2013;156(4):644-651.

52. Hara C, Sawa M, Sayanagi K, Nishida K. One-year results of intravitreal aflibercept for polypoidal choroidal vasculopathy. *Retina.* 2016;36(1):37-45.

53. Inoue M, Yamane S, Taoka R, Arakawa A, Kadonosono K. Aflibercept for polypoidal choroidal vasculopathy: as needed versus fixed interval dosing. *Retina.* 2016;36(8):1527-1534.

54. Koh A, Lee WK, Chen LJ, et al. EVEREST study: efficacy and safety of verteporfin photodynamic therapy in combination with ranibizumab or alone versus ranibizumab monotherapy in patients with symptomatic macular polypoidal choroidal vasculopathy. *Retina.* 2012;32(8):1453-1464.

55. Gomi F, Oshima Y, Mori R, et al. Initial versus delayed photodynamic therapy in combination with ranibizumab for treatment of polypoidal choroidal vasculopathy: the Fujisan study. *Retina.* 2015;35(8):1569-1576.

56. Wong IY, Shi X, Gangwani R, et al. 1-year results of combined half-dose photodynamic therapy and ranibizumab for polypoidal choroidal vasculopathy. *BMC Ophthalmol.* 2015;15:66.

57. Saito M, Kano M, Itagaki K, Oguchi Y, Sekiryu T. Switching to intravitreal aflibercept injection for polypoidal choroidal vasculopathy refractory to ranibizumab. *Retina.* 2014;34(11):2192-2201.

58. Cho HJ, Kim KM, Kim HS, et al. Intravitreal aflibercept and ranibizumab injections for polypoidal choroidal vasculopathy. *Am J Ophthalmol.* 2016;165:1-6.

59. Neri P, Salvolini S, Mariotti C, Mercanti L, Celani S, Giovannini A. Long-term control of choroidal neovascularisation secondary to angioid streaks treated with intravitreal bevacizumab (Avastin). *Br J Ophthalmol.* 2009;93(2):155-158.

60. Sawa M, Gomi F, Tsujikawa M, Sakaguchi H, Tano Y. Long-term results of intravitreal bevacizumab injection for choroidal neovascularization secondary to angioid streaks. *Am J Ophthalmol.* 2009;148(4):584-590.e582.

61. Wiegand TW, Rogers AH, McCabe F, Reichel E, Duker JS. Intravitreal bevacizumab (Avastin) treatment of choroidal neovascularisation in patients with angioid streaks. *Br J Ophthalmol.* 2009;93(1):47-51.

62. Mimoun G, Tilleul J, Leys A, Coscas G, Soubrane G, Souied EH. Intravitreal ranibizumab for choroidal neovascularization in angioid streaks. *Am J Ophthalmol.* 2010;150(5):692-700.e691.

63. Finger RP, Charbel Issa P, Hendig D, Scholl HP, Holz FG. Monthly ranibizumab for choroidal neovascularizations secondary to angioid streaks in pseudoxanthoma elasticum: a one-year prospective study. *Am J Ophthalmol.* 2011;152(4):695-703.

64. Browning AC, Chung AK, Ghanchi F, et al. Verteporfin photodynamic therapy of choroidal neovascularization in angioid streaks: one-year results of a prospective case series. *Ophthalmology.* 2005;112(7):1227-1231.

65. Gliem M, Finger RP, Fimmers R, Brinkmann CK, Holz FG, Charbel Issa P. Treatment of choroidal neovascularization due to angioid streaks: a comprehensive review. *Retina.* 2013;33(7):1300-1314.

66. Nicholson B, Noble J, Forooghian F, Meyerle C. Central serous chorioretinopathy: update on pathophysiology and treatment. *Surv Ophthalmol.* 2013;58(2):103-126.

67. Kitzmann AS, Pulido JS, Diehl NN, Hodge DO, Burke JP. The incidence of central serous chorioretinopathy in Olmsted County, Minnesota, 1980-2002. *Ophthalmology.* 2008;115(1):169-173.

68. Daruich A, Matet A, Dirani A, et al. Central serous chorioretinopathy: recent findings and new physiopathology hypothesis. *Prog Retin Eye Res.* 2015;48:82-118.

69. Spaide RF, Campeas L, Haas A, et al. Central serous chorioretinopathy in younger and older adults. *Ophthalmology.* 1996;103(12):2070-2079; discussion 2079-2080.

70. Lim JW, Kim MU, Shin MC. Aqueous humor and plasma levels of vascular endothelial growth factor and interleukin-8 in patients with central serous chorioretinopathy. *Retina.* 2010;30(9):1465-1471.

71. Artunay O, Yuzbasioglu E, Rasier R, Sengul A, Bahcecioglu H. Intravitreal bevacizumab in treatment of idiopathic persistent central serous chorioretinopathy: a prospective, controlled clinical study. *Curr Eye Res.* 2010;35(2):91-98.

72. Lim JW, Ryu SJ, Shin MC. The effect of intravitreal bevacizumab in patients with acute central serous chorioretinopathy. *Korean J Ophthalmol.* 2010;24(3):155-158.

73. Chung YR, Seo EJ, Lew HM, Lee KH. Lack of positive effect of intravitreal bevacizumab in central serous chorioretinopathy: meta-analysis and review. *Eye (Lond).* 2013;27(12):1339-1346.

74. Kim M, Lee SC, Lee SJ. Intravitreal ranibizumab for acute central serous chorioretinopathy. *Ophthalmologica.* 2013;229(3):152-157.

75. Bae SH, Heo J, Kim C, et al. Low-fluence photodynamic therapy versus ranibizumab for chronic central serous chorioretinopathy: one-year results of a randomized trial. *Ophthalmology.* 2014;121(2):558-565.

76. Pitcher JD III, Witkin AJ, DeCroos FC, Ho AC. A prospective pilot study of intravitreal aflibercept for the treatment of chronic central serous chorioretinopathy: the CONTAIN study. *Br J Ophthalmol.* 2015;99(6):848-852.

77. Kleiner RC, Ratner CM, Enger C, Fine SL. Subfoveal neovascularization in the ocular histoplasmosis syndrome. A natural history study. *Retina.* 1988;8(4):225-229.

78. Schadlu R, Blinder KJ, Shah GK, et al. Intravitreal bevacizumab for choroidal neovascularization in ocular histoplasmosis. *Am J Ophthalmol.* 2008;145(5):875-878.

79. Cionni DA, Lewis SA, Petersen MR, et al. Analysis of outcomes for intravitreal bevacizumab in the treatment of choroidal neovascularization secondary to ocular histoplasmosis. *Ophthalmology.* 2012;119(2):327-332.

80. Chang LK, Spaide RF, Brue C, Freund KB, Klancnik JM Jr, Slakter JS. Bevacizumab treatment for subfoveal choroidal neovascularization from causes other than age-related macular degeneration. *Arch Ophthalmol.* 2008;126(7):941-945.

81. Carneiro AM, Silva RM, Veludo MJ, et al. Ranibizumab treatment for choroidal neovascularization from causes other than age-related macular degeneration and pathological myopia. *Ophthalmologica.* 2011;225(2):81-88.

9

Diabetic Macular Edema

Emily D. Cole, BS; Eduardo A. Novais, MD; and
Nadia K. Waheed, MD, MPH

Diabetic retinopathy affects more than 90 million people worldwide and is the most frequent cause of legal blindness among working-age individuals in developed countries.[1-3] Although diabetes mellitus may cause vision loss by several means including optic neuropathy, cataract formation, macular ischemia, and proliferative retinopathy, diabetic macular edema (DME) is the most common reason for moderate visual loss in diabetes.[2,4]

The pathogenesis of DME is multifactorial and may include contributing factors such as mechanical traction, upregulation and downregulation of a variety of cytokines including vascular endothelial growth factor (VEGF), and inflammation.[5] Hyperglycemia leads to high intracellular levels of glucose, formation of free radicals, and protein kinase C activation,[6] which in turn leads to disruption of the blood-retinal barrier and increased accumulation of fluid into the retina.[7-10] Other influential factors include hypoxia, altered blood flow, and retinal ischemia.

The Early Treatment Diabetic Retinopathy Study (ETDRS) group established level-one guidelines for the use of macular laser photocoagulation to treat patients with clinically significant DME.[11] In the ETDRS, focal photocoagulation reduced the risk of moderate visual acuity loss (defined as a loss of 15 or more letters) by approximately 50%, from 24% to 12%, after 3 years.[12] However, these clinical laser treatment guidelines were established before the use of adjunctive pharmacologic agents.

In the past decade, novel pharmacologic therapies have shifted treatment paradigms away from laser photocoagulation. Of these, intravitreal anti-VEGF agents are the most widely used and have shown substantial improvements both in visual and anatomic outcomes (Figure 9-1).[13-19] However, one of the main drawbacks of anti-VEGF therapy is its short duration of action, requiring many patients to undergo repeated intravitreal injections.[20]

Duker JS, Liang MC, eds.
Anti-VEGF Use in
Ophthalmology (pp. 101-111).
© 2017 Taylor & Francis Group.

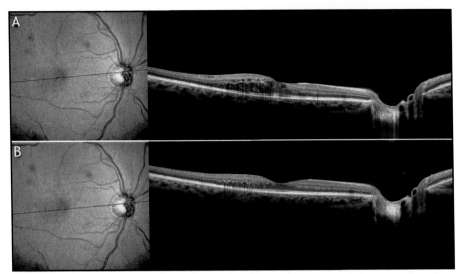

Figure 9-1. Optical coherence tomography of a 33-year-old woman with diabetic macular edema pre- and post-intravitreal anti-vascular endothelial growth factor (VEGF). (A) Pre-anti-VEGF intraocular injection, there are cystic structures extending from the outer nuclear layer to the inner nuclear layer and focal areas of hyper-reflective hard exudates throughout the external plexiform layers. (B) Post-anti-VEGF intraocular injection, there is a significant reduction in the size and number of intra-retinal cysts. The focal areas of hyper-reflective hard exudates are still present but to a lesser degree. (Reprinted with permission from Dr. Gabriel Andrade.)

Corticosteroid Treatments for Diabetic Macular Edema

Inflammatory factors have been associated with macular edema of different etiologies. Intraocular corticosteroids have been used as adjunctive or alternative treatments for DME, and work by inhibiting inflammatory cytokines and decreasing vascular permeability.[5,21] Intravitreal triamcinolone was evaluated previously as a treatment for DME in a randomized trial conducted by the Diabetic Retinopathy Clinical Research Network (DRCR.net).[22] Although the data suggested that intravitreal triamcinolone was superior to observation in the ETDRS, it was not superior to focal/grid photocoagulation.[23] The United States Food and Drug Administration (FDA) later approved a dexamethasone intravitreal implant (Ozurdex) for treating DME, in addition to macular edema associated with noninfectious posterior uveitis and retinal vein occlusion. This sustained-release formulation was designed to release dexamethasone for up to 6 months, eliminating the need for monthly injections.[24] Functional and anatomic improvements with Ozurdex have been reported in several case series of patients with persistent DME.[25-27] However, steroid-related adverse events such as cataract formation and increased intraocular pressure, as well as migration of implants into the anterior chamber requiring surgical removal, can complicate treatment.[28]

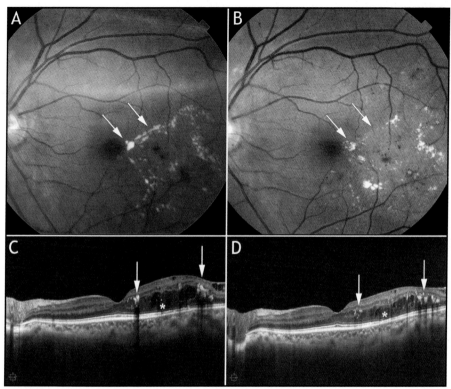

Figure 9-2. Color fundus imaging and optical coherence tomography of a 53-year-old diabetic woman with clinically significant macular edema pre- and post-intravitreal anti-vascular endothelium growth factor (VEGF). (A) Pre-anti-VEGF intraocular injection. Color fundus photography shows hard exudates associated with retinal thickening within 500 µm of the center of the fovea (arrows), microaneurysms, cotton wool spots, and dot hemorrhages. (B) Post-anti-VEGF intraocular injection. Retinal thickening is decreased and there is partial regression of intraretinal exudates (arrows). (C) Optical coherence tomography B-scan pre- and (D) post-anti-VEGF intraocular injection show partial regression of intra-retinal exudates (arrows) and decrease in size and number of intraretinal cysts (asterisks).

Anti-Vascular Endothelial Growth Factor Agents for the Treatment of Diabetic Macular Edema

VEGF blockade can be achieved by targeting extracellular anti-VEGF, inhibiting VEGF receptor expression, or via antibodies that bind to the VEGF molecule to prevent receptor binding. There are multiple agents used in the management of DME. Currently, ranibizumab, bevacizumab, and aflibercept are the most commonly used.[29-34] Ocular imaging, including color fundus photography, optical coherence tomography (OCT), and more recently OCT angiography, has been useful in the management of DME (Figures 9-2 and 9-3) and deciding when to treat with these anti-VEGF agents.

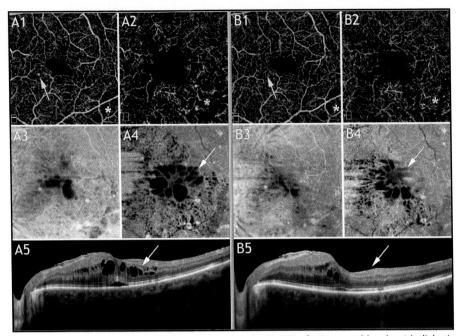

Figure 9-3. Optical coherence tomography angiography (OCTA) of a 74-year-old male with diabetic macular edema pre- and post-intravitreal anti-vascular endothelial growth factor (VEGF). (A1) Pre-treatment OCTA segmented at the superficial plexus shows areas of ischemia (white asterisk), micro-aneurysms (yellow arrow), and parafoveal areas of capillary flow impairment. (B1) Post-treatment OCTA segmented at the superficial plexus shows improvement of ischemia (white asterisk) and the microaneurysms previously seen are no longer visible (yellow arrow). (A2) Pre-treatment OCTA segmented at the deep plexus shows areas of diabetic macular edema that appear as cystoid, dark areas that correspond to cysts easily seen on the corresponding structural *en face* OCT (A3 and A4). The yellow asterisk corresponds to an area of decreased flow. (B2) Post-treatment OCTA segmented at the deep plexus shows improvement of ischemia (yellow asterisk) and decrease in size and number of intraretinal cysts on the corresponding structural *en face* OCT (B3 and B4). (A5) Corresponding OCT B-scan shows intra- and subretinal fluid. The white arrows correspond to the same intraretinal cyst on structural *en face* OCT (A4). (B5) Post-injection OCT B-scan, the cysts are markedly reduced in size, which is most apparent on the structural *en face* OCT B-scan (B4).

Pegaptanib

Pegaptanib, the first anti-VEGF agent approved for the treatment of neovascular age-related macular degeneration (AMD), is a 28-nucleotide aptamer that binds to and inactivates the extracellular $VEGF_{165}$ isomer. It has an intermediate level of diffusion ability and heparin binding ability, which corresponds to the ability to bind to cell surfaces and basement membranes.[30] It has been associated with improved visual outcomes and a reduction in mean central subfoveal thickness (CST) in patients with DME, with a comparable safety profile when compared to sham.[35]

In 2005, a phase II randomized trial compared multiple concentrations of pegaptanib to sham treatment for DME. The 0.3 mg group had significantly greater gains in visual acuity (VA), a reduction in the mean CST, and fewer patients requiring laser compared to sham.[35] The subsequent phase II/III trial also demonstrated benefit of pegaptanib over sham, with 36.8% of patients receiving pegaptanib gaining more than 10 letters compared to 19.7% in the sham group at week 54. At all points within the 2-year follow-up, the change in mean VA from baseline was significantly greater in patients treated with pegaptanib than sham. This study also looked at longer-term safety of the drug and found that the sham and treated groups had similar numbers of adverse events and frequency of discontinuation.[36] Today, pegaptanib is rarely used in clinical practice because the comparative efficacy of the drug is lower than other available treatment options.

Ranibizumab

Ranibizumab is a humanized monoclonal antibody fragment derived from bevacizumab, a full-length humanized antibody. It binds all isoforms of VEGF-A and active proteolytic fragments and was designed for better penetration into the retina because of its smaller size. It was first approved for the treatment of neovascular AMD and has also been extensively studied in clinical trials for the treatment of DME.[37-39]

The READ-2 study provided early evidence that ranibizumab was effective in the treatment of DME, and that combining focal and grid laser with ranibizumab may decrease the frequency of injections needed to control edema for at least 2 years. The READ-3 studies compared 2 different doses of ranibizumab (0.5 mg and 2 mg), and demonstrated that a higher dose did not show significant benefits over a 6-month period.[19,40,41] The RIDE and RISE studies were 2 identical phase III multicenter studies that led to the approval of 0.3 mg ranibizumab by the FDA for DME. Both studies showed that a significantly higher number of patients with center-involved DME treated with 0.3 mg ranibizumab gained 15 or more letters at month 24 compared to those treated with sham. These results were equivalent to those seen with 0.5 mg ranibizumab, thus leading to the approval of the lower dose. Treated patients also required fewer macular laser procedures. Improvements in macular edema on OCT as well as the degree of retinopathy were also found to improve. In the extension phase of both studies, patients could cross over from the sham group into the monthly treatment arm, creating a delayed treatment initiation group. These patients gained VA but not to the degree of those treated with early initiation of ranibizumab therapy.[42,43] This demonstrated that intraocular anti-VEGF treatment should be initiated early to maximize visual acuity outcomes.

The DRCR.net performed a randomized clinical trial comparing ranibizumab with prompt or deferred laser and found that ranibizumab combined with both prompt or deferred laser had greater VA gains than laser alone. Similar gains in VA were also seen in pseudophakic eyes treated with triamcinolone. In the expanded 2-year follow-up, compared to sham, the mean change in the VA letter score from baseline was 3.7 letters greater in the ranibizumab plus prompt laser group, 5.8 letters greater in the ranibizumab plus deferred laser group, and 1.5 letters less in the triamcinolone plus prompt laser group. This difference in the steroid-treated group was found to be due to the development of cataract, which was more frequent in the triamcinolone plus prompt laser group. Forty percent of the eyes in both ranibizumab groups still had central macular edema after 2 years.[44,45]

The RESTORE and REVEAL studies were phase III trials that demonstrated ranibizumab was superior to laser therapy alone. In the 3-year extension of the RESTORE study, ranibizumab improved VA and decreased CST on OCT on a pro re nata (PRN), or as-needed, treatment regimen.[17,46,47] The REVEAL study compared ranibizumab to laser in an Asian population, and found that ranibizumab monotherapy or ranibizumab combined with laser had superior VA improvements over laser treatment alone.[48] Furthermore, there was not an increased rate of ocular or nonocular severe adverse events compared to sham in the RESOLVE trial.[18]

Recently, Protocol T from the DRCR.net compared the effectiveness of ranibizumab, aflibercept, and bevacizumab for center-involved DME over 2 years. All 3 groups showed improvement in VA, decreased frequency of visits, and decreased requirement of laser photocoagulation after 2 years. In the first year, aflibercept was found to be associated with greater gains in VA compared to the other 2 agents when baseline vision was 20/50 or worse. In eyes with baseline vision better than 20/50, there was no difference in visual acuity gains over 1 or 2 years although patients treated with bevacizumab were less likely to have OCT findings of less than 250 μm CST.[49,50]

Bevacizumab

Bevacizumab is one of the most widely used anti-VEGF agents because of its low cost compared to the other agents. It is a full-length humanized antibody that is active against all isoforms of VEGF-A and competitively inhibits them in the extracellular space. It is FDA approved for the treatment of metastatic colon cancer but is used off-label for the treatment of AMD, DME, and several other ocular diseases. Michels et al[51] initially proposed the use of bevacizumab as an intravitreal treatment for neovascular AMD in 2005, when they noticed VA improvement in patients treated with systemic bevacizumab for metastatic colorectal cancer.[51]

Protocol H of the DRCR.net was a short-term pilot study designed to evaluate the short-term effects of bevacizumab (1.25 mg and 2.5 mg) compared to focal laser. There was a significant reduction in CST in both treatment groups over 3 weeks but no significant difference in functional or anatomic outcomes between the groups. However, the initial positive response to patients treated with bevacizumab was also seen in the focal laser group after 3 weeks. Data from this study provided limited early evidence that bevacizumab may be beneficial in some eyes with DME.[52]

Subsequent work by Ahmadiah, Faghihi, and Soheilian built on the DRCR.net findings and explored the combination of bevacizumab and triamcinolone. None of the studies found strong evidence that the addition of triamcinolone led to improved functional or visual outcomes. In a 2-year follow-up study comparing bevacizumab, bevacizumab plus triamcinolone, and macular photocoagulation, no significant differences in visual outcomes among the 3 groups were noted.[53-57]

The Bevacizumab or Laser Therapy (BOLT) trial was a randomized, controlled trial over 2 years that compared intravitreal bevacizumab to macular laser therapy in patients with a history of macular laser. After one year, patients treated with bevacizumab had significantly better VA, gained a mean of 8.6 letters compared to a loss of 0.5 letters in the laser-treated arm, and had no serious adverse events noted after 12 months. This prospective study supported the long-term use of bevacizumab for DME.[58]

Protocol T also found similar rates of serious adverse events, hospitalizations, and ocular adverse events between the anti-VEGF agents. Although a post hoc analysis showed a higher frequency of cardiac and vascular disorders in the ranibizumab group, this was thought to be secondary to other confounding factors and not to be of clinical significance.[59] Moreover, several other studies have failed to reproduce this difference in adverse events between the various different anti-VEGF agents.

Aflibercept

Aflibercept is a recombinant fusion protein that acts as a decoy receptor and binds VEGF-A, VEGF-B, and placental growth factor. It binds with much higher affinity than ranibizumab and bevacizumab. Also originally used as a chemotherapy agent, it has since been FDA approved for ocular use in DME, neovascular AMD, and macular edema due to retinal vein occlusion.[16,60-62]

The DA VINCI study was a phase II trial that demonstrated aflibercept to be superior to macular laser treatment for DME over a 24-week period. The study compared multiple dosages and dosing regimens and found that in all dosing groups, VA was significantly improved and there were greater reductions in retinal thickness compared with laser treatment. The study was not powered to detect differences between the dosage groups, but all showed superiority to laser.[63,64]

The VIVID and VISTA studies were 2 identical phase III trials that led to the approval of aflibercept by the FDA for the treatment of DME. In these studies, eyes were randomized to receive 2 mg aflibercept every 4 weeks, 2 mg aflibercept every 8 weeks after 5 initial monthly doses, or macular laser. The 1-year and 100-week follow-up demonstrated that aflibercept was more effective compared to laser. At month 12, the mean change in VA (+12.5 vs +0.2 letters) and CST values (−185.9 vs −73.3 μm) were significantly greater with aflibercept compared to laser therapy. The mean change in VA improvement was noted through the 100-week follow-up (+11.3 vs +0.8 letters), suggesting the drug was still effective with long-term administration. The only adverse event noted in these studies over the long-term follow-up was the development of cataract.[65]

The results from Protocol T suggested the importance of baseline visual acuity when comparing the 3 agents. In the first year, aflibercept was found to be associated with greater gains in VA compared to the other 2 agents when baseline vision was 20/50 or worse. In eyes with baseline vision better than 20/50, there was no difference in VA gains over 2 years. Patients treated with aflibercept, however, were less likely to require subsequent laser photocoagulation.[49,50,66] Results from Protocol T have sparked debate regarding which agent should be used to initiate treatment in patients with VA less than 20/50 and the role of bevacizumab and ranibizumab nonresponders in driving the results. One option is to initiate treatment with bevacizumab and subsequently switch to aflibercept if there is no treatment response. Another option is to initiate treatment with aflibercept then continue with a hybrid of multiple agents for more long-term treatment. Currently, there is no clear evidence-based recommendation on the best anti-VEGF to use.

Conclusion

The development of anti-VEGF agents has revolutionized the treatment of vision-threatening chorioretinal diseases such as DME and neovascular AMD. Prior to this, laser photocoagulation was the main treatment option and visual outcomes were not as promising. Today, anti-VEGF agents are often the first-line treatment of choice for clinicians with a better visual prognosis with treatment. Current treatment paradigms vary; some treat on a monthly basis until stable, then continue on an as-needed basis, while others use a treat-and-extend approach. OCT is used extensively to quantify the macular edema and assess the success or failure of anti-VEGF therapy in these eyes. Although most studies investigated monthly treatment regimens for DME, this can be costly and often imposes an unrealistic burden on the patient, their families, and society. However, the DRCR.net PRN protocols provide good evidence that aggressive treatment, especially at the initiation, can lead to a good prognosis and reduced need for treatment after 1 to 2 years of aggressive "initiation" treatment. Moreover, there is emerging evidence that treatment for DME with anti-VEGF therapy may be disease modifying, with a regression of diabetic retinopathy in patients treated with anti-VEGF agents.[67] This has led to a label change with the approval of ranibizumab and aflibercept for the treatment of diabetic retinopathy in the setting of DME. Anti-VEGF agents are now being studied in combination with other agents to try to increase the treatment interval and duration of action of these medications. Newer delivery systems are also being studied that would allow for slow release of the agent, requiring fewer invasive procedures and reducing side effects associated with intravitreal injections.

References

1. Yau JW, Rogers SL, Kawasaki R, et al. Global prevalence and major risk factors of diabetic retinopathy. *Diabetes Care*. 2012;35(3):556-564.
2. Moss SE, Klein R, Klein BE. The 14-year incidence of visual loss in a diabetic population. *Ophthalmology*. 1998;105(6):998-1003.
3. Klein R, Klein BE, Moss SE, Cruickshanks KJ. The Wisconsin Epidemiologic Study of Diabetic Retinopathy: XVII. The 14-year incidence and progression of diabetic retinopathy and associated risk factors in type 1 diabetes. *Ophthalmology*. 1998;105(10):1801-1815.
4. Klein R, Klein BE, Moss SE, Cruickshanks KJ. The Wisconsin Epidemiologic Study of Diabetic Retinopathy: XIV. Ten-year incidence and progression of diabetic retinopathy. *Arch Ophthalmol*. 1994;112(9):1217-1228.
5. Antcliff RJ, Marshall J. The pathogenesis of edema in diabetic maculopathy. *Semin Ophthalmol*. 1999;14(4):223-232.
6. Wolfensberger TJ, Gregor ZJ. Macular edema—rationale for therapy. *Dev Ophthalmol*. 2010;47:49-58.
7. Witmer AN, Vrensen GF, Van Noorden CJ, Schlingemann RO. Vascular endothelial growth factors and angiogenesis in eye disease. *Prog Retin Eye Res*. 2003;22(1):1-29.
8. Miyamoto K, Khosrof S, Bursell SE, et al. Prevention of leukostasis and vascular leakage in streptozotocin-induced diabetic retinopathy via intercellular adhesion molecule-1 inhibition. *Proc Natl Acad Sci U S A*. 1999;96(19):10836-10841.
9. Kim W, Hudson BI, Moser B, et al. Receptor for advanced glycation end products and its ligands: a journey from the complications of diabetes to its pathogenesis. *Ann N Y Acad Sci*. 2005;1043:553-561.
10. Ramasamy R, Vannucci SJ, Yan SS, Herold K, Yan SF, Schmidt AM. Advanced glycation end products and RAGE: a common thread in aging, diabetes, neurodegeneration, and inflammation. *Glycobiology*. 2005;15(7):16R-28R.
11. Photocoagulation for diabetic macular edema. Early Treatment Diabetic Retinopathy Study report number 1. Early Treatment Diabetic Retinopathy Study research group. *Arch Ophthalmol*. 1985;103(12):1796-1806.
12. Diabetic Retinopathy Clinical Research Network, Scott IU, Edwards AR, et al. A phase II randomized clinical trial of intravitreal bevacizumab for diabetic macular edema. *Ophthalmology*. 2007;114(10):1860-1867.
13. Boyer DS, Hopkins JJ, Sorof J, Ehrlich JS. Anti-vascular endothelial growth factor therapy for diabetic macular edema. *Ther Adv Endocrinol Metab*. 2013;4(6):151-169.
14. Nguyen QD, Brown DM, Marcus DM, et al. Ranibizumab for diabetic macular edema: results from 2 phase III randomized trials: RISE and RIDE. *Ophthalmology*. 2012;119(4):789-801.
15. Michaelides M, Kaines A, Hamilton RD, et al. A prospective randomized trial of intravitreal bevacizumab or laser therapy in the management of diabetic macular edema (BOLT study) 12-month data: report 2. *Ophthalmology*. 2010;117(6):1078-1086.e2.

16. Korobelnik JF, Do DV, Schmidt-Erfurth U, et al. Intravitreal aflibercept for diabetic macular edema. *Ophthalmology.* 2014;121(11):2247-2254.

17. Mitchell P, Bandello F, Schmidt-Erfurth U, et al. The RESTORE study: ranibizumab monotherapy or combined with laser versus laser monotherapy for diabetic macular edema. *Ophthalmology.* 2011;118(4):615-625.

18. Massin P, Bandello F, Garweg JG, et al. Safety and efficacy of ranibizumab in diabetic macular edema (RESOLVE Study): a 12-month, randomized, controlled, double-masked, multicenter phase II study. *Diabetes Care.* 2010;33(11):2399-2405.

19. Nguyen QD, Shah SM, Khwaja AA, et al. Two-year outcomes of the ranibizumab for edema of the mAcula in diabetes (READ-2) study. *Ophthalmology.* 2010;117(11):2146-2151.

20. Haller JA. Current anti-vascular endothelial growth factor dosing regimens: benefits and burden. *Ophthalmology.* 2013;120(5 Suppl):S3-S7.

21. Sarao V, Veritti D, Boscia F, Lanzetta P. Intravitreal steroids for the treatment of retinal diseases. *ScientificWorldJournal.* 2014;2014:989501.

22. Diabetic Retinopathy Clinical Research Network. A randomized trial comparing intravitreal triamcinolone acetonide and focal/grid photocoagulation for diabetic macular edema. *Ophthalmology.* 2008;115(9):1447-1449, 1449.e1-1449.e10.

23. Diabetic Retinopathy Clinical Research Network, Beck RW, Edwards AR, et al. Three-year follow-up of a randomized trial comparing focal/grid photocoagulation and intravitreal triamcinolone for diabetic macular edema. *Arch Ophthalmol.* 2009;127(3):245-251.

24. Chang-Lin JE, Attar M, Acheampong AA, et al. Pharmacokinetics and pharmacodynamics of a sustained-release dexamethasone intravitreal implant. *Invest Ophthalmol Vis Sci.* 2011;52(1):80-86.

25. Zalewski D, Raczynska D, Raczynska K. Five-month observation of persistent diabetic macular edema after intravitreal injection of Ozurdex implant. *Mediators Inflamm.* 2014;2014:364143.

26. Zucchiatti I, Lattanzio R, Querques G, et al. Intravitreal dexamethasone implant in patients with persistent diabetic macular edema. *Ophthalmologica.* 2012;228(2):117-122.

27. Medeiros MD, Alkabes M, Navarro R, Garcia-Arumí J, Mateo C, Corcóstegui B. Dexamethasone intravitreal implant in vitrectomized versus nonvitrectomized eyes for treatment of patients with persistent diabetic macular edema. *J Ocul Pharmacol Ther.* 2014;30(9):709-716.

28. Khurana RN, Appa SN, McCannel CA, et al. Dexamethasone implant anterior chamber migration: risk factors, complications, and management strategies. *Ophthalmology.* 2014;121(1):67-71.

29. Ho AC, Scott IU, Kim SJ, et al. Anti-vascular endothelial growth factor pharmacotherapy for diabetic macular edema: a report by the American Academy of Ophthalmology. *Ophthalmology.* 2012;119(10):2179-2188.

30. Salam A, DaCosta J, Sivaprasad S. Anti-vascular endothelial growth factor agents for diabetic maculopathy. *Br J Ophthalmol.* 2010;94(7):821-826.

31. Virgili G, Parravano M, Menchini F, Evans JR. Anti-vascular endothelial growth factor for diabetic macular oedema. *Cochrane Database Syst Rev.* 2014;10:CD007419.

32. Goyal S, Lavalley M, Subramanian ML. Meta-analysis and review on the effect of bevacizumab in diabetic macular edema. *Graefes Arch Clin Exp Ophthalmol.* 2011;249(1):15-27.

33. Nicholson BP, Schachat AP. A review of clinical trials of anti-VEGF agents for diabetic retinopathy. *Graefes Arch Clin Exp Ophthalmol.* 2010;248(7):915-930.

34. Demirel S, Argo C, Agarwal A, et al. Updates on the clinical trials in diabetic macular edema. *Middle East Afr J Ophthalmol.* 2016;23(1):3-12.

35. Cunningham ET Jr, Adamis AP, Altaweel M, et al. A phase II randomized double-masked trial of pegaptanib, an anti-vascular endothelial growth factor aptamer, for diabetic macular edema. *Ophthalmology.* 2005;112(10):1747-1757.

36. Sultan MB, Zhou D, Loftus J, Dombi T, Ice KS, Macugen 1013 Study Group. A phase 2/3, multicenter, randomized, double-masked, 2-year trial of pegaptanib sodium for the treatment of diabetic macular edema. *Ophthalmology.* 2011;118(6):1107-1118.

37. Bandello F, Berchicci L, La Spina C, Battaglia Parodi M, Iacono P. Evidence for anti-VEGF treatment of diabetic macular edema. *Ophthalmic Res.* 2012;48(Suppl 1):16-20.

38. Ferrara N, Damico L, Shams N, Lowman H, Kim R. Development of ranibizumab, an anti-vascular endothelial growth factor antigen binding fragment, as therapy for neovascular age-related macular degeneration. *Retina.* 2006;26(8):859-870.

39. Chun DW, Heier JS, Topping TM, Duker JS, Bankert JM. A pilot study of multiple intravitreal injections of ranibizumab in patients with center-involving clinically significant diabetic macular edema. *Ophthalmology.* 2006;113(10):1706-1712.

40. Do DV, Sepah YJ, Boyer D, et al. Month-6 primary outcomes of the READ-3 study (Ranibizumab for Edema of the mAcula in Diabetes-Protocol 3 with high dose). *Eye (Lond).* 2015;29(12):1538-1544.

41. Nguyen QD, Shah SM, Heier JS, et al. Primary end point (six months) results of the Ranibizumab for Edema of the mAcula in diabetes (READ-2) study. *Ophthalmology.* 2009;116(11):2175-2181.e1.

42. Brown DM, Nguyen QD, Marcus DM, et al. Long-term outcomes of ranibizumab therapy for diabetic macular edema: the 36-month results from two phase III trials: RISE and RIDE. *Ophthalmology.* 2013;120(10):2013-2022.

43. Do DV, Nguyen QD, Khwaja AA, et al. Ranibizumab for edema of the macula in diabetes study: 3-year outcomes and the need for prolonged frequent treatment. *JAMA Ophthalmol.* 2013;131(2):139-145.

44. Elman MJ, Bressler NM, Qin H, et al. Expanded 2-year follow-up of ranibizumab plus prompt or deferred laser or triamcinolone plus prompt laser for diabetic macular edema. *Ophthalmology.* 2011;118(4):609-614.

45. Diabetic Retinopathy Clinical Research Network, Elman MJ, Aiello LP, et al. Randomized trial evaluating ranibizumab plus prompt or deferred laser or triamcinolone plus prompt laser for diabetic macular edema. *Ophthalmology.* 2010;117(6):1064-1077.e35.

46. Schmidt-Erfurth U, Lang GE, Holz FG, et al. Three-year outcomes of individualized ranibizumab treatment in patients with diabetic macular edema: the RESTORE extension study. *Ophthalmology.* 2014;121(5):1045-1053.

47. Mitchell P, Massin P, Bressler S, et al. Three-year patient-reported visual function outcomes in diabetic macular edema managed with ranibizumab: the RESTORE extension study. *Curr Med Res Opin.* 2015;31(11):1967-1975.

48. Ishibashi T, Li X, Koh A, et al. The REVEAL Study: ranibizumab monotherapy or combined with laser versus laser monotherapy in Asian patients with diabetic macular edema. *Ophthalmology.* 2015;122(7):1402-1415.

49. Diabetic Retinopathy Clinical Research Network, Wells JA, Glassman AR, et al. Aflibercept, bevacizumab, or ranibizumab for diabetic macular edema. *N Engl J Med.* 2015;372(13):1193-1203.

50. Wells JA, Glassman AR, Ayala AR, et al. Aflibercept, bevacizumab, or ranibizumab for diabetic macular edema: two-year results from a comparative effectiveness randomized clinical trial. *Ophthalmology.* 2016;123(6):1351-1359.

51. Michels S, Rosenfeld PJ, Puliafito CA, Marcus EN, Venkatraman AS. Systemic bevacizumab (Avastin) therapy for neovascular age-related macular degeneration twelve-week results of an uncontrolled open-label clinical study. *Ophthalmology.* 2005;112(6):1035-1047.

52. Diabetic Retinopathy Clinical Research Network, Elman MJ, Qin H, et al. Intravitreal ranibizumab for diabetic macular edema with prompt versus deferred laser treatment: three-year randomized trial results. *Ophthalmology.* 2012;119(11):2312-2318.

53. Soheilian M, Ramezani A, Bijanzadeh B, et al. Intravitreal bevacizumab (Avastin) injection alone or combined with triamcinolone versus macular photocoagulation as primary treatment of diabetic macular edema. *Retina.* 2007;27(9):1187-1195.

54. Faghihi H, Roohipoor R, Mohammadi SF, et al. Intravitreal bevacizumab versus combined bevacizumab-triamcinolone versus macular laser photocoagulation in diabetic macular edema. *Eur J Ophthalmol.* 2008;18(6):941-948.

55. Ahmadieh H, Taei R, Riazi-Esfahani M, et al. Intravitreal bevacizumab versus combined intravitreal bevacizumab and triamcinolone for neovascular age-related macular degeneration: six-month results of a randomized clinical trial. *Retina.* 2011;31(9):1819-1826.

56. Ahmadieh H, Ramezani A, Shoeibi N, et al. Intravitreal bevacizumab with or without triamcinolone for refractory diabetic macular edema; a placebo-controlled, randomized clinical trial. *Graefes Arch Clin Exp Ophthalmol.* 2008;246(4):483-489.

57. Soheilian M, Ramezani A, Obudi A, et al. Randomized trial of intravitreal bevacizumab alone or combined with triamcinolone versus macular photocoagulation in diabetic macular edema. *Ophthalmology.* 2009;116(6):1142-1150.

58. Rajendram R, Fraser-Bell S, Kaines A, et al. A 2-year prospective randomized controlled trial of intravitreal bevacizumab or laser therapy (BOLT) in the management of diabetic macular edema: 24-month data: report 3. *Arch Ophthalmol.* 2012;130(8):972-979.

59. Comparison of Age-related Macular Degeneration Treatments Trials (CATT) Research Group, Martin DF, Maguire MG, et al. Ranibizumab and bevacizumab for treatment of neovascular age-related macular degeneration: two-year results. *Ophthalmology.* 2012;119(7):1388-1398.

60. Ciombor KK, Berlin J. Aflibercept—a decoy VEGF receptor. *Curr Oncol Rep.* 2014;16(2):368.

61. Papadopoulos N, Martin J, Ruan Q, et al. Binding and neutralization of vascular endothelial growth factor (VEGF) and related ligands by VEGF Trap, ranibizumab and bevacizumab. *Angiogenesis.* 2012;15(2):171-185.

62. Heier JS, Brown DM, Chong V, et al. Intravitreal aflibercept (VEGF trap-eye) in wet age-related macular degeneration. *Ophthalmology.* 2012;119(12):2537-2548.

63. Do DV, Schmidt-Erfurth U, Gonzalez VH, et al. The DA VINCI Study: phase 2 primary results of VEGF Trap-Eye in patients with diabetic macular edema. *Ophthalmology.* 2011;118(9):1819-1826.

64. Do DV, Nguyen QD, Boyer D, et al. One-year outcomes of the da Vinci Study of VEGF Trap-Eye in eyes with diabetic macular edema. *Ophthalmology.* 2012;119(8):1658-1665.

65. Brown DM, Schmidt-Erfurth U, Do DV, et al. Intravitreal aflibercept for diabetic macular edema: 100-week results from the VISTA and VIVID studies. *Ophthalmology.* 2015;122(10):2044-2052.

66. Heier JS, Bressler NM, Avery RL, et al. Comparison of aflibercept, bevacizumab, and ranibizumab for treatment of diabetic macular edema: extrapolation of data to clinical practice. *JAMA Ophthalmol.* 2016;134(1):95-99.

67. Osaadon P, Fagan XJ, Lifshitz T, Levy J. A review of anti-VEGF agents for proliferative diabetic retinopathy. *Eye (Lond).* 2014;28(5):510-520.

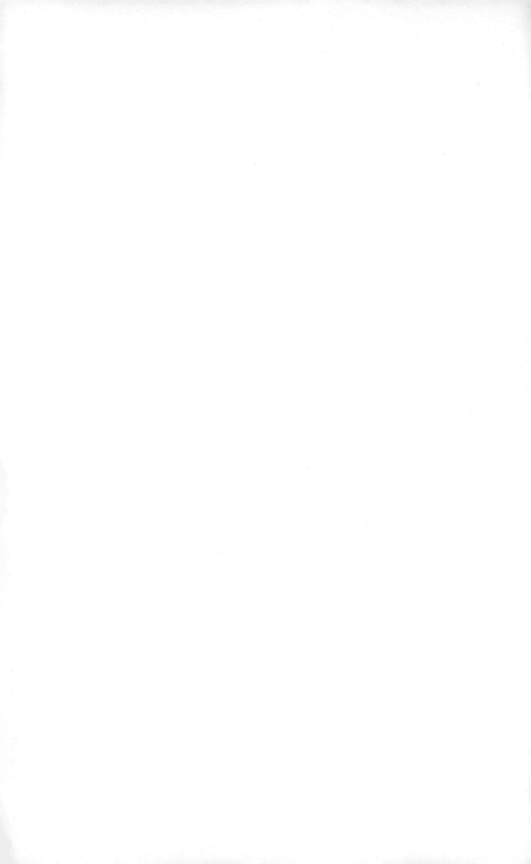

10

PROLIFERATIVE DIABETIC RETINOPATHY

Sabin Dang, MD and Chirag P. Shah, MD, MPH

Diabetic retinopathy is responsible for a significant amount of visual morbidity worldwide. Chronic insult to the retinal microcirculation induced by hyperglycemia can result in multiple pathologic processes that cause vision loss.[1] Among the most severe sequelae of this process is retinal neovascularization, the key feature of proliferative diabetic retinopathy (PDR) (Figure 10-1). Recent epidemiologic studies conducted in the United States have shown nearly 1.5% of Americans diagnosed with diabetes will progress to PDR.[2]

Patients with PDR develop new blood vessels that are derived from the existing retinal vasculature. These vessels are created in response to the hypoxic conditions of diabetic retinopathy; they do not follow normal vessel orientation and instead invade the vitreous cavity. In patients with PDR, there is significant risk of permanent vision loss without treatment. Neovascularization can lead to vitreous hemorrhage, tractional retinal detachment (TRD), and neovascular glaucoma.

Initial treatment of PDR was historically focused on the endocrine system, with pituitary ablation as the mainstay of treatment.[3] This procedure had significant morbidity and mortality associated with it and was quickly abandoned after the introduction of panretinal photocoagulation (PRP). Peripheral retinal laser destroys hypoxic retina, thus decreasing the metabolic requirements of the peripheral retina and allowing for more oxygenation of remaining tissue and reducing neovascular growth factors. This treatment reduces the risk of severe vision loss by 50% to 60%.[4] The advent of anti-vascular endothelial growth factor (VEGF) medications, however, has created new opportunities to treat PDR with a nondestructive treatment. This chapter reviews the evidence for anti-VEGF medications in the management of PDR and its associated complications.

Duker JS, Liang MC, eds.
Anti-VEGF Use in
Ophthalmology (pp. 113-120).
© 2017 Taylor & Francis Group.

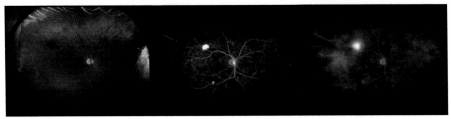

Figure 10-1. Features of proliferative diabetic retinopathy. (Left panel) A wide-field color fundus photo reveals retinal neovascularization. (Center panel) Fluorescein angiogram in the arterial-venous phase demonstrates early hyperfluorescence from the areas of neovascularization and hypofluorescence in the periphery in areas of capillary non-perfusion. (Right panel) Late-phase fluorescein angiogram shows further leakage in the areas of neovascularization. There is diffuse leakage of the peripheral retina with patchy filling.

Role of Vascular Endothelial Growth Factor in Development of Proliferative Diabetic Retinopathy

Much work has been performed to help understand the relationship between retinal ischemia and the development of neovascularization. In 1948, Michaelson proposed the presence of factor X, a hypothetical substance that diffused through ocular tissue in response to hypoxic states.[5] Forty years later, work by Senger et al[6] identified a glycoprotein candidate for factor X, a molecule that they named vascular permeability factor. Additional research by Jakeman et al[7] and Thieme et al[8] further characterized this glycoprotein into what is now known as VEGF.[8]

Since the discovery of VEGF, significant research has been conducted to establish its role in the development of neovascularization in diabetic retinopathy. Both in human and animal models, high levels of VEGF in the vitreous have been associated with PDR.[9-11] Injection of laboratory-derived VEGF into eyes of primates resulted in the creation of retinopathy similar to that seen in ischemic retinal disease. Furthermore, inhibition of VEGF in animal mouse models inhibited the development of retinal neovascularization. In humans, treatment of PDR with PRP has been shown to decrease intraocular VEGF levels.[2] This body of research strongly supported the role of VEGF as a key mediator in the development of diabetic retinopathy, and has led to numerous clinical trials evaluating treatment with anti-VEGF agents for the full spectrum of diabetic disease.

Given the strong association of VEGF and retinal vascular disease, questions arose regarding whether genetic variations could account for variability in retinal disease severity. Work in this area led to the discovery of several VEGF gene polymorphisms and their role in the development of retinal neovascularization. Ray et al[12] examined the $VEGF_{460}$ genotype in patients with diabetes with and without PDR and found increased rates of PDR in patients who carried the $VEGF_{460}$ allele. This research has interesting implications regarding the use of genetic screening to stratify patients and their risk for development of PDR. However, the clinical utility of such genetic screening has not yet been established.

Primary Treatment of Proliferative Diabetic Retinopathy Using Anti-Vascular Endothelial Growth Factor

Traditionally, PRP has been the main treatment choice for PDR used by retina physicians, with 98% reporting the use of laser for primary treatment.[13] While highly successful at reducing the risk of severe vision loss, PRP does have significant drawbacks. The application of PRP can induce or exacerbate diabetic macular edema, resulting in further vision loss. Additionally, ablation of the peripheral retina can lead to decreased contrast sensitivity, visual field loss, and decreased night vision.[14]

The observation of decreased proliferative retinopathy in patients receiving anti-VEGF treatments for diabetic macular edema led to multiple clinical trials. Arevalo et al[15] evaluated the effectiveness of bevacizumab (Avastin) on retinal neovascularization using dosages of 2.5 mg/0.1 mL and 1.25 mg/0.05 mg in patients with prior PRP as well as treatment-naïve eyes. Bevacizumab significantly improved vision and decreased retinal neovascularization, with similar effects between the PRP and treatment-naïve groups.

A randomized, controlled trial coordinated by the Diabetic Retinopathy Clinical Research Network (DRCR.net) aimed to evaluate the effectiveness of ranibizumab (Lucentis) relative to PRP. In this study, identified as Protocol S, patients were randomized to ranibizumab 0.5 mg/0.05 mL intravitreal injection monthly for 3 months. At 4 months, patients were reevaluated, and were followed monthly without further injections if neovascularization had completely resolved. If any neovascularization was still present, additional injections were given at months 4 and 5. Beginning month 6 of the treatment protocol, injections were performed as needed, ceasing further treatments if retinal neovascularization had completely resolved or if no improvement was noted after two consecutive injections. Any patient who developed progressive retinopathy despite monthly injections was allowed to receive PRP. Review of the data at 2 years demonstrated that monthly ranibizumab was noninferior to PRP for the primary treatment of PDR (Figure 10-2). Subanalysis revealed a clear benefit of ranibizumab treatment in regard to retention of peripheral visual field.[16]

One concern regarding the use of anti-VEGF agents as primary treatment for PDR has been reports of the "crunch" phenomenon, where existing fibrovascular membranes from PDR undergo contraction after anti-VEGF treatment and cause TRDs. However, no patients were reported to have this phenomenon within the DRCR.net Protocol S trial.[16] In comparison, a case series by Arevalo et al [15] found post-bevacizumab tractional detachments occurred in 5.2% of patients with severe PDR. This effect was seen on average 2 weeks after injection of bevacizumab, and thus was attributed to the administration of the anti-VEGF agent. Of note, in their case series, none of the eyes reported were treatment-naïve and all had refractory disease despite PRP, as well as poorly controlled hyperglycemia.

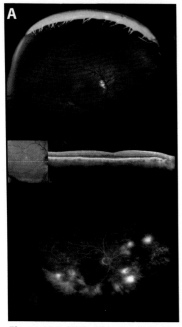
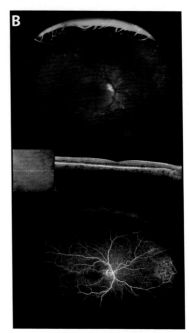

Figure 10-2. (A) Proliferative diabetic retinopathy prior to treatment with bevacizumab. Vision at presentation was 20/50. Color fundus photo (top panel) demonstrates subtle vascular changes. Optical coherence tomography of the macula (center panel) reveals a preserved foveal contour without significant macular edema. Fluorescein angiogram (bottom panel) better highlights the extent of neovascularization with multiple foci of hyperfluorescence. (B) Three months after injection with bevacizumab. Visual acuity improved to 20/16. Color fundus photo (top panel) demonstrates regression of prior neovascularization. Optical coherence tomography of the macula (center panel) remains stable without macular edema. Fluorescein angiogram (bottom panel) shows significant improvement in leakage from the prior areas of neovascularization.

Combination Therapy, Panretinal Photocoagulation + Anti-Vascular Endothelial Growth Factor

The current treatment paradigm for PDR appears to be evolving from PRP alone to treatment with anti-VEGF therapy with or without PRP. Some studies have evaluated the role of combination treatment with PRP and anti-VEGF medications given the theoretical benefits of coupling the long-term reductions in VEGF with PRP[17] with the short-term VEGF blockade of anti-VEGF injections.

Mirshahi et al[18] reported results of a double-masked clinical trial randomizing patients with high-risk PDR to bevacizumab vs sham injection at time of PRP. In this study, patients in the bevacizumab group demonstrated a rapid improvement, with 87.5% of patients having complete regression of their PDR by week 6, compared to only 25% of patients in the sham group. By 4 months, both groups were identical in their regression of proliferative retinopathy.[18] Another randomized trial by Tonello et al[19] also evaluated the role of anti-VEGF augmented PRP. In this study, all patients received PRP within

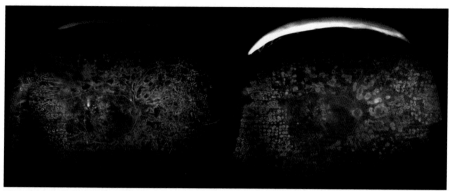

Figure 10-3. Proliferative diabetic retinopathy after panretinal photocoagulation and subsequent anti-vascular endothelial growth factor treatment. Prior to treatment with bevacizumab, fluorescein angiogram (left panel) demonstrates a few small areas of active neovascularization despite full treatment with previous laser. After treatment with bevacizumab, neovascularization has regressed (right panel).

2 sessions spaced 2 weeks apart. One group was randomized to receive bevacizumab 1.5 mg/0.05 mL after the second PRP session. Similar to the previous study, patients who received anti-VEGF treatment demonstrated a rapid improvement in their degree of neovascularization relative to the PRP-only group. These effects diminished with time, as the patients who received anti-VEGF therapy began aligning with the PRP-only group after several months. Of note, there was no statistical difference in the best corrected visual acuity between the groups.[19]

These studies support the short-term benefits of augmenting PRP with anti-VEGF medications (Figure 10-3). Other studies have also suggested a benefit in the prevention of VA loss and development of post-laser macular edema. Based on current limited evidence, there does not appear to be a role for one-time, anti-VEGF treatment in patients receiving PRP. There may be a role for multiple injections in these patients to provide more lasting effects; however, more research is needed.

Use of Anti-Vascular Endothelial Growth Factor in Diabetic Vitreous Hemorrhage

Patients presenting with dense vitreous hemorrhage secondary to severe PDR pose a specific challenge to retina specialists. First, the underlying disease progresses to proliferative retinopathy and then the subsequent hemorrhage prevents adequate visualization and treatment of the pathology. Traditionally, these patients are offered 1 of 2 management options: wait for spontaneous reabsorption of the vitreous hemorrhage followed by PRP, or go to the operating room for vitrectomy with endolaser PRP performed at the time of surgery.

A third option was proposed by Spaide and Fisher in 2006, where they described a small case series of 2 patients who were offered intravitreal bevacizumab for management of dense vitreous hemorrhage.[20] In this series, both patients had substantial and rapid resolution of their vitreous hemorrhages and avoided vitrectomy. The rapid resolution of the vitreous hemorrhage led to some interesting conclusions. They hypothesized that diabetic vitreous hemorrhages were progressive conditions, where blood is continually being cleared from the eye and replaced with new blood from areas of neovascularization. To support this theory, Spaide and Fisher pointed to the persistent red nature of vitreous hemorrhage in diabetics, whereas in other etiologies of vitreous hemorrhage, the blood can be seen to turn white with time. The persistent red nature of the vitreous hemorrhage suggests that some patients with PDR are continually replacing the blood in a constant manner. The use of anti-VEGF therapy in this instance is hypothesized to arrest the cycle of continued hemorrhage, allowing the existing blood to rapidly clear from the eye.[20]

DRCR.net further evaluated the role of anti-VEGF use in the management of diabetic vitreous hemorrhage in a clinical trial randomizing patients with diabetic vitreous hemorrhage to injection with ranibizumab or saline.[21] They found no statistically significant difference in the need for vitrectomy at 16 weeks between the 2 groups, with 12% of patients in the ranibizumab group requiring vitrectomy vs 17% of the saline controls. There was a statistical difference in the percentage of patients who were able to receive complete PRP at 16 weeks, with 44% of patients receiving ranibizumab able to complete laser treatment compared to 31% of controls. The biggest benefit to anti-VEGF use in these patients appeared to be in the prevention of recurrent vitreous hemorrhage; only 6% of patients in the ranibizumab group had recurrent hemorrhage compared to 17% of controls.

While the case series by Spaide and Fisher provided some initial promising results and a theoretical framework for the use of anti-VEGF in diabetic vitreous hemorrhage, the clinical benefit has not been established with a randomized clinical trial. Despite increasing the chance at receiving full PRP and decreasing the likelihood of recurrent hemorrhage, the rates of vitrectomy were not affected by the use of anti-VEGF in these patients. There has not been definitive data demonstrating vitreous hemorrhages clear more rapidly with the use of anti-VEGF, or that long-term vision improves with these treatments.

Anti-Vascular Endothelial Growth Factor Use as an Adjunct to Vitrectomy

Surgical management of TRDs with pars plana vitrectomy and membrane stripping can be a technically challenging procedure, and can be complicated by intraoperative and postoperative vitreous hemorrhage. The nature of broad neovascular membranes results in pre-retinal membranes with physical connections to the delicate abnormal retinal vasculature. Chen and Park proposed using bevacizumab as a preoperative adjunct therapy to TRD repair.[22] They hypothesized that administration of bevacizumab would promote regression of neovascularization, allowing for improved hemostasis and easier removal of pre-retinal membranes. Short-term regression of retinal neovascularization was noted in one patient they pretreated with bevacizumab. Intraoperatively, they noted improved hemostasis and easier removal of membranes with blunt dissection.

This case report provided anecdotal evidence for the possible benefits of preoperative adjunct treatment for TRD repair to minimize intraoperative vitreous hemorrhage. However, as discussed previously, one concern in severe PDR is contracture of fibrovascular membranes following treatment with anti-VEGF medication. In their report, Chen and Park followed the patient weekly after injection and promptly took the patient to the operating room upon regression of neovascularization. Had the authors not performed such close follow-up and prompt surgical intervention after regression, it is possible their patient could have had worsening contracture of fibrovascular membranes and subsequent worsening of the TRD. If anti-VEGF agents are used prior to TRD repair, it should be given with close follow-up and plans for prompt vitrectomy to avoid this complication.

The evidence for use of anti-VEGF agents in preventing early postoperative vitreous hemorrhage is much more robust. A meta-analysis performed by Smith and Steel demonstrated clear benefits to bevacizumab administration prior to or at the time of vitrectomy to avoid hemorrhage within the first 4 weeks after surgery. This meta-analysis reviewed 12 randomized, controlled trials involving vitrectomy for PDR.[23] The rates of postoperative vitreous hemorrhage were examined in patients who receive an intravitreal injection of bevacizumab prior to or at the time of vitrectomy. There was a statistically significant benefit for administration of bevacizumab on early (less than 4 weeks) postoperative vitreous hemorrhage, with a finding of 130 fewer hemorrhages/1000 vitrectomies performed. However, there was no benefit seen for the occurrence of late postoperative vitreous hemorrhage. An additional benefit identified with this analysis was the reduction of retinal detachment rates in those treated with bevacizumab. This was a weaker, but still statistically significant, effect with 49 fewer retinal detachments/1000 vitrectomies observed. It is important to note that these results were obtained from data combining all indications for vitrectomy in patients with PDR, including TRD, nonclearing vitreous hemorrhage, and combination tractional-rhegmatogenous retinal detachments.

At this time, there remains insufficient evidence to confirm the benefits of preoperative anti-VEGF use in the prevention of intraoperative vitreous hemorrhage during TRD repair. There is good evidence for its use in prevention of early postoperative vitreous hemorrhage, but these data are not specific to TRD repairs and also include patients who required vitrectomy for nonclearing vitreous hemorrhage. Ultimately, further studies are needed to clarify which indications for vitrectomy in a patient with PDR maximally benefit from adjunctive anti-VEGF medication.

Conclusion

With the introduction of intravitreal anti-VEGF agents, clinicians now have a nondestructive treatment modality with which to treat PDR, and treatment paradigms are shifting. Evidence has demonstrated the effectiveness anti-VEGF therapy has as a primary treatment for the neovascular complications of diabetes. Despite the benefits of anti-VEGF agents as a primary treatment of PDR, the use of these medications as an adjunct to PRP laser still requires further investigation. In addition, they have not been shown to decrease the need for vitrectomy in those patients with vitreous hemorrhage. However, treatment with anti-VEGF agents has shown benefit in the short-term risk of postoperative vitreous hemorrhage. Whether this affects long-term visual outcome remains to be seen. With additional research, the role of these agents as a nondestructive treatment modality for PDR will be further established.

References

1. Aiello LP. Angiogenic pathways in diabetic retinopathy. *N Engl J Med.* 2005;353(8):839-841.
2. Tremolada G, Del Turco C, Lattanzio R, et al. The role of angiogenesis in the development of proliferative diabetic retinopathy: impact of intravitreal anti-VEGF treatment. *Exp Diabetes Res.* 2012;2012:728325.

3.   Antonetti DA, Klein R, Gardner TW. Diabetic retinopathy. *N Engl J Med*. 2012;366(13):1227-1239.

4.   Photocoagulation treatment of proliferative diabetic retinopathy. Clinical application of Diabetic Retinopathy Study (DRS) findings, DRS Report Number 8. The Diabetic Retinopathy Study Research Group. *Ophthalmology*. 1981;88(7):583-600.

5.   Michaelson IC. The mode of development of the vascular system of the retina, with some observations on its significance for certain retinal diseases. *Trans Ophthalmol Vis Sci UK*. 1948;68:137-180.

6.   Senger DR, Perruzzi CA, Feder J, Dvorak HF. A highly conserved vascular permeability factor secreted by a variety of human and rodent tumor cell lines. *Cancer Res*. 1986;46:5629-5632.

7.   Jakeman LB, Winer J, Bennett GL, Altar CA, Ferrara N. Binding sites for vascular endothelial growth factor are localized on endothelial cells in adult rat tissues. *J Clin Invest*. 1992;89(1):244-253.

8.   Thieme H, Aiello LP, Takagi H, Ferrara N, King GL. Comparative analysis of vascular endothelial growth factor receptors on retinal and aortic vascular endothelial cells. *Diabetes*. 1995;44(1):98-103.

9.   Adamis AP, Miller JW, Bernal MT, et al. Increased vascular endothelial growth factor levels in the vitreous of eyes with proliferative diabetic retinopathy. *Am J Ophthalmol*. 1994;118(4):445-450.

10. Aiello LP, Avery RL, Arrigg PG, et al. Vascular endothelial growth factor in ocular fluid of patients with diabetic retinopathy and other retinal disorders. *N Engl J Med*. 1994;331(22):1480-1487.

11. Pe'er J, Folberg R, Itin A, Gnessin H, Hemo I, Keshet E. Upregulated expression of vascular endothelial growth factor in proliferative diabetic retinopathy. *Br J Ophthalmol*. 1996;80(3):241-245.

12. Ray D, Mishra M, Ralph S, Read I, Davies R, Brenchley P. Association of the VEGF gene with proliferative diabetic retinopathy but not proteinuria in diabetes. *Diabetes*. 2004;53(3):861-864.

13. Rezaei K, Stone TW. 2014 Global Trends in Retina Survey. Chicago, IL: American Society of Retina Specialists; 2014.

14. Diabetic Retinopathy Clinical Research Network, Brucker AJ, Qin H, et al. Observational study of the development of diabetic macular edema following panretinal (scatter) photocoagulation given in 1 or 4 sittings. *Arch Ophthalmol*. 2009;127(2):132-140.

15. Arevalo JF, Maia M, Flynn HW, et al. Tractional retinal detachment following intravitreal bevacizumab (Avastin) in patients with severe proliferative diabetic retinopathy. *Br J Ophthalmol*. 2008;92(2):213-216.

16. Writing Committee for the Diabetic Retinopathy Clinical Research Network, Gross JG, Glassman AR, et al. Panretinal photocoagulation vs intravitreous ranibizumab for proliferative diabetic retinopathy: a randomized clinical trial. *JAMA*. 2015;314(20):2137-2146.

17. Xiao M, McLeod D, Cranley J, Williams G, Boulton M. Growth factor staining patterns in the pig retina following retinal laser photocoagulation. *Br J Ophthalmol*. 1999;83(6):728-736.

18. Mirshahi A, Roohipoor R, Lashay A, Mohammadi SF, Abdoallahi A, Faghihi H. Bevacizumab-augmented retinal laser photocoagulation in proliferative diabetic retinopathy: a randomized double-masked clinical trial. *Eur J Ophthalmol*. 2008;18(2):263-269.

19. Tonello M, Costa RA, Almeida FP, Barbosa JC, Scott IU, Jorge R. Panretinal photocoagulation versus PRP plus intravitreal bevacizumab for high-risk proliferative diabetic retinopathy (IBeHi study). *Acta Ophthalmol*. 2008;86(4):385-389.

20. Spaide RF, Fisher YL. Intravitreal bevacizumab (Avastin) treatment of proliferative diabetic retinopathy complicated by vitreous hemorrhage. *Retina*. 2006;26(3):275-278.

21. Diabetic Retinopathy Clinical Research Network. Randomized clinical trial evaluating intravitreal ranibizumab or saline for vitreous hemorrhage from proliferative diabetic retinopathy. *JAMA Ophthalmol*. 2013;131(13):283-293.

22. Chen E, Park CH. Use of intravitreal bevacizumab as a preoperative adjunct for tractional retinal detachment repair in severe proliferative diabetic retinopathy. *Retina*. 2006;26(6):699-700.

23. Smith JM, Steel DH. Anti-vascular endothelial growth factor for prevention of postoperative vitreous cavity haemorrhage after vitrectomy for proliferative diabetic retinopathy. *Cochrane Database Syst Rev*. 2015;8:CD008214.

11

RETINAL VEIN OCCLUSION

Shilpa Desai, MD and Caroline R. Baumal, MD

Retinal vein occlusion (RVO) is the second most common retinal vascular disorder following diabetic retinopathy.[1] The incidence of RVO (branch [BRVO] and central combined [CRVO]) ranges from 0.8% to 1.8%.[2] RVO has an age- and sex-standardized prevalence of 4.42/1000 for BRVO and 0.80/1000 for CRVO. The prevalence of CRVO increases with age with 0.27 occurring/1000 in those from 0 to 49 years and 5.44 occurring/1000 in those 80 years and older.[3] Worldwide, an estimated 16.4 million adults are affected by RVO, with 2.5 million affected by CRVO and 13.9 million affected by BRVO.[4,5]

The etiology of RVO can be external compression of the vein by an atherosclerotic artery, intraluminal thrombosis, or inflammation of the vein.[6,7] Systemic risk factors include hypercoagulable state (hazard ratio [HR] 2.92), history of stroke (HR 1.4), hypertension-related end-organ damage (HR 1.92), and diabetes mellitus-related end-organ damage (HR 1.53). Cigarette smoking and both angle closure and primary open-angle glaucoma have also been identified as risk factors for vein occlusion.[8] Furthermore, in the United States (US), African Americans have a 58% increased risk of CRVO compared to Caucasians (HR 1.58) and women have a 25% decreased risk compared to men (HR 0.75) after adjustment for confounders.[5] After developing CRVO, there is a 10% chance/year of RVO occurring in the fellow eye.[9] There is also an increased risk of mortality because of its statistical association with comorbid diabetes and/or cardiovascular disease.[10]

The majority of individuals over age 65 have one or more of the following risk factors for RVO:

- Smoking
- Hypertension
- Diabetes mellitus
- Increased age
- Elevated lipids/cholesterol

Duker JS, Liang MC, eds.
*Anti-VEGF Use in
Ophthalmology* (pp. 121-135).
© 2017 Taylor & Francis Group.

Figure 11-1. Fundus photograph of central retinal vein occlusion. The patient's vision was 20/100.

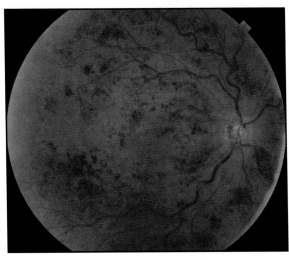

In these patients, optimizing systemic control of these risk factors is part of the therapeutic protocol and no additional systemic workup is required. In younger individuals, studies have shown that systemic hypertension, hyperlipidemia, and increased body mass index are important risk factors for vein occlusions.[11] In young patients without these risk factors, however, it is important to assess for hypercoagulable states or inflammatory disease as the underlying cause.

Medicare reimbursement accounting for resource use (fluorescein angiography [FA], optical coherence tomography, intravitreal injection, panretinal laser, vitrectomy) and direct medical costs for CRVO were $11,587 at 1 year and $31,585 at 3 years.[12] These costs excluded calculations for treatment of systemic hypertension and glaucoma.[13] Using the Beaver Dam Eye Study estimates of prevalence, the total cost to the US Medicare population is expected to be $1.3 billion annually for CRVO.[12] The cost/line of vision saved using therapies for cystoid macular edema (CME) range from $704 to $7611 for intravitreal triamcinolone and ranibizumab, respectively.[14] Patients treated with ranibizumab, the original anti-vascular endothelial growth factor (VEGF) agent tested in clinical trials, have shown improvements in vision-related quality of life at 1 and 6 months after anti-VEGF therapy.[15]

Diagnosis of Retinal Vein Occlusion

RVO presents with painless vision loss associated with retinal hemorrhages and retinal venous tortuosity in the quadrant(s) of the affected vein. Additional findings can include cotton wool spots, optic nerve edema, CME, lipid exudation, and concurrent signs of hypertensive retinopathy[16] (Figure 11-1). Optic nerve collateral vessels, neovascularization (NV) of the iris, and sheathed veins may develop after the acute event. RVO is classified as central, hemi-, or branch depending on the distribution of the occlusion. Presentation is typically acute, but may be subacute depending on patient symptoms and the quadrant(s) involved. On imaging, early-phase FA in acute RVO reveals a delay in the arteriovenous transit time (typically longer than 20 seconds); the late phase shows areas of capillary nonperfusion. The ischemic type of CRVO is defined as at least 10 disc areas

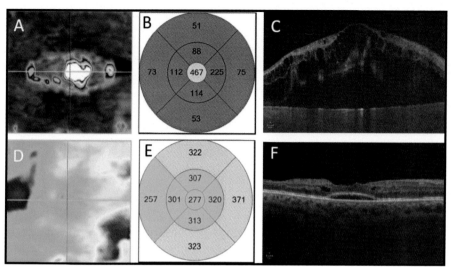

Figure 11-2. Patient with macular ischemia secondary to central retinal vein occlusion. (A-C) Macula cube, internal limiting membrane-retinal pigment epithelium thickness, and B scan optical coherence tomography prior to aflibercept. The color scheme of the cube appears abnormal due to the height of ischemia. (D-F) Macula cube, internal limiting membrane-retinal pigment epithelium thickness, and B scan optical coherence tomography after aflibercept. Despite dramatic improvement in subretinal and intraretinal fluid, the vision remained count fingers at 4 feet due to diffuse ischemia and retinal damage.

of retinal capillary nonperfusion on FA,[17] and is associated with more retinal venous engorgement, fluorescein leakage, retinal capillary dilation, and capillary nonperfusion than nonischemic CRVO. It accounts for 20% of acute presentations and is associated with worse baseline acuity, afferent papillary defect, and poorer visual outcomes compared to their nonischemic counterparts even after treatment.[10,18-20] FA may not be able to differentiate between ischemic and nonischemic RVO subtypes in up to 40% of cases because of masking of retinal vascular details by extensive retinal hemorrhages, media opacities (vitreous hemorrhage, lens changes), and limited assessment of the peripheral retina.[21] Furthermore, nonischemic RVO may convert to the ischemic subtype in one-third of cases.[10]

Vision loss in RVO can be secondary to ischemia of the macula, CME, ocular NV, or secondary glaucoma.[22,23] CME in RVO is characterized by fluid collection in the intercellular spaces within the outer plexiform layer of the retina. Pockets of fluid may also develop in the subretinal space secondary to breakdown of the capillary endothelium blood-retinal barrier and leakage of fluid from the vasculature.[24,25] In nonischemic CRVO, macular edema is strongly associated with vision loss. In ischemic CRVO, however, visual acuity may not be correlated with macular edema due to ischemia of the retinal ganglion cells (Figure 11-2). In addition, the underlying retinal ischemia in ischemic RVO leads to a large quantity of VEGF being released into the eye.[26] This excessively high level of VEGF leads to the proliferation of blood vessels causing NV of the retina and/or optic disc in BRVO and iris in CRVO. The risk of developing ischemia of the macula, macular edema, ocular NV, and secondary glaucoma is 16% in eyes with more than 5.5 disc areas of nonperfusion in contrast to 4.0% of eyes with less than 5.5 disc areas of nonperfusion.[27]

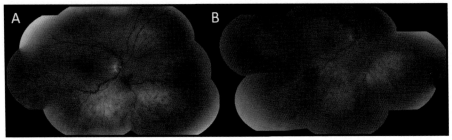

Figure 11-3. Color fundus photographs demonstrating spontaneous improvement in central retinal vein occlusion. (A) Initial presentation, vision 20/60. (B) One month after initial presentation, no treatment given, vision 20/40.

Natural history studies of RVO reveal that some patients will improve spontaneously without therapy[10] (Figure 11-3). In 714 CRVO eyes followed without treatment, 65% of patients with vision better than or equal to 20/40 maintained this level of vision. The degree of improvement varied based on the initial acuity. In patients with vision better than 20/200, 56% showed improvement without treatment. In patients with vision worse than 20/200, only 20% showed improvement without treatment. Overall, patients with nonischemic CRVO spontaneously improve more frequently than those with ischemic CRVO.[23,28-30] In hemi-retinal or BRVO, spontaneous improvement is more likely when the macula is not involved.

Treatment for Central Retina Vein Occlusion and Branch Retinal Vein Occlusion

It is hypothesized that acute vein occlusions also block arterial flow, leading to ischemia of the retina and release of VEGF, which then causes CME and NV of the retina (more common in BRVO) and iris (more common in CRVO). At some point after the acute event, the vein and thrombus become infiltrated with lymphocytes, causing a secondary inflammatory response.[6] With these concepts in mind, therapies to treat RVO have centered on reducing the release of VEGF (laser, anti-VEGF therapy) or reducing venous inflammation to improve blood flow (corticosteroid therapy). In all cases of RVO, treatment must involve management of the underlying systemic vascular risk factors in conjunction with the primary care provider. Low-dose aspirin (ASA) use is controversial as ASA has been shown to decrease the risk of cerebrovascular accident, but in RVO studies, ASA use was correlated with decreased visual recovery.[31]

Laser

Macular grid laser was introduced as a treatment for RVO as a method to decrease macular edema. The mechanism of grid laser-induced resolution of CME is unknown. Proposed mechanisms include laser-induced scarring of photoreceptors leading to better oxygen perfusion to the inner retina, enhanced proliferation of retinal pigment epithelial and endothelial cells restoring the blood-retina barrier, and laser-induced production of cytokines, which antagonize the effects of VEGF. Initial studies showed macular grid laser photocoagulation improved visual acuity in eyes with CME secondary to BRVO (BVOS)[32] but not CRVO (CVOS).[3,10] This may be due to the lower prevalence of ischemia in eyes with BRVO, making them more amenable to visual improvement with grid laser treatment as compared to CRVO eyes. As such, macular grid laser was the mainstay of treatment for CME in BRVO until anti-VEGF agents became available, and is still used in certain situations today.

Panretinal laser photocoagulation (PRP) is used to treat retinal or iris NV secondary to RVO. PRP is thought to work by destroying ischemic retina and reducing the overall amount of VEGF released into the eye. The BVOS study demonstrated that PRP reduces development of retinal NV and vitreous hemorrhage; however, it does not improve visual outcomes.[33,34] Hayreh et al[33] found that in CRVO, for those eyes without retinal NV, only 12% of PRP-treated eyes developed vitreous hemorrhage compared to 22% in the nontreated eyes. For eyes with NV, 29% developed vitreous hemorrhage in the treatment group vs 60% in the nontreated group. Side effects of PRP include peripheral vision loss and decreased night vision.

Corticosteroids

Intravitreal injection with corticosteroids has also been demonstrated to be efficacious in the treatment of CME secondary to RVO. It is thought to work by down-regulating inflammatory cytokines and reducing dysregulation of endothelial tight junction proteins that can lead to CME. Triamcinolone acetonide has also been shown to decrease the amount of VEGF measured in the vitreous.[35] The Standard Care vs COrticosteroid for REtinal Vein Occlusion (SCORE) trial evaluated treatment of intravitreal triamcinolone acetonide (IVTA) in RVO and concluded IVTA was better than observation in CRVO but recommended grid laser should still be used in BRVO as there was no difference in percentage of patients who gained 3 or more lines of vision and to avoid the risks of cataract and glaucoma associated with corticosteroid therapy.[36] Similarly, Avitabile et al[37] found that IVTA improved central macular thickness and vision in the CRVO group but not the BRVO group when compared with grid laser. In addition, the effectiveness of triamcinolone appears to wane by 3 months. Numerous studies have shown that macular edema returns and vision declines at 3 or 6 months post-treatment.[38-43]

Extended-release steroid therapy is also used in RVO for the treatment of CME. The extended-release formulation aims to provide a more uniform dose of corticosteroid to the eye and lengthen the time between treatments. The GENEVA trial compared a sustained-release dexamethasone implant (Ozurdex 0.7 mg or 0.35 mg) with sham treatment for CME secondary to BRVO and CRVO. For the CRVO group only, the time to improve 15 letters was significantly faster in the 2 Ozurdex treatment groups. There was a faster improvement in visual acuity and mean decrease in central subfield retinal thickness (CST) through the 90-day point, but this waned by the 180-day timepoint, at which point there was no significant difference in both the visual acuity and mean decrease in CST between treated and nontreated eyes. Ocular hypertension (treated successfully in almost all cases) was noted in 4 and 3.9% in the dexamethasone implant groups, respectively, as compared to 0.7% in the sham group.[44,45] The Retisert implant (Bausch + Lomb) and Iluvien (Alimera Sciences) are alternate intravitreal implants that contain extended-release fluocinolone acetonide. Both have been shown to improve macular edema in diabetes and may have applications in RVO in the future.

Adverse events related to any corticosteroid use include cataract and elevated intra-ocular pressure (IOP). The risk of these events may be specific to dose and vehicle-related effects. The SCORE study showed a dose-dependent increase in IOP with steroid use (35% of patients in the 4 mg group, 20% of patients in the 1 mg group, and 8% of patients in the observation group needed medication for increased IOP). In addition, the higher the steroid dose, the higher the rate of necessary cataract surgery (21% in the 4 mg group, 3% in the 1 mg group, and 0% in the observation group).[22] Suspension formulations of intravitreal corticosteroid (such as IVTA) include the additional risk of sterile endo-phthalmitis. On the other hand, solid sustained-release implants may migrate into the anterior chamber in aphakic eyes or eyes with an open posterior capsule, causing corneal edema and necessitating removal.

Alternative Treatments

Numerous other treatments of historical interest have been used in an attempt to directly counteract the primary event of the occlusion of the retinal vein rather than treat the secondary consequences of CME and NV. Isovolemic hemodilution was attempted to dilute the blood enough to bypass the RVO; however, this practice was abandoned because of significant systemic risk factors.[46-48] Radial optic neurotomy and pars plana sheathotomy have also been attempted to increase the potential space for venous flow at the level of the occlusion. Randomized studies demonstrated no visual benefit from these interventions.[49,50] Both practices were abandoned because they were considered high risk given the risk of retinal detachment and cataract.[51,52] Laser induction of a chorioretinal anastamosis was attempted to anatomically reestablish adequate venous drainage in CRVO with CME. The Central Retinal Bypass Study found that an anasto-mosis was created in 76% of treated eyes. The anastomosis group had a mean improve-ment of 11.7 letters as compared to loss of 8.1 letters in the control group at 18 months post-intervention. However, this therapy was not widely accepted because of procedure-related complications such as fibrovascular traction, macular traction, and vitreous hemorrhage.[53] Finally, retinal endovascular lysis was also attempted for CRVO. In this procedure, a fibrinolytic agent is injected into a cannulated retinal vein after pars plana vitrectomy to allow for blood flow through the vein. In the nonrandomized study of this technique in CRVO, there was no improvement in vision at one year and the complication rate was high, including neovascular glaucoma leading to phthisis, retinal detachment, and cataract.[54]

Anti-Vascular Endothelial Growth Factor Therapy

VEGF is produced by Müller cells, endothelial cells, astrocytes, retinal pigment epithe-lial cells, and ganglion cells in response to decreased oxygen and causes a time- and dose-dependent breakdown in the blood-retinal barrier.[25] Studies have shown that vitreous VEGF levels are higher in patients with any disorder that produces ischemia to the retina, including eyes with RVO.[55] VEGF levels have been correlated with the severity of retinal ischemia and macular edema in RVO.[56,57] Anti-VEGF therapy downregulates the level of VEGF in the vitreous, stabilizing the blood-retinal barrier and reducing intraretinal fluid

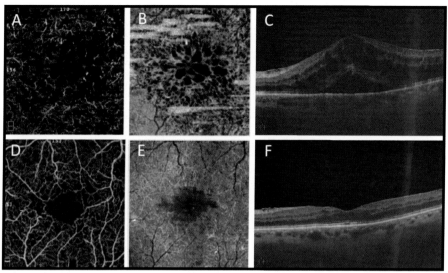

Figure 11-4. Improvement in macular edema and vision after treatment of vein occlusion with afliber-cept. (A-C) Optical coherence tomography angiography (OCTA) of the deep plexus, en face OCTA, and B scan OCT prior to treatment. (D-F) OCTA of the deep retina, en face OCTA, and B scan optical coherence tomography after treatment. The patient had a dramatic response after treatment with a commensurate improvement in vision from 20/200 to 20/40.

exudation (Figure 11-4). Anti-VEGF treatment for RVO is typically monthly, treat and extend, or pro re nata (PRN) based on patient symptoms, exam, and physician preference. Commonly used agents include ranibizumab, bevacizumab, and aflibercept.

Several large, multicenter trials have evaluated the efficacy of anti-VEGF therapy for CME secondary to RVO. Ranibizumab was US Food and Drug Administration approved in June 2010 to treat CME secondary to CRVO and BRVO on the basis of the Central Retinal vein occlUSion study (CRUISE) and BRAnch Vein Occlusion Study (BRAVO) trials, respectively (Table 11-1). In both studies, patients were randomized to receive monthly injections (sham, 0.3 mg ranibizumab, or 0.5 mg ranibizumab) for the first 6 months. The CRUISE study found a significant improvement in best-corrected visual acuity (BCVA) and CST in eyes treated with monthly ranibizumab (0.3 mg or 0.5 mg) compared to sham injection after 6 months.[58] The intravitreal ranibizumab group was associated with an increased rate of cataract development at 12 months in both the 0.3 mg (4%) and the 0.5 mg (7%) group as compared to sham eyes (0%). The BRAVO study was similar in design to the CRUISE study except that patients could receive focal/grid laser at month 3. BRAVO found a significant improvement in BCVA and CST in the ranibi-zumab treatment arms compared to the sham group.[59] Macular focal/grid laser treatment was given to 26 of 131 (20%) of patients treated with ranibizumab and 71 of 132 (54%) of patients treated with sham injection. The HORIZON study was an open-label extension of the CRUISE and BRAVO trials. During the extension, patients could receive ranibi-zumab for either central foveal thickness greater than or equal to 250 μm or persistent CME. This study found that improvement in swelling on optical coherence tomography was maintained with many fewer injections in BRVO, but not CRVO. On average, BCVA

Table 11-1. Studies Evaluating Anti-Vascular Endothelial
Growth Factor Therapy for Retinal Vein Occlusion

Study Name	Drug	Randomization	Study Patient	Number of Patients	Endpoint	Primary Outcomes	Secondary Outcomes
CRUISE	Ranibizumab	Phase III, multi-center, randomized, prospective, sham-injection controlled trial of ranibizumab	CRVO diagnosed in last 12 months, BCVA 20/40 to 0/320, mean CST > 205	392	6 months	Mean change BCVA +12.7 and +14.9 letters in 0.3 and 0.5 mg ranibizumab groups, respectively; −0.8 letters sham	Mean change in CST decreased by 434 μm and 452 μm in the 0.3 and 0.5 mg ranibizumab groups respectively; 168 μm in the sham group
BRAVO	Ranibizumab	Phase III, multi-center, randomized, prospective, sham-injection controlled trial of ranibizumab	BRVO diagnosed in last 12 months, BCVA 20/40 to 20/320, mean CST > 205	397	6 months	Mean change BCVA +16.6 and +18.3 letters in 0.3 and 0.5 mg ranibizumab groups, respectively; +7.3 letters sham	Mean change in CST decreased by 337 μm and 345 μm in the 0.3 and 0.5 mg ranibizumab groups, respectively; 158 μm in the sham group
HORIZON	Ranibizumab	Open-label extension of BRAVO/CRUISE with treatment Q3 months	BRAVO/CRUISE	608	12 months	Incidence of SAEs in treatment group was 1% to 9% across all groups	Vision stable or worsen in treatment and sham arms

All reported results are statistically significant.
BCVA = best-corrected visual acuity; CST = central subfield retinal thickness; CRVO = central retinal vein occlusion; BRVO = branch retinal vein occlusion.

(continued)

Table 11-1 (continued). Studies Evaluating Anti-Vascular Endothelial Growth Factor Therapy for Retinal Vein Occlusion

Study Name	Drug	Randomization	Study Patient	Number of Patients	Endpoint	Primary Outcomes	Secondary Outcomes
Epstein et al[60]	Bevacizumab	Prospective, randomized, sham injection-controlled, double-masked clinical trial	Macular edema secondary to CRVO	60	6 months	60% of patients in bevacizumab treated group gained ≥ 15 letters compared with 20% in the sham control group	BCVA improved 14.1 letters at 24 weeks in bevacizumab eyes compared to decrease of 2.0 letters in the sham eyes. CRT decreased 426 μm in bevacizumab eyes and 102 μm in sham. Zero patients in the bevacizumab group and 16.7% in the sham gr oup developed iris neovascularization
COPERNICUS	Aflibercept	Phase III, prospective, randomized controlled, double-masked, multi-center trial	Macular edema secondary to CRVO	187	52 weeks	The proportion of patients gaining ≥ 15 letters was 56.1% in the treatment arm versus 12.3% in the sham arm	The mean reduction from baseline in central retinal thickness was 457.2 μm in the treatment group vs 144.8 μm in the sham group

All reported results are statistically significant.
BCVA = best-corrected visual acuity; CST = central subfield retinal thickness; CRVO = central retinal vein occlusion; BRVO = branch retinal vein occlusion.

(continued)

Table 11-1 (continued). Studies Evaluating Anti-Vascular Endothelial
Growth Factor Therapy for Retinal Vein Occlusion

Study Name	Drug	Randomization	Study Patient	Number of Patients	Endpoint	Primary Outcomes	Secondary Outcomes
GALILEO	Aflibercept	Phase III, randomized, double-masked clinical trial	Macular edema secondary to CRVO	172	24 week	The proportion of patients who gained ≥ 15 letters in the intravitreal aflibercept and sham groups was 60.2% vs 22.1%	Mean μm change from baseline central retinal thickness was 448.6 in the treatment group vs 169.3 in the sham group
VIBRANT	Aflibercept	Phase III, randomized, double-masked	Macular edema secondary to BRVO	181	24 weeks	The proportion of patients who gained ≥ 15 letters in the intravitreal aflibercept and laser group was 52.7% vs 26.7%	The proportion of patients who gained ≥ 15 letters in the intravitreal aflibercept and laser group was 52.7% vs 26.7%

All reported results are statistically significant.
BCVA = best-corrected visual acuity; CST = central subfield retinal thickness; CRVO = central retinal vein occlusion; BRVO = branch retinal vein occlusion.

worsened over the 12-month HORIZON study, likely because of under-treatment of some patients on the PRN protocol.[60,61]

Bevacizumab is currently used off-label as intravitreal anti-VEGF therapy for CME in RVO. Epstein et al[60] conducted a prospective, sham-controlled clinical trial randomizing patients to either intravitreal bevacizumab 1.25 mg or sham injection every 4 weeks for 6 months for CME due to CRVO. Bevacizumab-treated eyes had a statistically significant improvement in BCVA, decrease in CST, and no incidence of iris NV.[60] Six months after study enrollment, sham eyes could receive bevacizumab treatment for CME. At one year, 60% of eyes in the bevacizumab group gained 15 letters compared to 33% of eyes in the sham crossover to bevacizumab group, suggesting the delay in anti-VEGF therapy may adversely affect final visual outcomes.[62] Many other studies have supported the beneficial visual and anatomical effect of bevacizumab for CME in RVO.[63-65] Bevacizumab has also been used successfully to treat NV of the iris and posterior pole in the setting of vein occlusion[66,67] and has been demonstrated to help treat elevated IOP in combination with panretinal photocoagulation in neovascular glaucoma secondary to CRVO.[68-70]

The COPERNICUS study evaluated monthly aflibercept injections to treat CME in CRVO. At the 24-week primary endpoint, statistically more patients gained 15 or more letters in the treatment group (56%) vs the sham injection group (12%). Treated eyes also had a significant decrease in central retinal thickness. In addition, there was 0% ocular neovascularization in the treatment group vs 7% in the sham group. After 24 weeks, eyes in the study arm were treated with aflibercept PRN. At the 52-week timepoint, 55% of eyes in the aflibercept group gained 15 or more letters compared to 30% in the sham group.[71,72] The GALILEO study was a similar study that also found a statistically significant improvement in BCVA and macular edema. In the VIBRANT study evaluating CME in BRVO, there was a statistically higher proportion of patients gaining 15 or more letters in the aflibercept monthly treatment group compared to the laser treatment group.[73] Based on these studies, aflibercept was approved by the Food and Drug Administration for use for macular edema in CRVO on September 21, 2012, and BRVO on February 24, 2014. Aside from CME, preliminary results of the ANDROID study suggest that aflibercept may also improve peripheral non-perfusion in retinal vein occlusion. Further study on this topic is forthcoming.

Comparisons of Treatment Modalities

Ding et al[74] conducted a study comparing intravitreal triamcinolone (4.0 mg/0.1 mL) with 1.25 mg bevacizumab for macular edema secondary to CRVO. Eyes were retreated after 3 months if there was macular edema or 2 or more lines of vision loss. Retreatment was required in 5 of 16 IVTA eyes and 12 of 16 bevacizumab eyes. Overall, the mean number of bevacizumab injections (2.4) was higher than the triamcinolone group (1.3 injections). There was no significant difference in BCVA between the groups at 1, 3, 6, and 9 months and both groups improved significantly.[74] Mayer et al[75] completed a nonrandomized prospective study comparing eyes treated with intravitreal bevacizumab followed by an Ozurdex implant vs an Ozurdex implant alone. Eyes receiving dexamethasone monotherapy gained 2.5 letters after 6 months, while eyes treated with combination bevacizumab and Ozurdex gained 5.9 letters. Narayanan et al[76] compared 0.5 mg ranibizumab to 1.25 mg bevacizumab for CME due to BRVO and found no significant difference between BCVA and central retinal thickness.

Conclusions

RVO is an important cause of ocular morbidity. Intravitreal anti-VEGF therapy effectively reduces macular edema and NV leading to improved BCVA, although this may ultimately be limited by retinal ischemia. Repeated injections may be necessary to sustain long-term visual benefits because of the short intraocular half-life of these drugs. Further research is necessary to determine which, if any, anti-VEGF agent leads to better visual outcomes and the role of combination therapy with laser and/or corticosteroid therapy in the treatment of RVO.

References

1. Cugati S, Wang JJ, Rochtchina E, Mitchell P. Ten-year incidence of retinal vein occlusion in an older population: the Blue Mountains Eye Study. *Arch Ophthalmol.* 2006;124(5):726-732.
2. Klein R, Moss SE, Meuer SM, Klein BE. The 15-year cumulative incidence of retinal vein occlusion: the Beaver Dam Eye Study. *Arch Ophthalmol.* 2008;126(4):513-518.
3. Rogers S, McIntosh RL, Cheung N, et al. The prevalence of retinal vein occlusion: pooled data from population studies from the United States, Europe, Asia, and Australia. *Ophthalmology.* 2010;117(2):313-319.e1.
4. Ho M, Liu DT, Lam DS, Jonas JB. Retinal vein occlusions, from basics to the latest treatment. *Retina.* 2016;36(3):432-448.
5. Stem MS, Talwar N, Comer GM, Stein JD. A longitudinal analysis of risk factors associated with central retinal vein occlusion. *Ophthalmology.* 2013;120(2):362-370.
6. Green WR, Chan CC, Hutchins GM, Terry JM. Central retinal vein occlusion: a prospective histopathologic study of 29 eyes in 28 cases. *Retina.* 1981;1(1):27-55.
7. Frangieh GT, Green WR, Barraquer-Somers E, Finkelstein D. Histopathologic study of nine branch retinal vein occlusions. *Arch Ophthalmol.* 1982;100(7):1132-1140.
8. Klein R, Klein BE, Moss SE, Meuer SM. The epidemiology of retinal vein occlusion: the Beaver Dam Eye study. *Trans Am Ophthalmol Soc.* 2000;98:133-141; discussion 141-143.
9. A randomized clinical trial of early panretinal photocoagulation for ischemic central vein occlusion. The Central Vein Occlusion Study Group N report. *Ophthalmology.* 1995;102(10):1434-1444.
10. Bertelsen M, Linneberg A, Christoffersen N, Vorum H, Gade E, Larsen M. Mortality in patients with central retinal vein occlusion. *Ophthalmology.* 2014;121(3):637-642.
11. Lam HD, Lahey JM, Kearney JJ, Ng RR, Lehmer JM, Tanaka SC. Young patients with branch retinal vein occlusion: a review of 60 cases. *Retina.* 2010;30(9):1520-1523.
12. Yeh S, Kim SJ, Ho AC, et al. Therapies for macular edema associated with central retinal vein occlusion: a report by the American Academy of Ophthalmology. *Ophthalmology.* 2015;122(4):769-778.
13. Fekrat S, Shea AM, Hammill BG, et al. Resource use and costs of branch and central retinal vein occlusion in the elderly. *Curr Med Res Opin.* 2010;26(1):223-230.
14. Smiddy WE. Economic considerations of macular edema therapies. *Ophthalmology.* 2011;118:1827-1833.
15. Varma R, Bressler NM, Suñer I, et al. Improved vision related function after ranibizumab for macular edema after retinal vein occlusion: results from the BRAVO and CRUISE trials. *Ophthalmology.* 2012;119(10):2108-2118.
16. Hayreh SS, Zimmerman MB. Fundus changes in central retinal vein occlusion. *Retina.* 2015;35(1):29-42.
17. Hayreh SS, Zimmerman MB. Fundus changes in branch retinal vein occlusion. *Retina.* 2015;35(5):1016-1027.
18. Hayreh SS. Classification of central retinal vein occlusion. *Ophthalmology.* 1983;90(5):458-474.
19. Hayreh SS, Zimmerman MB, Podhajsky P. Incidence of various types of retinal vein occlusion and their recurrence and demographic characteristics. *Am J Ophthalmol.* 1994;117(4):429-441.

20. Hayreh SS, Podhajsky PA, Zimmerman MB. Natural history of visual outcome in central retinal vein occlusion. *Ophthalmology*. 2011;118(1):119-133.

21. Hayreh SS, Klugman MR, Beri M, Kimura AE, Podhajsky P. Differentiation of ischemic from non-ischemic central retinal vein occlusion during the early acute phase. *Graefes Arch Clin Exp Ophthalmol*. 1990;228(3):201-217.

22. Scott IU, VanVeldhuisen PC, Oden NL, et al. SCORE study report 1: baseline associations between central retinal thickness and visual acuity in patients with retinal vein occlusion. *Ophthalmology*. 2009;116(3):504-512.

23. Campochiaro PA, Hafiz G, Shah SM, et al. Ranibizumab for macular edema due to retinal vein occlusions: implication of VEGF as a critical stimulator. *Mol Ther*. 2008;16(4):791-799.

24. Guex-Crosier Y. The pathogenesis and clinical presentation of macular edema in inflammatory diseases. *Doc Ophthalmol*. 1999;97(3-4):297-309.

25. Vinores SA, Derevjanik NL, Ozaki H, Okamoto N, Campochiaro PA. Cellular mechanisms of blood-retinal barrier dysfunction in macular edema. *Doc Ophthalmol*. 1999;97(3-4):217-228.

26. Funk M, Kriechbaum K, Prager F, et al. Intraocular concentrations of growth factors and cytokines in retinal vein occlusion and the effect of therapy with bevacizumab. *Invest Ophthalmol Vis Sci*. 2009;50(3):1025-1032.

27. Chan CK, Ip MS, Vanveldhuisen PC, et al. SCORE study report #11: incidences of neovascular events in eyes with retinal vein occlusion. *Ophthalmology*. 2011;118(7):1364-1372.

28. Hayreh SS. Ocular vascular occlusive disorders: natural history of visual outcome. *Prog Retin Eye Res*. 2014;41:1-25.

29. Hayreh SS, Zimmerman MB. Branch retinal vein occlusion natural history of visual outcome. *JAMA Ophthalmol*. 2014;132(1):13-22.

30. Hayreh SS, Zimmerman MB. Hemicentral retinal vein occlusion: natural history of visual outcome. *Retina*. 2012;32(1):68-76.

31. Hayreh SS, Podhasky PA, Zimmerman MB. Central and hemicentral retinal vein occlusion: role of anti-platelet aggregation agents and anticoagulants. *Ophthalmology*. 2011;118(8):1603-1611.

32. Argon laser photocoagulation for macular edema in branch vein occlusion. The Branch Retinal Vein Occlusion Study Group. *Am J Ophthalmol*. 1984;98(3):271-282.

33. Hayreh SS, Rojas P, Podhajsky P, Montague P, Woolson RF. Ocular neovascularization with retinal vascular occlusion-III. Incidence of ocular neovascularization with retinal vein occlusion. *Ophthalmology*. 1983;90(5):488-506.

34. Shilling JS, Jones CA. Retinal branch vein occlusion: a study of argon laser photocoagulation in the treatment of macular oedema. *Br J Ophthalmol*. 1984;68:196-198.

35. McAllister IL, Vijayasekaran S, Chen SD, Yu DY. Effect of triamcinolone acetonide on vascular endothelial growth factor and occluding levels in branch retinal vein occlusion. *Am J Ophthalmol*. 2009;147(5):838-846.

36. Ip MS, Scott IU, VanVeldhuisen PC, et al. A randomized trial comparing the efficacy and safety of intravitreal triamcinolone with observation to treat vision loss associated with macular edema secondary to central retinal vein occlusion: the Standard Care vs Corticosteroid for Retinal Vein Occlusion (SCORE) study report 5. *Arch Ophthalmol*. 2009;127(9):1101-1114.

37. Avitabile T, Longo A, Reibaldi A. Intravitreal triamcinolone compared with macular laser grid photocoagulation for the treatment of cystoids macular edema. *Am J Ophthalmol*. 2005;140(4):695-702.

38. Krepler K, Ergun E, Sacu S, et al. Intravitreal triamcinolone acetonide in patients with macular oedema due to branch retinal vein occlusion: a pilot study. *Acta Ophthalmol Scand*. 2005;83(5):600-604.

39. Krepler K, Ergun E, Sacu S, et al. Intravitreal triamcinolone acetonide in patients with macular oedema due to central retinal vein occlusion. *Acta Ophthalmol Scand*. 2005;83(1):71-75.

40. Bakri SJ, Shah A, Falk NS, Beer PM. Intravitreal preservative-free triamcinolone acetonide for the treatment of macular oedema. *Eye (Lond)*. 2005;19(6):686-688.

41. Tewari HK, Sony P, Chawla R, Garg SP, Venkatesh P. Prospective evaluation of intravitreal triamcinolone acetonide injection in macular edema associated with retinal vascular disorders. *Eur J Ophthalmol*. 2005;15(5):619-626.

42. Yepremyan M, Wertz FD, Tivnan T, Eversman L, Marx JL. Early treatment of cystoid macular edema secondary to branch retinal vein occlusion with intravitreal triamcinolone acetonide. *Ophthalmic Surg Lasers Imaging.* 2005;36(1):30-36.

43. Karacorlu M, Ozdemir H, Karacorlu SA. Resolution of serous macular detachment after intravitreal triamcinolone acetonide treatment of patients with branch retinal vein occlusion. *Retina.* 2005;25(7):856-860.

44. Haller JA, Bandello F, Belfort R Jr, et al. Randomized, sham controlled trial of dexamethasone intravitreal implant in patients with macular edema due to retinal vein occlusion. *Ophthalmology.* 2010;117(6):1134-1146.

45. Haller JA, Bandello F, Belfort R Jr, et al. Dexamethasone intravitreal implant in patients with macular edema related to branch or central retinal vein occlusion twelve-month study results. *Ophthalmology.* 2011;118(12):2453-2460.

46. Chen HC, Wiek J, Gupta A, Luckie A, Kohner EM. Effect of isovolaemic haemodilution on visual outcome in branch retinal vein occlusion. *Br J Ophthalmol.* 1998;82(2):162-167.

47. Hansen LL, Wiek J, Arntz R. Randomized study of the effect of isovolemic hemodilution in retinal branch vein occlusion [article in German]. *Fortschr Ophthalmol.* 1988;85(5):514-516.

48. Poupard P Eledjam JJ, Dupeyron G, et al. Role of acute normovolemic hemodilution in treating retinal venous occlusions [article in French]. *Ann Fr Anesth Reanim.* 1986;5(3):229-233.

49. Shah GK, Sharma S, Fineman MS, Federman J, Brown MM, Brown GC. Arteriovenous adventitial sheathotomy for the treatment of macular edema associated with branch retinal vein occlusion. *Am J Ophthalmol.* 2000;129(1):104-106.

50. Mason J III, Feist R, White M Jr, Swanner J, McGwin G Jr, Emond T. Sheathotomy to decompress branch retinal vein occlusion. *Ophthalmology.* 2004;111(3):540-545.

51. Aggermann T, Brunner S, Krebs I, et al. A prospective, randomised, multicenter trial for surgical treatment of central retinal vein occlusion: results of the Radial Optic Neurotomy for Central Vein Occlusion (ROVO) study group. *Graefes Arch Clin Exp Ophthalmol.* 2013;251(4):1065-1072.

52. Kumagai K, Furukawa M, Ogino N, Uemura A, Larson E. Long-term outcomes of vitrectomy with or without arteriovenous sheathotomy in branch retinal vein occlusion. *Retina.* 2007;27(1):49-54.

53. Ehlers JP, Fekrat S. Retinal vein occlusion: beyond the acute event. *Surv Ophthalmol.* 2011;56(4):281-299.

54. Feltgen N, Junker B, Agostini H, Hansen LL. Retinal endovascular lysis in ischemic central retinal vein occlusion: one-year results of a pilot study. *Ophthalmology.* 2007;114(4):716-723.

55. Noma H, Funatsu H, Mimura T, Eguchi S, Shimada K, Hori S. Vitreous levels of pigment epithelium-derived factor and vascular endothelial growth factor in macular edema with central retinal vein occlusion. *Curr Eye Res.* 2011;36(3):256-263

56. Noma H, Funatsu H, Yamasaki M, et al. Pathogenesis of macular edema with branch retinal vein occlusion and intraocular levels of vascular endothelial growth factor and interleukin-6. *Am J Ophthal.* 2005;140(2):256-261.

57. Noma H, Funatsu H, Mimura T, Harino S, Hori S. Vitreous levels of interleukin-6 and vascular endothelial growth factor in macular edema with central retinal vein occlusion. *Ophthalmology.* 2009;116(1):87-93.

58. Brown DM, Campochiaro PA, Singh RP, et al. Ranibizumab for macular edema following central retinal vein occlusion: six-month primary end point results of a phase III study. *Ophthalmology.* 2010;117(6):1124-1133.

59. Campochiaro PA, Brown DM, Awh CC, et al. Sustained benefits from ranibizumab for macular edema following central retinal vein occlusion: twelve-month outcomes of a phase III study. *Ophthalmology.* 2011;118(10):2041-2049.

60. Epstein DL, Algvere PV, von Wendt G, Seregard S, Kvanta A. Bevacizumab for macular edema in central retinal vein occlusion: a prospective, randomized, double-masked clinical study. *Ophthalmology.* 2012;119(6):1184-1189.

61. Heier JS, Campochiaro PA, Yau L, et al. Ranibizumab for macular edema due to retinal vein occlusions: long-term follow-up in the HORIZON trial. *Ophthalmology.* 2012;119(4):802-809.

62. Epstein DL, Algvere PV, von Wendt G, Seregard S, Kvanta A. Benefit from bevacizumab for macular edema in central retinal vein occlusion: twelve-month results of a prospective, randomized study. *Ophthalmology.* 2012;119(12):2587-2591.

63. Algvere PV, Epstein D, von Wendt G, Seregard S, Kvanta A. Intravitreal bevacizumab in central retinal vein occlusion: 18-month results of a prospective clinical trial. *Eur J Ophthalmol.* 2011;21(6):789-795.

64. Loukianou E, Brouzas D, Chatzistefanou K, Koutsandrea C. Clinical, anatomical, and electrophysiological assessments of central retina following intravitreal bevacizumab for macular edema secondary to retinal vein occlusion. *Int Ophthalmol.* 2016;36(1):21-36.

65. Demir M, Oba E, Gulkilik G, Obadasi M, Ozdal E. Intravitreal bevacizumab for macular edema due to branch retinal vein occlusion: 12-month results. *Clin Ophthalmol.* 2011;5:745-749.

66. Ahmadieh H, Moradian S, Malihi M. Rapid regression of extensive retinovitreal neovascularization secondary to branch retinal vein occlusion after single intravitreal injection of bevacizumab. *Int Ophthalmol.* 2005;26(4-5):191-193.

67. Grisanti S, Biester S, Peters S, et al. Intracameral bevacizumab for iris rubeosis. *Am J Ophthalmol.* 2006;142(1):158-160.

68. Brouzas D, Charakidas A, Moschos M, Koutsandrea C, Apostolopoulos M, Baltatzis S. Bevacizumab (Avastin) for the management of anterior chamber neovascularization and neovascular glaucoma. *Clin Ophthalmol.* 2009;3:685-688.

69. Ciftci S, Sakalar YB, Unlu K, Keklikci U, Caca I, Dogan E. Intravitreal bevacizumab combined with panretinal photocoagulation in the treatment of open angle neovascular glaucoma. *Eur J Ophthalmol.* 2009;19(6):1028-1033.

70. Iliev ME, Domig D, Wolf-Schnurrbursch U, Wolf S, Sarra GM. Intravitreal bevacizumab (Avastin) in the treatment of neovascular glaucoma. *Am J Ophthalmol.* 2006;142(6):1054-1056.

71. Boyer D, Heier J, Brown DM, et al. Vascular endothelial growth factor Trap-Eye for macular edema secondary to central retinal vein occlusion: six-month results of the phase 3 COPERNICUS study. *Ophthalmology.* 2012;119(5):1024-1032.

72. Brown DM, Heier JS, Clark WL, et al. Intravitreal aflibercept injection for macular edema secondary to central retinal vein occlusion: 1-year results from the phase 3 COPERNICUS study. *Am J Ophthalmol.* 2013;155(3):429-437.

73. Campochiaro PA, Clark WL, Boyer DS, et al. Intravitreal aflibercept for macular edema following branch retinal vein occlusion: the 24-week results of the VIBRANT study. *Ophthalmology.* 2015;122(3):538-544.

74. Ding X, Li J, Hu X, Yu S, Pan J, Tang S. Prospective study of intravitreal triamcinolone acetonide versus bevacizumab for macular edema secondary to central retinal vein occlusion. *Retina.* 2011;31(5):838-845.

75. Mayer WJ, Remy M, Wolf A, et al. Comparison of intravitreal bevacizumab upload followed by a dexamethasone implant versus dexamethasone implant monotherapy for retinal vein occlusion with macular edema. *Ophthalmologica.* 2012;228(2):110-116.

76. Narayanan R, Panchal B, Das T, et al. A randomized, double-masked, controlled study of the efficacy and safety of intravitreal bevacizumab versus ranibizumab in the treatment of macular oedema due to branch retinal vein occlusion: MARVEL report No. 1. *Br J Ophthalmol.* 2015;99(7):954-959.

12

UVEITIS

Lana M. Rifkin, MD

Uveitis is defined as intraocular inflammation with potentially various causes. It is classified as anterior, intermediate, posterior, or panuveitis, based on the location of inflammation. Uveitis accounts for about 10% of legal blindness in the United States.[1] The most common cause of significant vision loss in patients with intraocular inflammatory disease is cystoid macular edema (CME), which occurs in more than 30% of uveitis patients.[2] Choroidal neovascularization (CNV) can also occur as a consequence of uveitis, but less commonly, in 2% to 3% of uveitis patients.[3]

Uveitic CME can occur in any type of uveitis. It is most commonly a sequelae of panuveitis, where more than 60% of patients get CME, followed by intermediate uveitis, which causes approximately 30% of uveitic CME. Ten percent to 15% of patients with anterior uveitis can also suffer from CME.[4] CME may persist despite quiescence of uveitis and can lead to irreversible visual compromise if not adequately treated. The current gold standard for treating CME is corticosteroids. Topical steroids and nonsteroidal anti-inflammatory agents may not be effective in uveitic macular edema. Thus, oral steroids or injection of steroid into the subtenon or intravitreal space are often offered. Common side effects of steroid injection, which may be limiting for some patients, are intraocular pressure elevation and cataract progression.[5] Oral steroids may cause significant side effects of weight gain, blood sugar fluctuations, psychiatric side effects, bruising, and osteoporosis, among others.[6]

The pathophysiology of uveitic CME is not completely understood but is postulated to be a consequence of increased vascular permeability. It has been suggested that vascular endothelial growth factor (VEGF) may be implicated in the pathogenesis of uveitic CME. Indeed, increased VEGF concentration has been observed in the aqueous humor of patients with uveitic CME when compared to uveitis patients without CME.[7] Intravitreal VEGF levels have also been measured in uveitis patients and, in comparison, the mean concentrations of VEGF in the vitreous of diabetic patients are 5.5 times greater than that of patients with uveitis, as compared to a healthy control group, in whom the levels

Duker JS, Liang MC, eds.
*Anti-VEGF Use in
Ophthalmology (pp. 137-141).*
© 2017 Taylor & Francis Group.

Figure 12-1. (A) Spectral domain-optical coherence tomography of a 24-year-old male with cystoid macular edema secondary to pars planitis and decreased vision to 20/60. (B) Spectral domain-optical coherence tomography of the same patient showing near-complete resolution of cystoid macular edema after one injection of intravitreal bevacizumab. Visual acuity improved to 20/25. (Reprinted with permission from Debra Goldstein, MD.)

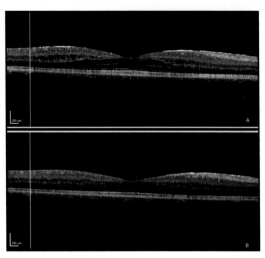

of VEGF are zero. Intraocular VEGF levels detected in the vitreous of patients with uveitis are similar to those described in patients with neovascular age-related macular degeneration.[8]

With these discoveries, anti-VEGF agents such as bevacizumab, ranibizumab, and aflibercept have begun to be employed in resistant cases of uveitic CME or CNV or in cases where corticosteroids are otherwise contraindicated. Large multicenter trials evaluating the safety and efficacy of intravitreal anti-VEGF, particularly when compared to triamcinolone injection, for uveitic CME and CNV have not yet been undertaken but several small studies and case reports do exist, noting the use of anti-VEGF agents as an alternative or perhaps adjunct to steroid therapy. However, these reports and series are retrospective in nature and have various limitations.

Bevacizumab in Uveitic Cystoid Macular Edema and Choroidal Neovascularization

Bevacizumab (Avastin), a recombinant humanized monoclonal antibody, was the first clinically available anti-VEGF agent used, albeit off-label, for the treatment of resistant-to-standard-therapy CME and CNV secondary to ocular inflammatory disease.

The earliest report of intravitreal bevacizumab for the treatment of uveitic macular edema (Figure 12-1) was in 2007, with Cordero Coma et al[9] reporting that 62% of patients with CME secondary to intraocular inflammation showed an improvement in visual acuity after a single injection of bevacizumab. Intravitreal bevacizumab treatment was also shown to be fast acting and effective in the treatment of refractory macular edema in uveitis patients in another small pilot study.[10] A decrease in central retinal thickness was seen within 2 weeks in some patients; however, improvement in visual acuity did not always correlate as these patients had long-standing CME, causing photoreceptor damage, and intravitreal bevacizumab was used as a last-resort measure. Additionally, the effect was transient and repeat injections were necessary. In contrast, that same year, Ziemssen et al[11] indicated that the response to intravitreal bevacizumab was weak

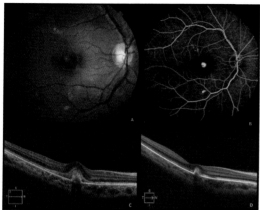

Figure 12-2. (A) Color photo of a 20-year-old female with choroidal neovascularization (CNV) secondary to punctate inner choroiditis and decreased vision to 20/40. (B) Fluorescein angiography demonstrating leakage into the macula, confirming presence of CNV. (C) Spectral domain-optical coherence tomography showing an elevated choroidal lesion corresponding with a CNV. (D) Spectral domain-optical coherence tomography of the same patient, after 3 monthly injections of bevacizumab, showing reduction of CNV. Visual acuity improved to 20/25. (Photo provided courtesy of Andre Witkin.)

and transient. In their report, none of their 6 patients with chronic macular edema as a sequelae of uveitis had significant improvement in visual acuity or a decrease in central retinal thickness. It was postulated that perhaps acute and previously untreated uveitic CME may respond more favorably.

Inflammatory CNV is fairly rare but can also be a significant cause of visual compromise in uveitis patients. It can occur in 2% to 3% of posterior or panuveitis, and has been shown to be more likely in patients with uveitis secondary to Vogt-Koyanagi-Harada disease or punctate inner choroiditis. Laser photocoagulation and photodynamic therapy, as well as local or systemic corticosteroids, have been tried as potential treatments in uveitic CNV[12] and more recently, uveitic CNV has been treated off-label with anti-VEGF agents (Figure 12-2). One study of 84 eyes in 79 patients with CNV secondary to various diseases including multifocal choroiditis with panuveitis, punctate inner choroidopathy, ocular histoplasmosis, idiopathic uveitis, Vogt-Koyanagi-Harada disease, serpiginous choroiditis, retinal vasculitis, pars planitis, ocular toxoplasmosis, ocular tuberculosis, ocular sarcoid, and birdshot choroiditis showed significant gains in visual acuity in the short term and regression of inflammatory CNV.[13] The 5-year follow-up of this study showed sustained, significant improvement in visual acuity without major complications after a median of 5 intravitreal injections of bevacizumab.[14] Eyes with inflammatory CNV may show an initial improvement in visual acuity after anti-VEGF injection, but these results may not be sustained long term as photoreceptor disruption or fibrosis may limit further improvement in visual acuity.

Retinal edema seems to respond more favorably to intravitreal anti-VEGF therapy in eyes with uveitic CNV than in eyes with uveitic CME, indicating that anti-VEGF may be more efficacious in patients with inflammatory CNV rather than inflammatory CME.[15] When compared to traditional treatments of periocular and intravitreal steroid injection, although intravitreal bevacizumab was found to have a significant decrease in central foveal thickness, it was less so than in triamcinolone-injected eyes. Interestingly, in patients with Behçet's uveitis-associated CME, intravitreal bevacizumab initially showed a greater improvement in visual acuity than patients who underwent steroid injection; however, the difference was not sustained past 12 weeks of follow-up.[16]

Ranibizumab in Uveitic Cystoid Macular Edema and Choroidal Neovascularization

Ranibizumab (Lucentis), the monoclonal antibody fragment created from the same mouse antibody as bevacizumab, has also been used clinically off-label for the treatment of CME and CNV in ocular inflammatory disease. There have been some promising data indicating that intravitreal ranibizumab injections may lead to an increase in visual acuity and cause a regression of persistent uveitic CME.[17] Although there have not been comparative studies of ranibizumab to bevacizumab for uveitic CME or CNV, it is plausible that ranibizumab may have some advantages as it has been shown to be 5 to 20 times more potent in bioassays measuring human VEGF-induced endothelial cell mitogenesis.

Aflibercept in Uveitic Cystoid Macular Edema and Choroidal Neovascularization

Aflibercept (Eylea) is the most recent anti-VEGF agent to be used in the treatment of eye disease. It is currently approved for use in neovascular age-related macular degeneration, macular edema as a result of retinal vein occlusion, and diabetic macular edema as well as diabetic retinopathy. Although aflibercept is not approved for use in uveitic macular edema or CNV, it has been tried off-label and a few published case reports do exist.[18,19] One such case report showed that a single intravitreal injection of aflibercept in a patient with idiopathic intermediate uveitis previously treated with multiple intravitreal injections of ranibizumab and bevacizumab was effective in completely and permanently causing regression of chronic uveitic CME.[18] In another report of 3 patients with multifocal choroiditis and secondary choroidal neovascular membranes not responsive to multiple intravitreal injections of ranibizumab, an improvement in visual acuity and decrease in central retinal thickness was seen after 3 to 4 intravitreal injections of aflibercept. Long-term follow-up is yet unknown.[19]

Conclusion

Anti-VEGF injection may be an alternative option for the treatment of uveitic CME and CNV but is currently typically reserved for recalcitrant or unresponsive-to-standard-therapy ocular inflammatory disease. Particularly in cases of macular edema or CNV secondary to infectious uveitis (ie, ocular tuberculosis, for which immunosuppression would not be a feasible option), intravitreal anti-VEGF injection may be considered. There is no consensus on efficacy as large studies do not yet exist, but several small retrospective case reports and case series do indicate a favorable response to bevacizumab, ranibizumab, and aflibercept. Thus far, all reports have been retrospective in nature and with relatively small sample sizes so the level of supportive evidence for the use of these agents in uveitis is low. Furthermore, blockage of VEGF has not been shown to have any anti-inflammatory effects and thus, the role of anti-VEGF therapy in uveitis remains not fully understood. The treatment of the underlying etiology of inflammation with corticosteroids and/or immunosuppression remains the key to the management of uveitis, although anti-VEGF therapies can be helpful in treating the complications of CME and/or CNV that may result.

References

1. Acharya NR, Tham VM, Esterberg E, et al. Incidence and prevalence of uveitis: results from the Pacific Ocular Inflammation Study. *JAMA Ophthalmol.* 2013;131(11):1405-1402.

2. Rothova A, Suttorp-van Schulten MS, Frits Treffers W, Kijlstra A. Causes and frequency of blindness in patients with intraocular inflammatory disease. *Br J Ophthalmol.* 1996;80:332-336.

3. Baxter SL, Pistilli M, Pujari SS, et al. Risk of choroidal neovascularization among uveitides. *Am J Ophthalmol.* 2013;156(3):468-477.

4. Lardenoye CW, van Kooii B, Rothova A. Impact of macular edema on visual acuity in uveitis. *Ophthalmology.* 2006;113(8):1446-1449.

5. Sen HN, Vitale S, Gangaputra SS, et al. Periocular corticosteroid injections in uveitis: effects and complications. *Ophthalmology.* 2014;121(11):2275-2286.

6. Manson SC, Brown RE, Cerulli A, Vidaurre CF. The cumulative burden of oral corticosteroid side effects and the economic implications of steroid use. *Respir Med.* 2009;103(7):975-994.

7. Fine HF, Baffi J, Reed GF, Csaky KG, Nussenblatt RB. Aqueous humor and plasma vascular endothelial growth factor in uveitis-associated cystoid macular edema. *Am J Ophthalmol.* 2001;132(5):794-796.

8. Weiss K, Steinbrugger I, Weger M, et al. Intravitreal VEGF levels in uveitis patients and treatment of uveitic macular oedema with intravitreal bevacizumab. *Eye (Lond).* 2009;23(9):1812-1818.

9. Cordero Coma M, Sobrin L, Onal S, Christen W, Foster CS. Intravitreal bevacizumab for treatment of uveitic macular edema. *Ophthalmology.* 2007;114(8):1574-1579.e1.

10. Mackensen F, Heinz C, Becker MD, Heilingenhaus A. Intravitreal bevacizumab (Avastin) as a treatment for refractory macular edema in patients with uveitis: a pilot study. *Retina.* 2008;28(1):41-45.

11. Ziemssen F, Deuter CM, Stuebinger N, Zierhut M. Weak transient response of chronic uveitic macular edema to intravitreal bevacizumab (Avastin). *Graefes Arch Clin Exp Ophthalmol.* 2007;245(6):917-918.

12. Rogers AH, Duker JS, Nichols N, Baker BJ. Photodynamic therapy of idiopathic and inflammatory choroidal neovascularization in young adults. *Ophthalmology.* 2003;110(7):1315-1320.

13. Mansour AM, Mackensen F, Arevalo JF, et al. Intravitreal bevacizumab in inflammatory ocular neovascularization. *Am J Ophthalmol.* 2008;146(3):410-416.

14. Mansour AM, Mackensen F, Mahendradas P, Khairallah M, Lai TY, Bashshur Z. Five-year visual results of intravitreal bevacizumab in refractory inflammatory ocular neovascularization. *Clin Ophthalmol.* 2012;6:1233-1237.

15. Lott MN, Schiffman JC, Davis JL. Bevacizumab in inflammatory eye disease. *Am J Ophthalmol.* 2009;148(5):711-717.

16. Bae HJ, Lee, CS, Lee SC. Efficacy and safety of intravitreal bevacizumab compared with intravitreal and posterior sub-tenon triamcinolone acetonide for treatment of uveitic cystoid macular edema. *Retina.* 2011;31(1):111-118.

17. Acharya NR, Hong KC, Lee SM. Ranibizumab for refractory uveitis-related macular edema. *Am J Ophthalmol.* 2009;148(2):303-309.

18. Swituła M. Complete and permanent regression of persistent uveitic cystoid macular edema after single intravitreal injection of aflibercept in patient previously treated with multiple intravitreal injections of ranibizumab and bevacizumab [article in Polish]. *Klin Oczna.* 2015;117(1):31-34.

19. Hernández-Martínez P, Dolz-Marco R, Alonso-Plasencia M, Abreu-Gonzalez R. Aflibercept for inflammatory choroidal neovascularization with persistent fluid on intravitreal ranibizumab therapy. *Graefes Arch Clin Exp Ophthalmol.* 2014;252(8):1337-1339.

13

RETINOPATHY OF PREMATURITY

Nikisha A. Kothari, MD and Audina M. Berrocal, MD

Retinopathy of prematurity (ROP), a disease of very low birth-weight premature infants, is characterized by abnormal vascularization and angiogenesis of the retina. ROP is a leading cause of vision loss and blindness evoked by retinal detachment and temporal dragging of the macula.[1] The prevalence of blindness from ROP is estimated to be 50,000 worldwide. Because of the survival of more low birth-weight infants, the absolute number of infants with ROP has consequently increased.[1]

Retinal vascularization begins at 16 weeks gestation from the optic nerve and completes temporally at 40 weeks gestation. Infants born prior to 40 weeks may have abnormal avascular peripheral retina or ROP. The location of retinal vascularization defines the zone; zone 1 is a circle twice the distance from the center of the disc and center of the macula extending from the disc; zone 2 encircles zone 1 extending to the nasal ora; and zone 3 is the remaining crescent shaped temporal retina. The severity of disease, or staging, is determined by the appearance of the vasculature at the interface between the avascular and vascular retina. The interface is a line in stage 1, a ridge in stage 2, and a ridge with extraretinal neovascularization in stage 3. Furthermore, partial retinal detachment is classified as stage 4 disease and complete retinal detachment as stage 5.[2] Plus disease is the presence of 2 or more quadrants with dilated and tortuous vessels, which current guidelines emphasize when determining the threshold to treat.[2,3] Aggressive posterior ROP (AP-ROP) is defined as tortuous blood vessels in all 4 quadrants out of proportion to the extent of peripheral retinopathy and implies a poorer prognosis.[2] This classification of ROP is important to understand as it gives us a common language and guides management and the threshold to treat.

Treatment

Based on the Early Treatment of ROP study, treatment should be initiated in eyes with zone 1 ROP, any stage, with plus disease, zone 1 ROP that is stage 3 without plus

Duker JS, Liang MC, eds.
Anti-VEGF Use in Ophthalmology (pp. 143-149).
© 2017 Taylor & Francis Group.

disease, and zone 2 ROP that is stage 2 or 3 with plus disease.[3] Conventional treatment is peripheral retinal ablation by laser therapy, which has largely replaced cryotherapy over the years. Laser photocoagulation results in reduced rates of retinal detachment and improvement in visual acuity outcomes.[4] However, photocoagulation therapy has limitations, particularly in zone 1 and AP-ROP cases that require treatment adjacent to the macula and progress rapidly.[5] Because of limitations of conventional therapy, anti-vascular endothelial growth factor (VEGF) agents have been proposed as an alternative therapy with early, promising results.[5]

In normal retinal development, VEGF is released in response to increased oxygen demand in order to facilitate vascularization of the peripheral retina. In ROP, the imbalance of VEGF levels divided into 2 phases is the cause of disease development and progression. In the vaso-obliterative phase, 22 to 30 weeks postmenstrual stage, hyperoxia caused by increased postnatal arterial oxygen levels and supplemental oxygen results in failure of the peripheral retinal vasculature to develop. In the vaso-proliferative phase, 31 to 40 weeks postmenstrual stage, ischemia in the avascular retina results in angiogenesis and the production of VEGF.[6] While abnormal vasculature in ROP often spontaneously regresses without intervention, it can progress to traction and retinal detachment. Extremely high levels of VEGF are found in the vitreous of eyes with stage 4 disease, confirming the upregulation of VEGF as a marker of disease progression and severity.[7] Thus, treatment is aimed at reducing VEGF levels either by ablating the peripheral avascular retina producing VEGF or pharmacologically inhibiting VEGF. As anti-VEGF agents have become more widely used in other retinal neovascular processes such as neovascular age-related macular degeneration, their use in ROP was explored. Multiple case reports and consecutive case series have been published; however, very limited data come from randomized, controlled clinical trials.

Anti-Vascular Endothelial Growth Factor Therapy

The Bevacizumab Eliminates the Angiogenic Threat of Retinopathy of Prematurity (BEAT-ROP) study was the first multicenter randomized unmasked study that compared monotherapy with intravitreal bevacizumab to conventional diode laser photocoagulation. Study criteria included a birth weight of 1500 grams or less and 30 weeks gestational age or less with stage 3+ disease in zone 1 or 2. Bevacizumab (0.625 mg in 0.025 mL) was injected in the vitreous 2.5 mm posterior to the limbus with a 31-gauge needle. Infants, not eyes, were randomly assigned to injection or laser to avoid the potential risk of amblyopia from possible poor visual acuity in the eye treated with laser photocoagulation. The primary outcome of the study was recurrence of retinal neovascularization requiring treatment by 54 weeks. Eyes treated with intravitreal bevacizumab had lower rates of recurrence compared to those treated with conventional laser (6% vs 26%, respectively). However, this finding was statistically significant only in the eyes with zone 1 disease treated with bevacizumab, not zone 2 disease. An important consideration regarding the primary outcome in this study is that recurrence is typically later with anti-VEGF therapy compared to laser (19.2 weeks + 8.6 weeks vs 6.4 weeks + 6.7 weeks, respectively).[5] Moreover, recurrence after the 54-week follow-up period after treatment with intravitreal bevacizumab is not uncommon.[8] A similar randomized, controlled trial performed in Europe compared conventional laser therapy with and without adjuvant intravitreal pegaptanib (0.3 mg in 0.02 mL). The rate of recurrence was significantly higher in the conventional laser therapy group compared to the combination intravitreal pegaptanib and conventional laser therapy group (38% vs 11.7%, respectively).[9]

Another clinical trial, RAnibizumab Compared with Laser Therapy for the Treatment of INfants BOrn Prematurely with Retinopathy of Prematurity (RAINBOW), is currently underway to determine if intravitreal ranibizumab is superior to laser ablation therapy for the treatment of ROP. Primary outcome measures include the absence of active ROP and unfavorable structural outcome 24 weeks starting after study treatment. Secondary outcome measures include recurrence of ROP and requirement and timing for intervention with a second modality. It will also examine the systemic levels of ranibizumab and VEGF (NCT02375971).

Advantages Over Ablative Therapy

A potential pitfall of conventional laser therapy is the increased risk of high myopia, particularly very high myopia as demonstrated by the BEAT-ROP study group.[10] Both the presence and severity of ROP are independent risk factors for the development of high myopia.[3,4] Interestingly, the difference in cycloplegic refraction was not statistically significant between zone 1 and zone 2 eyes in the BEAT-ROP study. Therefore, the authors concluded that laser therapy, not the severity of disease, was the primary etiology for myopia. Thus, treatment with anti-VEGF and possible avoidance of any laser therapy may reduce the incidence of laser-associated myopia.

Another major consequence of ablative therapy is the reduction of peripheral vision.[5] Particularly in zone 1-treated eyes, the application of laser photocoagulation adjacent to the macula is technically challenging and causes constricted visual fields. In the Early Treatment of ROP study, zone 1 eyes had a 55.2% unfavorable outcome rate, representing a subset that has the capacity to greatly improve outcomes. An advantage of anti-VEGF monotherapy is the potential for normal retinal revascularization to develop in the periphery where it was previously avascular (Figure 13-1) and preservation of the peripheral field.

Anti-VEGF therapy is typically administered under local anesthesia at the bedside, compared to laser treatment, which often requires general anesthesia.[5] Both administration of anti-VEGF and application of laser therapy require proper training and mentoring, although anti-VEGF treatment may arguably be easier for most clinicians than conventional laser. Intravitreal injections do carry other risks including endophthalmitis, cataract, and postinjection intraocular inflammation, rare in the neonate population.

Concerns

One consideration is the potential systemic effect and safety profile of anti-VEGF agents in infants. The authors of the BEAT-ROP study argue that minimal bevacizumab enters the systemic circulation because of its large molecular size. However, Sato et al[11] found serum levels of bevacizumab were higher and levels of VEGF were lower one week after injection with anti-VEGF. Also, while the BEAT-ROP study used half the adult dose of bevacizumab, there is a lack of understanding regarding the appropriate dosing in infants. Systemic anti-VEGF may affect organogenesis such as pulmonary, renal, neuronal, and skeletal development. In the BEAT-ROP study, 7 infants died, 5 of whom were

Figure 13-1. Increased retinal vascularization after intravitreal bevacizumab monotherapy. (A,B) Fundus photography and fluorescein angiography prior to treatment demonstrates an avascular peripheral retina. (C) Fundus photography over 80 weeks after initial treatment with intravitreal bevacizumab shows slightly tortuous vessels with normal vascularization of the peripheral retina.

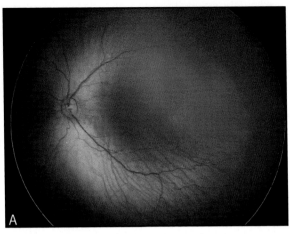

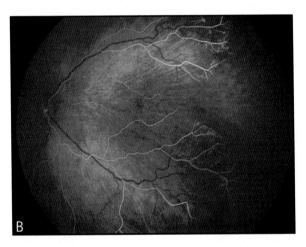

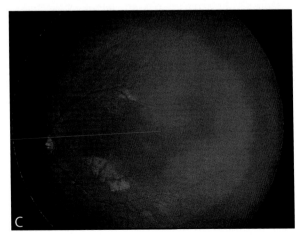

in the bevacizumab group, though the difference between the groups was not statistically significant. All deaths in the bevacizumab group were secondary to respiratory arrest. The study concluded that a larger sample size would be needed to make an assessment regarding morbidity, mortality, and systemic or local toxicity. In general, when administering anti-VEGF agents in infants, one should err on the side of caution with lack of definitive evidence regarding their safety.

Conclusion

While more information is being gathered, it is not clearly defined which ROP eyes should be treated and what the optimal dosing regimen with anti-VEGF therapy is. Furthermore, no guidelines exist based on the current evidence regarding timing, frequency, and extent of follow-up. With the risk of late recurrence, however, compliance is an important factor in deciding what treatment an infant should receive. Anti-VEGF treatment requires longer follow-up compared to conventional laser, with reported late recurrence up to 80 weeks potentially requiring treatment (Figure 13-2).[12] Poor compliance once the infant leaves the neonatal intensive care unit may portend a poor prognosis with progression to retinal detachment. Moreover, evaluation of the peripheral retina and detection of late recurrences becomes more challenging in older infants in clinic without performing an exam under anesthesia.

With the current data available, anti-VEGF treatment appears to be most advantageous over conventional laser for eyes with zone 1 disease and AP-ROP, in which application of laser is challenging and often results in failure for ROP to regress with late progression of the disease. However, additional research with larger sample sizes and longer follow-up is required to be certain of long-term systemic side effects of anti-VEGF agents in infants.

Figure 13-2. Recurrence of retinopathy of prematurity after intravitreal bevacizumab. (A) Fundus photography reveals tortuous vessels and an avascular peripheral retina. (B) Fluorescein angiography highlights a frond of neovascularization in an area of avascular retina around 75 weeks after the last treatment with intravitreal bevacizumab. (C) Fundus photography after laser treatment demonstrates regression of neovascularization.

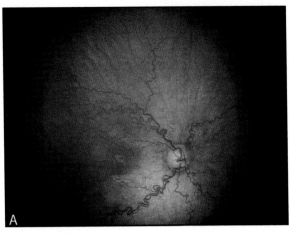

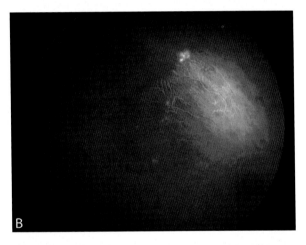

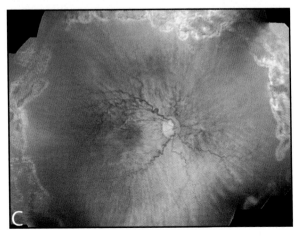

References

1. Gilbert C. Retinopathy of prematurity: a global perspective of the epidemics, population of babies at risk and implications for control. *Early Hum Dev.* 2008;84(2):77-82.
2. International Committee for the Classification of Retinopathy of Prematurity. The International Classification of Retinopathy of Prematurity revisited. *Arch Ophthalmol.* 2005;123(7):991-999.
3. Early Treatment for Retinopathy of Prematurity Cooperative Group. Revised indications for the treatment of retinopathy of prematurity: results of the early treatment for retinopathy of prematurity randomized trial. *Arch Ophthalmol.* 2003;121(12):1684-1694.
4. The natural ocular outcome of premature birth and retinopathy. Status at 1 year. Cryotherapy for Retinopathy of Prematurity Cooperative Group. *Arch Ophthalmol.* 1994;112(7):903-912.
5. Mintz-Hittner HA, Kennedy KA, Chuang AZ, BEAT-ROP Cooperative Group. Efficacy of intravitreal bevacizumab for stage 3+ retinopathy of prematurity. *N Engl J Med.* 2011;364(7):603-615.
6. Ashton N, Ward B, Serpell G. Effect of oxygen on developing retinal vessels with particular reference to the problem of retrolental fibroplasia. *Br J Ophthalmol.* 1954;38(7):397-432.
7. Lashkari K, Hirose T, Yazdany J, McMeel JW, Kazlauskas A, Rahimi N. Vascular endothelial growth factor and hepatocyte growth factor levels are differentially elevated in patients with advanced retinopathy of prematurity. *Am J Pathol.* 2000;156(4):1337-1344.
8. Hu J, Blair MP, Shapiro MJ, Lichtenstein SJ, Galasso JM, Kapur R. Reactivation of retinopathy of prematurity after bevacizumab injection. *Arch Ophthalmol.* 2012;130(8):1000-1006.
9. Autrata R, Krejčírová I, Senková K, Holoušová M, Doležel Z, Borek I. Intravitreal pegaptanib combined with diode laser therapy for stage 3+ retinopathy of prematurity in zone I and posterior zone II. *Eur J Ophthalmol.* 2012;22(5):687-694.
10. Geloneck MM, Chuang AZ, Clark WL, et al. Refractive outcomes following bevacizumab monotherapy compared with conventional laser treatment: a randomized clinical trial. *JAMA Ophthalmol.* 2014;132(11):1327-1333.
11. Sato T, Wada K, Arahori H, et al. Serum concentrations of bevacizumab (Avastin) and vascular endothelial growth factor in infants with retinopathy of prematurity. *Am J Ophthalmol.* 2012;153(2):327-333.e1.
12. Snyder LL, Garcia-Gonzalez JM, Shapiro MJ, Blair MP. Very late reactivation of retinopathy of prematurity after monotherapy with intravitreal bevacizumab. *Ophthalmic Surg Lasers Imaging Retina.* 2016;47(3):280-283.

14

MISCELLANEOUS RETINAL AND CHOROIDAL DISEASES

Michael D. Tibbetts, MD

Vitelliform Macular Dystrophy

Vitelliform macular dystrophy is an inherited disease associated with deposition of lipofuscin in the central macula.[1] The condition is described as Best disease when present early in life and as adult-onset vitelliform dystrophy (AOVD) when present in middle age or later.[2] Lipofuscin deposition can lead to progressive central vision loss when atrophy and scarring occur. The clinical phenotype can be highly variable. Men and women are equally affected but the incidence of Best disease and AOVD are not known. Best disease is caused by an autosomal dominant mutation in the bestrophin (VMD2) gene[3] and AOVD is associated with mutations of VMD2, retinal degeneration slow (RDS), interphotoreceptor matrix 1 and 2 (IMPG1 and IMPG2), as well as a polymorphism in the HtrA Serine Peptidase 1 gene (HTRA1).[4,5] However, the causative gene cannot be found in most AOVD patients.

Vitelliform dystrophies are characterized by central yolk-like (vitelliform), yellow macular lesions (Figures 14-1 and 14-2). In patients with Best disease, the macular lesion progresses to cause scarring and atrophy, which contribute to vision loss. Most patients will maintain sufficient central visual acuity to read and drive but vision can decrease to the 20/200 range. AOVD typically results in metamorphopsia and mildly blurred vision with vision loss only occurring with atrophy and scarring. In both diseases, choroidal neovascular membranes (CNVM) may develop from macular scarring.[6,7] Best disease is diagnosed based on clinical examination, fluorescein angiography (FA), optical coherence tomography (OCT), and electro-oculogram (EOG). Patients with Best disease will have a light-to-dark Arden ratio of less than 1.5 on EOG. In contrast, patients with AOVD will have a near normal EOG with Arden ratio greater than 1.7.

In Best disease, the macular lesions evolve from a previtelliform stage to vitelliform stage to the "scrambled egg" stage with pseudohypopyon (Figure 14-1) to the atrophic stage. The macular OCT in Best disease demonstrates a dome-shaped, hyper-reflective,

Duker JS, Liang MC, eds.
Anti-VEGF Use in
Ophthalmology (pp. 151-165).
© 2017 Taylor & Francis Group.

Figure 14-1. Pseudohypopyon stage of Best disease. (A) Fundus photograph shows an elevated yellowish lesion in the macula. (B) Spectral domain-optical coherence tomography demonstrates a subfoveal lesion with elevation of the foveal contour and areas of both hyper-reflectivity and lucency. (Reprinted with permission from Jay S. Duker, MD.)

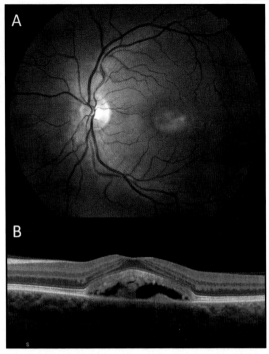

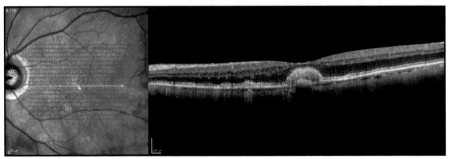

Figure 14-2. Vitelliform lesion of adult-onset vitelliform dystrophy. Spectral domain-optical coherence tomography image through the fovea shows a hyper-reflective subretinal deposit with resulting flattening of the foveal contour. (Reprinted with permission from Jay S. Duker, MD.)

and homogenous lesion located below the hyper-reflective photoreceptor layer.[8] In AOVD, the lesions are localized to the photoreceptor-retinal pigment epithelium complex. OCT also demonstrates a dome-shaped hyper-reflective lesion and there may be overlying loss of the photoreceptor layer (Figure 14-2).

There is no validated therapy for preventing the development of a vitelliform lesion or reducing the size of the subfoveal vitelliform deposit. The use of anti-vascular endothelial growth factor (VEGF) therapy for vitelliform macular dystrophy is limited to the treatment of choroidal neovascularization.[2] Anti-VEGF agents have been used to successfully treat CNVM secondary to Best disease in children as young as 6 years old.[9] In a case series of 11 eyes with CNVM secondary to AOVD treated with intravitreal bevacizumab, there was a reduction in foveal thickness but a guarded visual outcome.[10] Further studies are needed to determine the optimal choice of therapy and duration of treatment for CNVM secondary to vitelliform dystrophy.

Anti-VEGF treatment of vitelliform dystrophy macular lesions with associated vision loss but without evidence of CNVM has been reported with variable functional and anatomic responses. In 1 small case series of 6 patients, there was an improvement in visual acuity after 3 consecutive monthly injections of ranibizumab, but no improvement on OCT thickness analysis.[11] The lack of structural correlation to the functional findings is not consistent with the response to anti-VEGF therapy in multiple diseases studied in randomized clinical trials. In another case, 3 consecutive monthly injections of 0.5 mg intravitreal ranibizumab were given to treat a 72-year-old female patient with central vision loss secondary to AOVD.[12] There was no improvement in visual acuity or in the size of the vitelliform detachment as measured by spectral-domain (SD)-OCT. Currently, the treatment of Best disease or AOVD in the absence of CNVM is not justified by the medical literature.

Ocular Tumors

Malignant neoplasms can arise from primary sites in the eye or metastatic invasion from distant primary tumors. The most common primary intraocular malignancy in children is retinoblastoma and the most common primary intraocular malignancy in adults is uveal melanoma. However, metastatic cancer to the eye is the most common intraocular malignant neoplasm. A review of all intraocular tumors is beyond the scope of this chapter. We will briefly review those neoplasms for which anti-VEGF therapy has been studied and may have a role in the treatment paradigm including choroidal osteoma, capillary hemangioma of the retina, choroidal hemangioma, and choroidal metastasis.

Choroidal Osteoma

Choroidal osteoma is an uncommon, benign, acquired bony tumor of the choroid.[13,14] They typically appear in the second and third decades of life with more than 90% occurring in women. The typical choroidal osteoma is yellowish to orange, juxtapapillary or circumpapillary, and has well-defined margins (Figure 14-3[A]). Patients may present with painless, progressive loss of vision or the sudden onset of visual distortion. Visual acuity can be impaired if there is degeneration of the overlying photoreceptors and sensory retina or from the formation of a CNVM. The diagnosis of a choroidal osteoma is made based on fundus examination in combination with ancillary testing (Figure 14-3). B-scan ultrasonography demonstrates shadowing due to the composition of dense bone (Figure 14-3[C]) and computed tomography scan shows thickening of the posterior ocular wall that is isodense with normal skeletal bone.[13] Some patients may have hyperparathyroidism with alterations of serum calcium and phosphorus levels, but most patients have no systemic abnormalities.

CNVM secondary to choroidal osteomas can be treated with intravitreal anti-VEGF injection (Figure 14-4). This therapy is sometimes used in combination with focal laser photocoagulation or photodynamic therapy (PDT) depending on the location of the CNVM. In a series of 8 eyes in 8 patients with CNVM secondary to choroidal osteomas treated with monthly ranibizumab or bevacizumab with or without PDT, there was resolution of subretinal fluid on OCT in all but one patient.[15] Fifty percent of patients had a

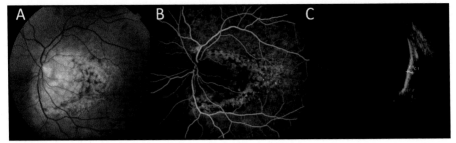

Figure 14-3. Choroidal neovascularization caused by choroidal osteoma. (A) Fundus photograph demonstrates a choroidal lesion extending from the optic nerve to the temporal macula with overlying pigment clumping and small retinal hemorrhages in the inferior macula. (B) Fluorescein angiogram shows patches of hyperfluorescence along the edge of the lesion and hypofluorescence caused by blockage from the pigment clumps. (C) B-scan ultrasonography reveals hyper-reflectivity and blocking consistent with calcification. (Reprinted with permission from Jay S. Duker, MD.)

Figure 14-4. Anti-VEGF treatment of choroidal neovascularization caused by choroidal osteoma. (A) Spectral domain-optical coherence tomography (SD-OCT) image shows a choroidal lesion with overlying subretinal fluid on presentation. (B) SD-OCT image after initial treatment with intravitreal bevacizumab shows a small reduction in subretinal fluid. (C) SD-OCT image after treatment with intravitreal aflibercept demonstrates elimination of subretinal fluid. (Reprinted with permission from Jay S. Duker, MD.)

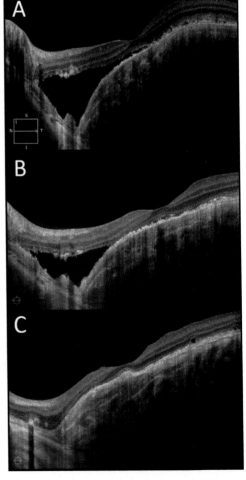

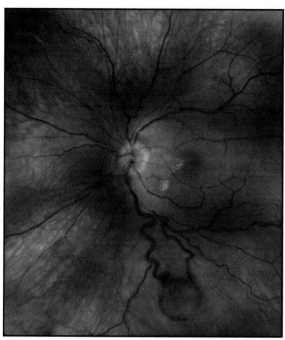

Figure 14-5. Retinal capillary hemangioma in a patient with von Hippel-Lindau syndrome. The classic spherical, elevated reddish lesion with large feeding and draining vessels is located inferior to the inferior arcade. There are exudates tracking into the macula. (Reprinted with permission from Jay S. Duker, MD.)

recurrence of exudation requiring further therapy. In this uncontrolled study, there was a modest increase in visual acuity at a mean of 32 months follow-up. Further studies are needed to determine the choice of anti-VEGF agents and optimum number of treatments for CNVM secondary to choroidal osteomas.

Capillary Hemangiomas of the Retina

The retinal capillary hemangioma is a benign vascular tumor that can arise from the retina or optic disc.[16] They may occur unilaterally or bilaterally and may be unifocal or multifocal, sometimes associated with von Hippel-Lindau syndrome.[17] The lesions tend to enlarge progressively and can lead to exudative or tractional retinal detachment. Capillary hemangiomas are uncommon but the exact frequency is not known. Most patients are diagnosed between the ages of 15 and 35.[17] The typical retinal capillary hemangioma appears as a reddish-orange, spherical lesion fed and drained by dilated tortuous retinal vessels (Figure 14-5). Intraretinal and subretinal exudation may surround the lesion and exudates may accumulate in the macula even when the lesion is located in the retinal periphery. Diagnosis can be made by dilated fundus examination in combination with ancillary testing. FA demonstrates rapid filling of the afferent artery, brisk filling of the tumor with intense hyperfluorescence, and rapid filling of the efferent vein.

The use of anti-VEGF therapy for the treatment of retinal capillary hemangiomas has been reported in small case series. In 1 study of 5 patients with retinal capillary hemangiomas associated with von Hippel-Lindau syndrome, patients received an average of 10 injections over an average period of 47 weeks.[18] The study concluded that anti-VEGF therapy had minimal beneficial effects on most lesions.[18] However, there was possible evidence of effect on a small lesion with less exudation, raising the question as to whether anti-VEGF therapy may be effective if given earlier in the disease course. Isolated case reports have demonstrated a reduction of tumor-associated exudation with intravitreal bevacizumab treatment in combination with PDT.[19,20] Further studies are needed to define the role of anti-VEGF therapy in the management of capillary hemangiomas of the retina.

Choroidal Hemangiomas

Choroidal hemangiomas are benign vascular tumors of the choroid.[21] There are 2 distinct forms: a circumscribed form that is isolated and not associated with a systemic syndrome, and a diffuse form that is associated with Sturge-Weber syndrome of encephalofacial hemangiomatosis.[22] Choroidal hemangiomas are uncommon and affect both sexes and all ethnic groups. The lesions are not hereditary but are probably congenital in most patients. Choroidal hemangiomas are typically not detected until the second to fourth decades of life. The visual impairment from both types of lesions can range from completely asymptomatic to total vision loss. The diffuse choroidal hemangioma is usually identified ipsilateral to the facial nevus flammeus in patients with Sturge-Weber syndrome.

There are case reports in the literature documenting the use of intravitreal anti-VEGF injections for the treatment of both circumscribed and diffuse choroidal hemangiomas. In 1 study, 9 patients with circumscribed choroidal hemangiomas were treated with intravitreal bevacizumab.[23] Five of the 9 patients were also treated with transpupillary thermotherapy and therefore the response to bevacizumab alone was not well defined. In another report, 3 patients with circumscribed choroidal hemangiomas were treated with bevacizumab with 2 patients treated in combination with PDT.[24] Other reports showed a response to PDT after an initial failure to respond to ranibizumab.[25] In a report of a diffuse choroidal hemangioma in a patient with Sturge-Weber syndrome, an associated exudative detachment was treated with intravitreal bevacizumab and found to resolve after 4 treatments over a 6-month period.[26] As there have been variable results with the studies published thus far, further research is needed to elucidate the role of anti-VEGF therapy alone or in combination with other treatments both for circumscribed choroidal hemangiomas and diffuse choroidal hemangiomas.

Metastatic Cancer

Metastatic cancer to the eye arises from the implantation of tumor cells spreading from another bodily organ or tissue.[27] There are estimates that 1% to 2.5% of all people have metastatic carcinoma in at least one eye at the time of death though many of these tumors may never be clinically apparent.[28] The most common site of metastatic invasion is the choroid, but metastases can also invade the iris, ciliary body, optic nerve, and retina.[29,30] The most common primary cancer to cause metastatic disease in the eye is breast cancer in women and lung cancer in men. Overall, the presence of metastasis to the eye bodes a poor prognosis for long-term survival.

Metastatic cancer to the eye can be detected by slit lamp and funduscopic examination. Typical metastatic choroidal tumors arising from the breast, lung, or gastrointestinal tract are yellow to white in color and round or oval in shape (Figure 14-6). They may also be associated with an overlying serous retinal detachment. B-scan ultrasonography typically demonstrates lesions with high internal reflectivity as compared to uveal melanomas.

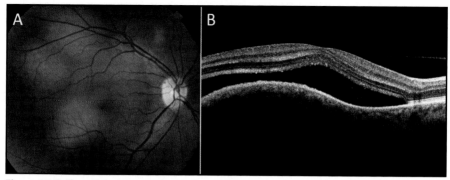

Figure 14-6. Choroidal metastases in a patient with metastatic lung cancer. (A) Fundus photography demonstrates multiple large, creamy, elevated choroidal lesions. (B) Spectral domain-optical coherence tomography through the macula reveals subretinal fluid and choroidal elevation from a metastatic lesion. (Reprinted with permission from Jay S. Duker, MD.)

Published studies are inconclusive on the role of anti-VEGF therapy in the treatment of metastatic cancer to the eye. In 1 series of 3 patients with choroidal metastases who developed vision loss during systemic chemotherapy, at least 2 doses of intravitreal bevacizumab were administered to the affected eye.[31] All 3 patients had improvement in vision, resolution of subretinal fluid, and regression of the choroidal tumor. Other case series have demonstrated similar results for the treatment of choroidal metastasis from cancers arising from the colon, lung, and breast with intravitreal anti-VEGF therapy often administered concurrently with systemic chemotherapy.[32-34] However, another case series of 5 patients with choroidal metastases from varying primary cancers demonstrated no observable response.[35] Four of the five tumors progressed despite intravitreal bevacizumab treatment. The authors concluded that intravitreal anti-VEGF therapy for choroidal metastasis alone is not recommended and should not delay more effective treatments. Others have argued, however, that intravitreal anti-VEGF agents must be given concurrently with systemic chemotherapy to be maximally effective.[36] The role of anti-VEGF therapy in the management of metastatic cancers to the eye requires further study before recommendations can be made on the choice, timing, and duration of treatment.

Radiation Retinopathy

Radiation retinopathy is a progressive occlusive vasculopathy caused by microvascular damage to retinal and choroidal vessels.[37-39] Radiation causes endothelial cell loss and capillary closure, which in turn can lead to macular edema, optic neuropathy, and neovascularization with a delayed onset after irradiation. Radiation retinopathy is a significant cause of visual morbidity in patients receiving radiation therapy for globe, orbit, head, and neck malignancies.[40] Clinically evident retinopathy most commonly occurs 6 months to 3 years after radiation. The diagnosis of radiation retinopathy is made by the presence of characteristic fundus findings in patients with a history of radiation exposure. The clinical course is similar to diabetic retinopathy with nonproliferative retinopathy, radiation maculopathy, and proliferative radiation retinopathy. Similar to diabetic retinopathy, radiation retinopathy may present with retinal hemorrhages, macular edema, hard exudates, cotton-wool spots, and vascular sheathing. In addition, widespread capillary nonperfusion may lead to proliferative radiation retinopathy. OCT and FA are the most useful diagnostic modalities to evaluate radiation retinopathy. OCT can quantitatively assess macular edema and the response to treatment, and FA can demonstrate retinal and disc neovascularization, capillary nonperfusion, and leakage consistent with macular edema.[38,41] FA can also differentiate between ischemic maculopathy in which there is little potential for visual recovery and nonischemic maculopathy.

VEGF has been implicated in the pathogenesis of radiation retinopathy.[42] There are multiple reports of radiation-induced macular edema, neovascularization, and optic neuropathy treated with intravitreal anti-VEGF therapy (Figures 14-7 and 14-8).[42-48] In an early case series, 6 patients with radiation retinopathy including retinal edema were treated with intravitreal bevacizumab every 6 to 8 weeks.[42] Reductions in retinal hemorrhages, exudates, cotton-wool spots, and macular edema were noted. All patients had stabilization or improvement of visual acuity. Other reports suggest the prompt diagnosis of radiation maculopathy by SD-OCT may help maintain functional visual acuity by initiating early treatment with bevacizumab[49] and that treatment with a single anti-VEGF agent may induce tachyphylaxis and switching to an alternative anti-VEGF medication may decrease persistent edema and improve vision.[50] Nonetheless, not all patients improve with anti-VEGF therapy alone and visual acuity outcomes may be limited, especially when the radiation treatment directly targeted a macular lesion. Other studies suggest there may be a role for anti-VEGF therapy in combination with intravitreal steroids.[51,52] These reports point to a role for anti-VEGF therapy in the treatment of radiation retinopathy but further studies are needed to compare the available anti-VEGF agents and determine the optimum frequency and duration of treatment. Given the pathologic similarities between diabetic retinopathy and radiation retinopathy, future studies are needed to determine if there are differences in outcomes between the available anti-VEGF agents as studies suggest for the treatment of diabetic macular edema.[53]

Other reports have examined the role for anti-VEGF therapy to prevent or delay the onset of radiation retinopathy after radiation treatment. A large, retrospective, nonrandomized study evaluated prophylactic treatment with intravitreal bevacizumab for the prevention of macular edema by OCT and clinically evident radiation retinopathy.[54] Patients treated for uveal melanoma with plaque brachytherapy were given an initial dose of intravitreal bevacizumab at the time of plaque removal and then 6 additional doses every 4 months until year 2. A control group with a similar median dose of foveolar radiation was chosen for comparison. At 2 years, there were significantly reduced rates of OCT-evident macular edema, clinically evident radiation retinopathy, moderate vision loss, and poor visual acuity.[54] Future prospective studies should further elucidate the role of anti-VEGF therapy to prevent or delay the onset of radiation retinopathy in these patients.

Sickle Cell Retinopathy

Sickle cell disease is caused by mutations in hemoglobin, an iron-containing globular protein in red blood cells that transports oxygen.[55] If the hemoglobin is mutated at the sixth position of the beta chain from the amino acid glutamic acid to valine, hemoglobin S is formed. A mutation from glutamic acid to lysine in the same position results in hemoglobin C. Decreased synthesis of hemoglobin causes thalassemia (Thal). The hemoglobin SS genotype causes more severe systemic disease while the hemoglobin SC and S-Thal genotypes are associated with more severe ocular manifestations.[56,57] Sickle

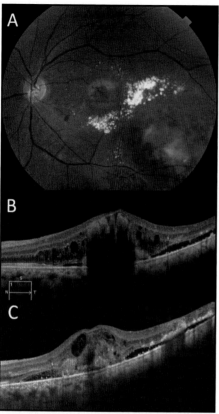

Figure 14-7. Radiation retinopathy treated with anti-vascular endothelial growth factor therapy. The affected eye was treated for a choroidal melanoma by gamma knife stereotactic radiotherapy. The patient developed radiation retinopathy 14 months after treatment. (A) Fundus photograph shows the choroidal melanoma in the temporal macula with exudates encroaching into the fovea and macular hemorrhages. (B) Spectral domain-optical coherence tomography image through the macula demonstrates intraretinal and subretinal fluid with intraretinal hyper-reflective material. (C) Spectral domain-optical coherence tomography image through the macula after multiple intravitreal anti-vascular endothelial growth factor therapy treatments including intravitreal bevacizumab and ranibizumab. The patient had no improvement in vision. (Reprinted with permission from Jay S. Duker, MD.)

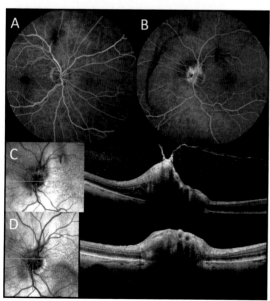

Figure 14-8. Radiation optic neuropathy before and after treatment with intravitreal bevacizumab. (A) Fluorescein angiogram of the right eye demonstrates no evidence of optic disc hyperfluorescence. (B) Fluorescein angiogram of the left eye shows hyperfluorescence of the optic disc with leakage consistent with neovascularization. (C) Spectral domain-optical coherence tomography image of the optic nerve in the left eye demonstrates edema with neovascularization of the optic disc. (D) Spectral domain-optical coherence tomography image of the optic nerve in the left eye 2 months after treatment with intravitreal bevacizumab reveals reduced edema and no neovascularization.

cell retinopathy is caused by the occlusion of small retinal vessels by sickled erythrocytes under hypoxic conditions. In patients with the SC genotype, approximately 40% to 43% will develop proliferative sickle cell retinopathy as compared to 14% to 20% of patients with the SS genotype.[56,57]

Sickle cell retinopathy occurs because of vaso-occlusion and retinal nonperfusion.[55] Vascular occlusion can cause retinal hemorrhages termed *salmon patches* for their orange-red color, and patients may experience decreased visual acuity if the occlusion occurs in perifoveal capillaries. Occlusions in the choroidal circulation may cause breaks in Bruch's membrane, which appear as angioid streaks. Chronic hypoxia and ischemia leads to the upregulation of vascular growth factors including VEGF and can lead to neo-vascularization, vitreous hemorrhage, and tractional retinal detachment (Figure 14-9). FA is the most useful diagnostic modality to evaluate capillary nonperfusion, ischemia, and neovascularization. OCT can also document macular atrophy caused by occlusive vasculopathy.

There are limited case reports documenting the use of intravitreal anti-VEGF medi-cations to treat proliferative sickle cell retinopathy. The first case report described a patient with proliferative sickle cell retinopathy with neovascularization and vitreous hemorrhage.[58] The patient declined vitrectomy and was given an injection of intravitreal bevacizumab. His vision improved from 20/60 to 20/20, the neovascularization regressed, and the vitreous hemorrhage cleared by 4 weeks postinjection. Similar findings were noted in a patient with sea fan neovascularization and vitreous hemorrhage treated with 1 intravitreal ranibizumab; exam findings were stable after 6 months of follow-up.[59] In another report, intravitreal bevacizumab was administered prior to planned vitrectomy for the management of tractional retinal detachment due to proliferative disease, and the authors found a subjective reduction in the expected amount of intraoperative hemor-rhage.[60] It is difficult to draw any conclusions from these uncontrolled reports as retinal neovascularization and vitreous hemorrhage may spontaneously clear in some patients without these therapies. The current preferred treatment modality for proliferative sickle cell retinopathy remains to be scatter laser photocoagulation, but additional studies are needed to determine the role of anti-VEGF therapy.

Retinal Artery Macroaneurysm

A retinal artery macroaneurysm (RAM) is an acquired, focal dilation of a retinal artery branch. RAMs are saccular or fusiform in shape and range in size from 100 μm to 250 μm in diameter, which differentiates them from capillary microaneurysms that are less than 100 μm. RAMs can cause vision loss when there is associated macular edema, end-arteriole occlusion from thrombosis, or hemorrhage due to rupture of the aneu-rysm.[61] The aneurysms form at the site of atherosclerotic damage to a vessel wall, which predisposes to vessel dilation. They most commonly occur in patients over 60 years of age and are more common in women.[62] Hypertension and other arteriolar risk factors are the primary cause.[62] Diagnosis is made by fundoscopic examination in conjunction with FA and OCT.

There are limited studies examining the benefits of intravitreal anti-VEGF therapy for symptomatic RAM (Figure 14-10). In a retrospective study comparing untreated patients to those treated with intravitreal bevacizumab for symptomatic RAM, the eyes treated with bevacizumab had a greater reduction in macular edema at one month postinjec-tion, but the final visual acuity and macular thickness were not significantly different

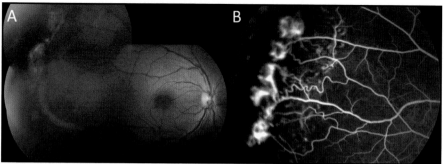

Figure 14-9. Sickle cell retinopathy in a patient with S-Thalassemia disease. (A) Mosaic fundus photograph demonstrates retinal hemorrhage temporal to the macula with elevated preretinal hemorrhage and temporal neovascularization. (B) Fluorescein angiogram of the temporal periphery shows leakage at the edge of retinal capillary nonperfusion consistent with sea fan neovascularization. (Reprinted with permission from Elias Reichel, MD.)

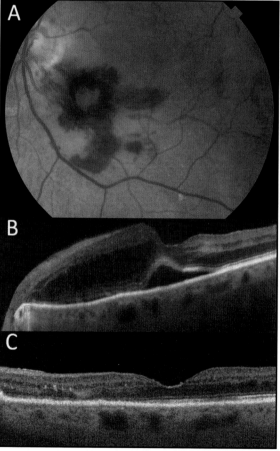

Figure 14-10. Retinal artery macroaneurysm with associated macular edema treated with intravitreal anti-vascular endothelial growth factor therapy. (A) Fundus photograph demonstrates retinal hemorrhage extending from the retinal artery macroaneurysm. (B) Spectral domain-optical coherence tomography image of the macula reveals intraretinal and subretinal fluid. (C) Spectral domain-optical coherence tomography image after treatment with intravitreal bevacizumab shows elimination of intraretinal and subretinal fluid. (Reprinted with permission from Michelle C. Liang, MD.)

in the treated and untreated groups.[63] In another uncontrolled study of 38 eyes with symptomatic RAM treated with 3 consecutive monthly doses of intravitreal bevacizumab, the macular edema resolved in all patients at 4 months and the average visual acuity improved.[64] Intravitreal anti-VEGF therapy may have a role in the treatment of symptomatic RAM with macular edema, but further controlled studies are needed to compare with observation and laser photocoagulation to determine the optimal treatment paradigm.

Conclusions

The evidence for the role of anti-VEGF therapy in miscellaneous retinal and choroidal diseases is varied. The role of anti-VEGF therapy for Best disease, AOVD, and choroidal osteoma is currently limited to those cases complicated by CNVM. The use of anti-VEGF therapy for ocular tumors including retinal capillary hemangiomas, choroidal hemangiomas, and choroidal metastases warrants further study as there are conflicting reports in the literature for each of these tumors. There are limited studies to support the routine use of anti-VEGF therapy for sickle cell retinopathy; however, there does seem to be a role for anti-VEGF therapy in the treatment of radiation retinopathy and retinal artery macroaneurysms. Overall, the low prevalence of these "miscellaneous" ocular disorders limits our evidence for use of anti-VEGF treatments to case reports and a few retrospective case series. It is hoped that further research and experience will be gathered to better elucidate the indications and benefits of treatment.

References

1. O'Gorman S, Flaherty WA, Fishman GA, Berson EL. Histopathologic findings in Best's vitelliform macular dystrophy. *Arch Ophthalmol.* 1988;106(9):1261-1268.

2. Chowers I, Tiosano L, Audo I, Grunin M, Boon CJ. Adult-onset foveomacular vitelliform dystrophy: a fresh perspective. *Prog Retin Eye Res.* 2015;47:64-85.

3. Stone EM, Nichols BE, Streb LM, Kimura AE, Sheffield VC. Genetic linkage of vitelliform macular degeneration (Best's disease) to chromosome 11q13. *Nat Genet.* 1992;1:246-250.

4. Bakall B, Marknell T, Ingvast S, et al. The mutation spectrum of the bestrophin protein—functional implications. *Hum Genet.* 1999;104(5):383-389.

5. Felbor U, Schilling H, Weber BH. Adult vitelliform macular dystrophy is frequently associated with mutations in the peripherin/RDS gene. *Hum Mutat.* 1997;10(4):301-309.

6. Ergun E, Costa D, Slakter J, Yannuzzi LA, Stur M. Photodynamic therapy and vitelliform lesions. *Retina.* 2004;24(3):399-406.

7. Mohler CW, Fine SL. Long-term evaluation of patients with Best's vitelliform dystrophy. *Ophthalmology.* 1981;88(7):688-692.

8. Ferrara DC, Costa RA, Tsang S, Calucci D, Jorge R, Freund KB. Multimodal fundus imaging in Best vitelliform macular dystrophy. *Graefes Arch Clin Exp Ophthalmol.* 2010;248:1377-1386.

9. Iannaccone A, Kerr NC, Kinnick TR, Calzada JI, Stone EM. Autosomal recessive best vitelliform macular dystrophy: report of a family and management of early-onset neovascular complications. *Arch Ophthalmol.* 2011;129:211-217.

10. Tiosano L, Jaouni T, Averbukh E, Grunin M, Banin E, Chowers I. Bevacizumab treatment for choroidal neovascularization associated with adult-onset foveomacular vitelliform dystrophy. *Eur J Ophthalmol.* 2014;24:890-896.

11. Gallego-Pinazo R, Dolz-Marco R, Pardo-López D, Arevalo JF, Díaz-Llopis M. Primary intravitreal ranibizumab for adult-onset foveomacular vitelliform dystrophy. *Graefes Arch Clin Exp Ophthalmol.* 2011;249(3):455-458.

12. Kandula S, Zweifel S, Freund KB. Adult-onset vitelliform detachment unresponsive to monthly intravitreal ranibizumab. *Ophthalmic Surg Lasers Imaging.* 2010;41(Suppl):S81-S84.

13. Shields CL, Shields JA, Augsburger JJ. Choroidal osteoma. *Surv Ophthalmol.* 1988;33(1):17-27.

14. Shields CL, Sun H, Demirci H, Shields JA. Factors predictive of tumor growth, tumor decalcification, choroidal neovascularization, and visual outcome in 74 eyes with choroidal osteoma. *Arch Ophthalmol.* 2005;123:1658-1666.

15. Khan MA, DeCroos FC, Storey PP, Shields JA, Garg SJ, Shields CL. Outcomes of anti-vascular endothelial growth factor therapy in the management of choroidal neovascularization associated with choroidal osteoma. *Retina.* 2014;34:1750-1756.

16. Schmidt D, Neumann HP. Retinal vascular hamartoma in von Hippel-Lindau disease. *Arch Ophthalmol.* 1995;113:1163-1167.

17. Hardwig P, Robertson DM. von Hippel-Lindau disease: a familial, often lethal, multi-system phakomatosis. *Ophthalmology.* 1984;91(3):263-270.

18. Wong WT, Liang KJ, Hammel K, Coleman HR, Chew EY. Intravitreal ranibizumab therapy for retinal capillary hemangioblastoma related to von Hippel-Lindau disease. *Ophthalmology.* 2008;115:1957-1964.

19. Mennel S, Meyer CH, Callizo J. Combined intravitreal anti-vascular endothelial growth factor (Avastin) and photodynamic therapy to treat retinal juxtapapillary capillary haemangioma. *Acta Ophthalmol.* 2010;88(5):610-613.

20. Ziemssen F, Voelker M, Inhoffen W, Bartz-Schmidt KU, Gelisken F. Combined treatment of a juxtapapillary retinal capillary haemangioma with intravitreal bevacizumab and photodynamic therapy. *Eye (Lond).* 2007;21(8):1125-1126.

21. Anand R, Augsburger JJ, Shields JA. Circumscribed choroidal hemangiomas. *Arch Ophthalmol.* 1989;107:1338-1342.

22. Witschel H, Font RL. Hemangioma of the choroid. A clinicopathologic study of 71 cases and a review of the literature. *Surv Ophthalmol.* 1976;20(6):415-431.

23. Kwon HJ, Kim M, Lee CS, Lee SC. Treatment of serous macular detachment associated with circumscribed choroidal hemangioma. *Am J Ophthalmol.* 2012;154:137-145.e1.

24. Sagong M, Lee J, Chang W. Application of intravitreal bevacizumab for circumscribed choroidal hemangioma. *Korean J Ophthalmol.* 2009;23:127-131.

25. Chan LW, Hsieh YT. Photodynamic therapy for choroidal hemangioma unresponsive to ranibizumab. *Optom Vis Sci.* 2014;91(9):e226-e229.

26. Bach A, Gold AS, Villegas VM, Wildner AC, Ehlies FJ, Murray TG. Spontaneous exudative retinal detachment in a patient with Sturge-Weber syndrome after taking arginine, a supplement for erectile dysfunction. *Eye Vis (Lond).* 2014;1:7.

27. Arepalli S, Kaliki S, Shields CL. Choroidal metastases: origin, features, and therapy. *Indian J Ophthalmol.* 2015;63:122-127.

28. Nelson CC, Hertzberg BS, Klintworth GK. A histopathologic study of 716 unselected eyes in patients with cancer at the time of death. *Am J Ophthalmol.* 1983;95:788-793.

29. Shields CL, Kaliki S, Crabtree GS, et al. Iris metastasis from systemic cancer in 104 patients: the 2014 Jerry A. Shields Lecture. *Cornea.* 2015;34:42-48.

30. Shields CL, McMahon JF, Atalay HT, Hasanreisoglu M, Shields JA. Retinal metastasis from systemic cancer in 8 cases. *JAMA Ophthalmol.* 2014;132(11):1303-1308.

31. Fenicia V, Abdolrahimzadeh S, Mannino G, Verrilli S, Balestrieri M, Recupero SM. Intravitreal bevacizumab in the successful management of choroidal metastases secondary to lung and breast cancer unresponsive to systemic therapy: a case series. *Eye (Lond).* 2014;28:888-891.

32. Augustine H, Munro M, Adatia F, Webster M, Fielden M. Treatment of ocular metastasis with anti-VEGF: a literature review and case report. *Can J Ophthalmol.* 2014;49(5):458-463.

33. Detorakis ET, Agorogiannis G, Drakonaki EE, Tsilimbaris MK, Pallikaris IG. Successful management of choroidal metastasis with intravitreal ranibizumab injections. *Ophthalmic Surg Lasers Imaging.* 2012;43(Online):e47-e51.

34. Kuo IC, Haller JA, Maffrand R, Sambuelli RH, Reviglio VE. Regression of a subfoveal choroidal metastasis of colorectal carcinoma after intravitreous bevacizumab treatment. *Arch Ophthalmol.* 2008;126:1311-1313.

35. Maudgil A, Sears KS, Rundle PA, Rennie IG, Salvi SM. Failure of intravitreal bevacizumab in the treatment of choroidal metastasis. *Eye (Lond).* 2015;29:707-711.

36. Singh N, Bansal R, Behera D, Gupta A. Intravitreal bevacizumab for choroidal metastases: the key to efficacy is simultaneous administration of systemic therapy. *Eye (Lond).* 2015;29:1629.

37. Midena E, Segato T, Valenti M, Degli Angeli C, Bertoja E, Piermarocchi S. The effect of external eye irradiation on choroidal circulation. *Ophthalmology.* 1996;103:1651-1660.

38. Brown GC, Shields JA, Sanborn G, Augsburger JJ, Savino PJ, Schatz NJ. Radiation retinopathy. *Ophthalmology.* 1982;89(12):1494-1501.

39. Archer DB. Doyne Lecture. Responses of retinal and choroidal vessels to ionising radiation. *Eye (Lond).* 1993;7(Pt 1):1-13.

40. Reichstein D. Current treatments and preventive strategies for radiation retinopathy. *Curr Opin Ophthalmol.* 2015;26:157-166.

41. Gündüz K, Shields CL, Shields JA, Cater J, Freire JE, Brady LW. Radiation retinopathy following plaque radiotherapy for posterior uveal melanoma. *Arch Ophthalmol.* 1999;117(5):609-614.

42. Finger PT, Chin K. Anti-vascular endothelial growth factor bevacizumab (Avastin) for radiation retinopathy. *Arch Ophthalmol.* 2007;125:751-756.

43. Finger PT, Chin KJ. Intravitreous ranibizumab (Lucentis) for radiation maculopathy. *Arch Ophthalmol.* 2010;128:249-252.

44. Gupta A, Muecke JS. Treatment of radiation maculopathy with intravitreal injection of bevacizumab (Avastin). *Retina.* 2008;28(7):964-968.

45. Mason JO III, Albert MA Jr, Persaud TO, Vail RS. Intravitreal bevacizumab treatment for radiation macular edema after plaque radiotherapy for choroidal melanoma. Retina. 2007;27(7):903-907.

46. Finger PT. Anti-VEGF bevacizumab (Avastin) for radiation optic neuropathy. *Am J Ophthalmol.* 2007;143:335-338.

47. Arriola-Villalobos P, Donate-López J, Calvo-González C, Reche-Frutos J, Alejandre-Alba N, Díaz-Valle D. Intravitreal bevacizumab (Avastin) for radiation retinopathy neovascularization. *Acta Ophthalmol.* 2008;86(1):115-116.

48. Yeung SN, Paton KE, Waite C, Maberley DA. Intravitreal bevacizumab for iris neovascularization following proton beam irradiation for choroidal melanoma. *Can J Ophthalmol.* 2010;45:269-273.

49. Shah NV, Houston SK, Markoe AM, Feuer W, Murray TG. Early SD-OCT diagnosis followed by prompt treatment of radiation maculopathy using intravitreal bevacizumab maintains functional visual acuity. *Clin Ophthalmol.* 2012;6:1739-1748.

50. Jutley G, Shona OA, Leen RC, Lee N, Olver JM, George SM. Response to ranibizumab following tachyphylaxis to bevacizumab in a patient with radiation maculopathy following stereotactic fractionated radiotherapy for optic nerve meningioma. *Arch Ophthalmol.* 2012;130:1466-1470.

51. Bakri SJ, Larson TA. The variable efficacy of intravitreal bevacizumab and triamcinolone acetonide for cystoid macular edema due to radiation retinopathy. *Semin Ophthalmol.* 2015;30:276-280.

52. Shah NV, Houston SK, Markoe A, Murray TG. Combination therapy with triamcinolone acetonide and bevacizumab for the treatment of severe radiation maculopathy in patients with posterior uveal melanoma. *Clin Ophthalmol.* 2013;7:1877-1882.

53. Wells JA, Glassman AR, Ayala AR, et al. Aflibercept, bevacizumab, or ranibizumab for diabetic macular edema: two-year results from a comparative effectiveness randomized clinical trial. *Ophthalmology.* 2016;123(6):1351-1359.

54. Shah SU, Shields CL, Bianciotto CG, et al. Intravitreal bevacizumab at 4-month intervals for prevention of macular edema after plaque radiotherapy of uveal melanoma. *Ophthalmology.* 2014;121:269-275.

55. Elagouz M, Jyothi S, Gupta B, Sivaprasad S. Sickle cell disease and the eye: old and new concepts. *Surv Ophthalmol.* 2010;55:359-377.

56. Downes SM, Hambleton IR, Chuang EL, Lois N, Serjeant GR, Bird AC. Incidence and natural history of proliferative sickle cell retinopathy: observations from a cohort study. *Ophthalmology.* 2005;112:1869-1875.

57. Fox PD, Dunn DT, Morris JS, Serjeant GR. Risk factors for proliferative sickle retinopathy. *Br J Ophthalmol.* 1990;74:172-176.

58. Siqueira RC, Costa RA, Scott IU, Cintra LP, Jorge R. Intravitreal bevacizumab (Avastin) injection associated with regression of retinal neovascularization caused by sickle cell retinopathy. *Acta Ophthalmol Scand.* 2006;84(6):834-835.

59. Mitropoulos PG, Chatziralli IP, Parikakis EA, Peponis VG, Amariotakis GA, Moschos MM. Intravitreal ranibizumab for stage IV proliferative sickle cell retinopathy: a first case report. *Case Rep Ophthalmol Med.* 2014;2014:682583.

60. Moshiri A, Ha NK, Ko FS, Scott AW. Bevacizumab presurgical treatment for proliferative sickle-cell retinopathy-related retinal detachment. *Retin Cases Brief Rep.* 2013;7(3):204-205.

61. Moosavi RA, Fong KC, Chopdar A. Retinal artery macroaneurysms: clinical and fluorescein angiographic features in 34 patients. *Eye (Lond).* 2006;20:1011-1020.

62. Panton RW, Goldberg MF, Farber MD. Retinal arterial macroaneurysms: risk factors and natural history. *Br J Ophthalmol.* 1990;74:595-600.

63. Cho HJ, Rhee TK, Kim HS, et al. Intravitreal bevacizumab for symptomatic retinal arterial macroaneurysm. *Am J Ophthalmol.* 2013;155:898-904.

64. Pichi F, Morara M, Torrazza C, et al. Intravitreal bevacizumab for macular complications from retinal arterial macroaneurysms. *Am J Ophthalmol.* 2013;155(2):287-294.

15

Neovascular Glaucoma

Manik Goel, MD and Joel S. Schuman, MD, FACS

Neovascular glaucoma (NVG), a form of secondary angle closure glaucoma, is characterized by the development of new vessels in the anterior segment, namely the iris and anterior chamber angle. The inciting event for new vessel formation and NVG is believed to be retinal hypoxia of any cause. The growth of new vessels leads to the formation of fibrovascular membranes across the anterior chamber angle and subsequently synechial angle closure and elevated intraocular pressure (IOP). NVG can be refractory to treatment and optimal control of IOP is often difficult. The lack of adequate IOP control puts the patient at risk of rapid and severe vision loss; thus, timely recognition and treatment of NVG is critical in preserving useful vision for the patient. Many different treatment modalities have been used in IOP management, including topical and oral hypotensives, cyclophotocoagulation, and filtering surgery. Recently, with the recognition of the role of angiopoietic factors like vascular endothelial growth factor (VEGF) in the pathogenesis of NVG, anti-VEGF agents are being used to achieve better outcomes.

Epidemiology and Pathogenesis

Angiogenesis is the formation of new blood vessels from existing blood vessels. The process of angiogenesis has an important physiologic role in growth, reproduction, and repair after injury.[1] Aberrant angiogenesis plays a critical part in pathological conditions both systemic, like tumor growth and metastases,[2,3] and pertaining to the eye, like diabetic retinopathy, age-related macular degeneration, and retinopathy of prematurity.[4-6] VEGF is involved both in physiologic and aberrant angiogenesis;[2-6] hypoxic tissues upregulate VEGF transcription to promote new vessel formation and maintain an adequate supply of essential nutrients.[7,8] As intravitreal administration of anti-VEGF agents have been highly successful in treating ocular neovascular disorders like proliferative diabetic retinopathy and neovacular age-related macular degeneration, they are also being used with good results in the treatment of neovascular glaucoma.

Duker JS, Liang MC, eds.
Anti-VEGF Use in
Ophthalmology (pp. 167-176).
© 2017 Taylor & Francis Group.

Coats provided the first description of iris neovascularization (NVI) in 1906 in patients with central retinal vein occlusion.[9] Weiss et al[10] later coined the term *neovascular glaucoma*. The primary factor responsible for NVI and the development of NVG is retinal hypoxia (97% of cases). The other 3% is secondary to intraocular inflammation without associated retinal ischemia.[11] The 3 most common causes of NVG are central retinal vein occlusion (36%), proliferative diabetic retinopathy (32%), and ocular ischemic syndrome (13%) (Table 15-1).[11] In these patients, hypoxia or ischemia induces increased expression of proangiogenic factors like VEGF from the retina.[12] VEGF then diffuses into the anterior segment, causing neovascularization of the iris and angle. This rate is increased in patients after removal of the crystalline lens and even more in those without an intact posterior capsule.[13-15] Elevated levels of VEGF have been detected in the aqueous humor and vitreous of patients with NVG.[16,17] It is reported to be 40 and 113 times higher than that of primary open-angle glaucoma and cataract patients, respectively.[12,16]

Many chemokines, other than VEGF, have also been suspected to play a part in angiogenesis. These substances include insulin-like growth factors I and II,[18] platelet-derived growth factor,[19] and basic fibroblast growth factor.[13] Inflammatory mediators such as angiopoietin 1 and 2 also play a role in new vessel formation.[20] At present, the evidence for the role of these other mediators is not as strongly established as for VEGF. However, with more research, the pathway for ocular angiogenesis is being elucidated in more detail and the role of other factors will become more obvious. This may lead to the development of new, more-effective therapeutic agents to target the angiogenic cascade.

Ocular Manifestations and Diagnosis

It is critical to identify and diagnose NVG at the earliest stage to give the patient the best chance at preserving vision. The clinician must have a high index of suspicion in any patient presenting with high IOP and risk factors as outlined in Table 15-1.

NVG is a clinical diagnosis. It is important to obtain a detailed history (including systemic risk factors and history of recent surgeries). A thorough slit lamp examination is warranted in any patient at risk for developing NVG. It is helpful to start with a nondilated pupil to identify new vessels at the pupil margin and perform gonioscopy. However, the importance of performing a dilated posterior segment exam to look for signs of retinal ischemia cannot be overemphasized.

Neovascularization of the anterior segment usually starts with fine vascular tufts at the pupillary margin that then extend radially across the iris surface toward the angle. As the vessels continue to proliferate, they grow across the angle recess extending from the root of the iris to the ciliary body band, scleral spur, and trabecular meshwork. This imparts the characteristic reddish hue to the angle seen in patients with NVG. Although initially the angle may appear open on gonioscopy, the growth of this fibrovascular membrane across the angle impedes aqueous outflow and IOP begins to rise. Eventually, myofibroblasts in the fibrovascular membrane contract causing contracture of the membrane and synechial angle closure.[21] Corneal endothelial proliferation may also occur across the angle recess.[22] At this point, patients may present with severe pain, markedly elevated IOP, and loss of vision. In addition, anterior chamber examination may reveal cells and flare with or without hyphema or ectropion uveae from radial traction on the iris pulling the posterior pigmented epithelial layer of the iris anteriorly. Aqueous humor dynamics[23] dictates that neovascularization makes its first appearance at the pupillary

Table 15-1. Disorders Predisposing to Rubeosis

Vasculopathies Affecting the Eye

- Diabetic retinopathy
- Central retinal vein occlusion
- Central retinal artery occlusion
- Branch retinal vein occlusion
- Coats disease
- Eales disease
- Retinopathy of prematurity
- Sickle cell retinopathy
- Persistent fetal vasculature
- Inflammatory or infectious retinal vasculitis

Systemic Vascular Disorders

- Ocular ischemic syndrome
- Carotid-cavernous fistula
- Carotid artery ligation
- Giant cell arteritis
- Takayasu arteritis

Other Ocular Disorders

- Chronic uveitis
- Endophthalmitis
- Retinal detachment
- Stickler syndrome
- Leber congenital amaurosis
- X-linked retinoschisis

Tumors

- Retinoblastoma
- Intraocular lymphoma
- Uveal melanoma
- Metastatic carcinoma

Ocular Therapy

- External beam radiation
- Radioactive plaques
- Charged particle therapy
- Scleral buckle

Trauma

margin; however, NVG may occur without NVI in 6% to 12% of cases of central retinal vein occlusion.[24-26]

Studying pupillary reactions can help predict the development of rubeosis. Research has shown that patients with central retinal vein occlusion with a relative afferent pupillary defect ≥ 0.6 log units have high sensitivity and specificity in predicting the development of rubeosis.[27] Although NVG is a clinical diagnosis, ancillary investigative modalities like angiography and electroretinography can be helpful in detecting subclinical cases.[12,28] Iris fluorescein angiography is able to detect NVI in 97% of eyes and in 36% of eyes before being clinically evident.[29] Fluorescein angiography of the angle with the Goldmann gonioscopy lens (fluorescein gonioangiography) may be useful in the diagnosis and management of NVG,[30] allowing clinicians to follow vascularization both before and after treatment of retinal ischemia. Electroretinography has been proposed as a surrogate marker to assess retinal ischemia and predict the likelihood of developing rubeosis in patients with central retinal vein occlusion.[31] However, there is a lack of consensus on what electroretinogram parameter (30 Hz implicit time, R_{max}, b/a wave ratio) is the best predictor for retinal ischemia.[31,32] In one study, the average b/a wave ratio in cases in which NVG developed was 0.84 and greater than 1 when this complication did not develop.[31] The use of iris angiography, gonioangiography, and electroretinogram may be helpful in predicting, and early detection, of rubeosis but their role needs to be validated further in controlled studies before they can be recommended for routine use in these patients.

Treatment

To ensure a successful outcome and to preserve maximal vision, it is crucial to identify NVG and institute treatment early on. Timely intervention can prevent synechial angle closure and a blind painful eye. Treatment of NVG has 2 critical aims: first, the underlying disease process driving the angiogenic cascade and second, controlling the intraocular pressure.[12]

Ischemic retina is responsible for producing pro-angiogenic factors like VEGF in the vast majority of NVG cases. Primary treatment of rubeosis is thus directed at the retina. Panretinal photocoagulation (PRP) is the current gold-standard treatment for almost all NVG patients and is recommended at the earliest sign of rubeosis. PRP reduces the stimulus for VEGF production by destroying the ischemic retina responsible for VEGF production.[33,34] It leads to the reduction of VEGF levels,[35] regression of new vessels in both the anterior and posterior segments,[30,36] and normalization of IOP in up to 42% of patients.[30] The improvement in IOP is more likely true for patients who have not yet suffered from angle closure due to fibrovascular membrane formation. PRP also improves the success rate of subsequent filtering surgeries.[37]

In patients with cloudy media or poor visualization of the retina, panretinal cryotherapy or transscleral diode laser photocoagulation may be performed. Panretinal cryotherapy has been shown to be equally effective as laser in controlling rubeosis.[38] It also leads to relief of pain and regression of anterior chamber inflammation in 93.5% of patients.[39] Some authors recommend anterior retinal cryotherapy in eyes with media opacities as a preliminary procedure for filtering surgery in eyes with NVG. Other studies have reported similar success with panretinal cryotherapy.[40,41] Another methodology, transscleral diode laser photocoagulation, also ablates peripheral retina and can be used in eyes with poor visualization preventing PRP. Reports in the literature show control and regression of rubeosis with diode laser photocoagulation.[42,43]

Although retinal ablative procedures are crucial in eliminating the source of vasoproliferative factors, these treatments lead to death of retinal cells and cause permanent visual field defects.[44] Treatment with anti-VEGF agents, however, can both regress neovascularization and preserve retinal function. Furthermore, it can be performed in eyes with no view to the posterior segment. Its use in the management of NVG is early, although encouraging. Bevacizumab has been used most commonly and is given intravit-really in the same dose as used to treat diseases of the posterior segment.

PRP and other retinal ablative procedures cause regression of new vessels in the angle and help control IOP. However, most patients will need additional medical or surgical treatment to provide adequate control. Pharmacotherapy with beta-blockers, alpha ago-nists, and carbonic anhydrase inhibitors is used to further decrease IOP. Prostaglandin analogs may also be used, but their efficacy can be limited because of decreased access of the aqueous to the uveoscleral pathway.[12] Miotics are best avoided because of the risk of enticing intraocular inflammation in eyes with an already compromised blood aqueous barrier. In addition, miotics may worsen synechial angle closure and thus IOP control. Other topical treatments include topical steroids to help improve intraocular inflamma-tion and cycloplegic drops to increase uveoscleral outflow. Both steroids and cyclopegics may also help with improving patient comfort.

In a significant percentage of patients, medical therapy alone will not provide adequate long-term IOP control. In these patients, additional intervention is needed and the choice of treatment may be guided by the visual potential of the patient. Patients with useful visual potential are usually treated with glaucoma-filtering surgeries (trabeculectomy or glaucoma drainage implant surgery); patients with poor visual potential often undergo cyclodestructive procedures.

Trabeculectomy or glaucoma drainage implant surgery in patients with NVG should be preceded by PRP to improve success rates. In general, trabeculectomies have a poorer success rate in NVG. Attempts have been made to improve outcomes with use of antime-tabolites such as 5-fluorouracil and mitomycin-C (MMC).[45,46] However, the long-term outcomes still remain poor. One reason for this is hemorrhage at the time of surgery and/or in the postoperative period.[45,47] Judicious use of cautery during the surgery to achieve hemostasis is recommended, and some authors advise direct cauterization of the periph-eral iris before performing iridectomy. Other risk factors associated with a poor surgical outcome after trabeculectomy include younger age, prior pars plana vitrectomy, type 1 diabetes, and extensive peripheral anterior synechiae.[45,47,48] The success rate 2 to 3 years after trabeculectomy with MMC in NVG patients is reported to be 61%.[47]

As our understanding of the pathophysiology of NVG has improved and the role of VEGF in the disease has been better defined, anti-VEGF agents are being used as adjuncts to trabeculectomy.[49-52] The use of intravitreal bevacizumab prior to trabeculec-tomy has been reported to decrease postoperative hyphema and improve IOP outcomes after trabeculectomy. This is attributed to rapid regression of NVI after anti-VEGF therapy.[53] Improved ischemia and wound healing are other proposed mechanisms by which anti-VEGF agents improve surgical outcomes. However, in a study comparing patients undergoing trabeculectomy with and without intravitreal bevacizumab, the success rate 1 year after surgery was not statistically different between the 2 groups.[51] In a another retrospective review, the reported surgical success rate for trabeculectomy with MMC and adjunctive intravitreal bevacizumab was 86.9% at 1 year and 51.3% at 5 years.[54] Lower preoperative IOP (<30 mmHg) indicating compromised aqueous produc-tion due to underlying ischemia and vitrectomy after trabeculectomy were identified as risk factors for surgical failure. Other studies report a success rate of 65% to 85% when trabeculectomy is combined with preoperative intravitreal bevacizumab as compared to 30% to 75% with trabeculectomy alone.[55-57] Furthermore, the mean IOP was found to be reduced by almost 66% 3 years after trabeculectomy with preoperative bevacizumab, although there was no significant change in visual acuity.[56] Similar to bevacizumab, use of intravitreal ranibizumab as an adjunct to trabeculectomy has also shown improvement in surgical outcomes.[58]

Glaucoma-drainage implants are commonly used in the management of patients with NVG as their success rate is less dependent on control of intraocular inflammation and presence of a filtering bleb. Success rates have ranged from 22% up to 97% with these devices.[59] In a retrospective study designed to assess the effectiveness of the Baerveldt glaucoma implant, there was adequate control of IOP, but postoperative visual loss was still common.[60] They reported a success rate of 79% at one year; 31% of patients remained stable or showed improvement in visual acuity, another 31% lost light perception vision. Younger age and poor preoperative visual acuity were associated with worse prognosis. In another report evaluating the Molteno implant for the same indication, success rates were reported to be 62% at 1 year and 10.3% at 5 years.[61] Almost half of the patients lost light perception vision and 18% went into phthisis. The Ahmed valve was evaluated similarly in patients with NVG from proliferative diabetic retinopathy with a reported 3-year success rate of 62.5% in patients with a prior history of vitrectomy and 68.5% in patients with no prior history of vitrectomy.[62] Intraocular silicone oil tamponade was noted as a risk factor for surgical failure.

As with trabeculectomy, use of preoperative anti-VEGF agents has been described to improve surgical results. In a comparison of preoperative intravitreal ranibizumab with Ahmed valve implantation vs Ahmed valve implantation alone, the success rate was 72.2% vs 68.4% at 12 months, respectively.[63] There were no significant differences in the 2 groups with respect to IOP control, visual acuity, and postoperative complications at 12 months. The authors concluded that a single intravitreal injection of ranibizumab (0.5 mg) before surgery had no significant effect on the medium- or long-term outcomes of Ahmed glaucoma valve implantation. However, in a meta-analysis of controlled clinical trials comparing Ahmed glaucoma valve implantation with or without preoperative intravitreal bevacizumab, the adjunctive treatment was found to be a safe and effective step associated with a numerically greater but not statistically significant IOP-lowering efficacy.[64] Additionally, the bevacizumab group was associated with significantly greater complete success rates and lower frequency of hyphema compared to the control group. Both groups were comparable in the reduction of glaucoma medication.

As trabeculectomy with mitomycin C and glaucoma drainage implants are the 2 most common procedures performed in patients with NVG, studies have compared surgical outcomes between the two. In a retrospective comparative case series, there was no statistically significant difference between trabeculectomy and Ahmed glaucoma valve in postoperative visual acuity, number of glaucoma medications, and IOP. Success was 60% and 55% at 2 years after Ahmed glaucoma valve implantation and trabeculectomy, respectively.[65] Similar findings were also reported in another study comparing the 2 surgical procedures.[66]

In patients not controlled on topical therapy alone and who are poor surgical candidates because of limited visual potential or systemic reasons, cyclodestructive procedures offer a good alternative. Transscleral cyclophotocoagulation was first described in 1972.[67] Since then, the technique has evolved and most surgeons prefer to use diode laser compared to neodymium:yttrium-aluminum-garnet laser because of lower rates of phthisis (10% with neodymium:yttrium-aluminum-garnet laser and 0% with diode laser).[68] IOP reduction in the range of more than 50% may be achieved with diode laser cyclophotocoagulation;[69] however, postoperative pain and inflammation are common and need to be managed with topical steroids and cycloplegics. In addition, long-term hypotony and loss of light perception vision[70] are possible, and hence, this procedure is generally reserved for patients with poor visual potential. A new laser modality called micropulse cyclophotocoagulation has recently become available. It is proposed to reduce the risk of postoperative pain, inflammation, and hypotony compared to traditional diode laser. Micropulse laser may potentially be used in eyes with good visual potential because of fewer postoperative complications, but there are no studies yet evaluating the effects of this laser long term. Direct application of laser to the ciliary processes with an endoscope has also been attempted, and in one study showed IOP lowering of up to 65%.[71,72] Alternatively, cyclocryotherapy can reduce IOP 50%, but there is a high incidence of vision loss, hypotony, inflammation, pain, retinal detachment, anterior segment ischemia, and phthisis bulbi.[73-75] In one study, 58% of patients lost light perception vision and 34% went into phthisis.[75] Surgical removal of part of the ciliary body has also been described but is associated with a high rate of complications.[76] In patients with painful eyes and no light perception vision, retrobulbar alcohol injection and enucleation can be attempted as a last resort.

Conclusion

NVG is a disease with potentially disastrous visual consequences. Early recognition and institution of treatment provides the patient with the best chance at preserving vision. Performing an undilated pupillary and iris exam with undilated gonioscopy is extremely important. A dilated retinal exam then needs to be performed to manage the source of the neovascularization. All efforts must be made to identify the disease before the angle is completely closed by the fibrovascular membrane. Performing PRP to eliminate the production of VEGF by ischemic retina is critical to the success of any antiglaucoma therapy, and intravitreal anti-VEGF therapies have more recently had a role in this process. Thereafter, one can start with topical and oral hypotensives, although most patients will end up requiring surgical intervention. Combining trabeculectomy or tube shunt surgery with preoperative anti-VEGF agents may help improve surgical outcomes, although more studies are required to substantiate these findings.

References

1. Adair TH, Montani JP. *Angiogenesis*. San Rafael, CA: Morgan & Claypool Life Sciences; 2010.
2. Bergers G, Benjamin LE. Tumorigenesis and the angiogenic switch. *Nat Rev Cancer*. 2003;3(6):401-410.
3. Folkman J. Role of angiogenesis in tumor growth and metastasis. *Semin Oncol*. 2002;29(6 Suppl 16):15-18.
4. Crawford TN, Alfaro DV III, Kerrison JB, Jablon EP. Diabetic retinopathy and angiogenesis. *Curr Diabetes Rev*. 2009;5(1):8-13.
5. Fruttiger M. Development of the retinal vasculature. *Angiogenesis*. 2007;10(2):77-88.
6. Witmer AN, Vrensen GF, Van Noorden CJ, Schlingemann RO. Vascular endothelial growth factors and angiogenesis in eye disease. *Prog Retin Eye Res*. 2003;22(1):1-29.
7. Ramakrishnan S, Anand V, Roy S. Vascular endothelial growth factor signaling in hypoxia and inflammation. *J Neuroimmune Pharmacol*. 2014;9(2):142-160.
8. Wu Y, Lucia K, Lange M, Kuhlen D, Stalla GK, Renner U. Hypoxia inducible factor-1 is involved in growth factor, glucocorticoid and hypoxia mediated regulation of vascular endothelial growth factor-A in human meningiomas. *J Neurooncol*. 2014;119(2):263-273.

9. Coats G. Further cases of thrombosis of central vein. *Roy London Ophthalmol Hosp Rep.* 1906;16:516-564.

10. Weiss DI, Shaffner RN, Nehrenberg TR. Neovascular glaucoma complicating carotid-cavernous fistula. *Arch Ophthalmol.* 1963;69:304-307.

11. Brown GC, Magargal LE, Schachat A, Shah H. Neovascular glaucoma. Etiologic considerations. *Ophthalmology.* 1984;91(4):315-320.

12. Sivak-Callcott JA, O'Day DM, Gass JD, Tsai JC. Evidence-based recommendations for the diagnosis and treatment of neovascular glaucoma. *Ophthalmology.* 2001;108(10):1767-1776.

13. Aiello LM, Wand M, Liang G. Neovascular glaucoma and vitreous hemorrhage after cataract surgery in patients with diabetes mellitus. *Ophthalmology.* 1983;90(7):814-820.

14. Rice TA, Michels RG, Maguire MG, Rice EF. The effect of lensectomy on the incidence of iris neovascularization and neovascular glaucoma after vitrectomy for diabetic retinopathy. *Am J Ophthalmol.* 1983;95(1):1-11.

15. Weinreb RN, Wasserstrom JP, Parker W. Neovascular glaucoma following neodymium-YAG laser posterior capsulotomy. *Arch Ophthalmol.* 1986;104(5):730-731.

16. Tripathi RC, Li J, Tripathi BJ, Chalam KV, Adamis AP. Increased level of vascular endothelial growth factor in aqueous humor of patients with neovascular glaucoma. *Ophthalmology.* 1998;105(2):232-237.

17. Sone H, Okuda Y, Kawakami Y, et al. Vascular endothelial growth factor level in aqueous humor of diabetic patients with rubeotic glaucoma is markedly elevated. *Diabetes Care.* 1996;19(11):1306-1307.

18. Meyer-Schwickerath R, Pfeiffer A, Blum WF, et al. Vitreous levels of the insulin-like growth factors I and II, and the insulin-like growth factor binding proteins 2 and 3, increase in neovascular eye diseases. Studies in nondiabetic and diabetic subjects. *J Clin Invest.* 1993;92(6):2620-2625.

19. Chen, KH, Wu CC, Roy S, Lee SM, Liu JH. Increased interleukin-6 in aqueous humor of neovascular glaucoma. *Invest Ophthalmol Vis Sci.* 1999;40(11):2627-2632.

20. Fiedler U, Reiss Y, Scharpfenecker M, et al. Angiopoietin-2 sensitizes endothelial cells to TNF-alpha and has a crucial role in the induction of inflammation. *Nat Med.* 2006;12(2):235-239.

21. John T, Sassani JW, Eagle RC Jr. The myofibroblastic component of rubeosis iridis. *Ophthalmology.* 1983;90(6):721-728.

22. Gartner S, Taffet S, Friedman AH. The association of rubeosis iridis with endothelialisation of the anterior chamber: report of a clinical case with histopathological review of 16 additional cases. *Br J Ophthalmol.* 1977;61(4):267-271.

23. Goel M, Picciani RG, Lee RK, Bhattacharya SK. Aqueous humor dynamics: a review. *Open Ophthalmol J.* 2010;4:52-59.

24. Browning DJ, Scott AQ, Peterson CB, Warnock J, Zhang Z. The risk of missing angle neovascularization by omitting screening gonioscopy in acute central retinal vein occlusion. *Ophthalmology.* 1998;105(5):776-784.

25. Baseline and early natural history report. The Central Vein Occlusion Study. Central Vein Occlusion Study Group. *Arch Ophthalmol.* 1993;11(8):1087-1095.

26. Blinder KJ, Friedman SM, Mames RN. Diabetic iris neovascularization. *Am J Ophthalmol.* 1995;120(3):393-395.

27. Bloom PA, Papakostopoulos D, Gogolitsyn Y, Leenderz JA, Papakostopoulos S, Grey RH. Clinical and infrared pupillometry in central retinal vein occlusion. *Br J Ophthalmol.* 1993;77(2):75-80.

28. Maruyama Y, Kishi S, Kamei Y, Shimizu R, Kimura Y. Infrared angiography of the anterior ocular segment. *Surv Ophthalmol.* 1995;39(Suppl 1): S40-S48.

29. Sanborn GE, Symes DJ, Magargal LE. Fundus iris fluorescein angiography: evaluation of its use in the diagnosis of rubeosis iridis [published erratum appears in *Ann Ophthalmol.* 1986;18(4):155]. *Ann Ophthalmol.* 1986;18(2):52-58.

30. Ohnishi Y, Ishibashi T, Sagawa T. Fluorescein gonioangiography in diabetic neovascularisation. *Graefes Arch Clin Exp Ophthalmol.* 1994;232(4):199-204.

31. Sabates R, Hirose T, McMeel JW. Electroretinography in the prognosis and classification of central retinal vein occlusion. *Arch Ophthalmol.* 1983;101(2):232-235.

32. Larsson J, Andreasson S, Bauer B. Cone b-wave implicit time as an early predictor of rubeosis in central retinal vein occlusion. *Am J Ophthalmol.* 1998;125(2):247-249.

33. Anchala AR, Pasquale LR. Neovascular glaucoma: a historical perspective on modulating angiogenesis. *Semin Ophthalmol.* 2009;24(2):106-112.

34. Kim M, Lee C, Payne R, Yue BY, Chang JH, Ying H. Angiogenesis in glaucoma filtration surgery and neovascular glaucoma: a review. *Surv Ophthalmol.* 2015;60(6):524-535.

35. Chalam KV, Brar VS, Murthy RK. Human ciliary epithelium as a source of synthesis and secretion of vascular endothelial growth factor in neovascular glaucoma. *JAMA Ophthalmol.* 2014;132(11):1350-1354.

36. Cashwell LF, Marks WP. Panretinal photocoagulation in the management of neovascular glaucoma. *South Med J.* 1988;81(11):1364-1368.

37. Allen RC, Bellows AR, Hutchinson BT, Murphy SD. Filtration surgery in the treatment of neovascular glaucoma. *Ophthalmology.* 1982;89(10):1181-1187.

38. Fernández-Vigo J, Castro J, Macarro A. Diabetic iris neovascularization. Natural history and treatment. *Acta Ophthalmol Scand.* 1997;75(1):89-93.

39. Sihota R, Sandramouli S, Sood NN. A prospective evaluation of anterior retinal cryoablation in neovascular glaucoma. *Ophthalmic Surg.* 1991;22(5):256-259.

40. Stefaniotou M, Paschides CA, Psilas K. Panretinal cryopexy for the management of neovascularization of the iris. *Ophthalmologica.* 1995;209(3):141-144.

41. Vernon SA, Cheng H. Panretinal cryotherapy in neovascular disease. *Br J Ophthalmol.* 1988;72(6):401-405.

42. Tsai JC, Bloom PA, Franks WA, Khaw PT. Combined transscleral diode laser cyclophotocoagulation and transscleral retinal photocoagulation for refractory neovascular glaucoma. *Retina.* 1996;16(2):164-166.

43. Flaxel CJ, Larkin GB, Broadway DB, Allen PJ, Leaver PK. Peripheral transscleral retinal diode laser for rubeosis iridis. *Retina.* 1997;17(5):421-429.

44. Fong DS, Girach A, Boney A. Visual side effects of successful scatter laser photocoagulation surgery for proliferative diabetic retinopathy: a literature review. *Retina.* 2007;27(7):816-824.

45. Tsai JC, Feuer WJ, Parrish RK II, Grajewski AL. 5-Fluorouracil filtering surgery and neovascular glaucoma. Long-term follow-up of the original pilot study. *Ophthalmology.* 1995;102(6):887-892; discussion 892-893.

46. Katz GJ, Higginbotham EJ, Lichter PR, et al. Mitomycin C versus 5-fluorouracil in high-risk glaucoma filtering surgery. Extended follow-up. *Ophthalmology.* 1995;102(9):1263-1269.

47. Kiuchi Y, Sugimoto R, Nakae K, Saito Y, Ito S. Trabeculectomy with mitomycin C for treatment of neovascular glaucoma in diabetic patients. *Ophthalmologica.* 2006;220(6):383-388.

48. Takihara Y, Inatani M, Fukushima M, Iwao K, Iwao M, Tanihara H. Trabeculectomy with mitomycin C for neovascular glaucoma: prognostic factors for surgical failure. *Am J Ophthalmol.* 2009;147(5):912-918.

49. Saito Y, Higashide T, Takeda H, Ohkubo S, Sugiyama K. Beneficial effects of preoperative intravitreal bevacizumab on trabeculectomy outcomes in neovascular glaucoma. *Acta Ophthalmol.* 2010;88(1):96-102.

50. Chen CH, Lai IC, Wu PC, et al. Adjunctive intravitreal bevacizumab-combined trabeculectomy versus trabeculectomy alone in the treatment of neovascular glaucoma. *J Ocul Pharmacol Ther.* 2010;26(1):111-118.

51. Takihara Y, Inatani M, Kawaji T, et al. Combined intravitreal bevacizumab and trabeculectomy with mitomycin C versus trabeculectomy with mitomycin C alone for neovascular glaucoma. *J Glaucoma.* 2011;20(3):196-201.

52. Gupta V, Jha R, Rao A, Kong G, Sihota R. The effect of different doses of intracameral bevacizumab on surgical outcomes of trabeculectomy for neovascular glaucoma. *Eur J Ophthalmol.* 2009;19(3):435-441.

53. Davidorf FH, Mouser JG, Derick RJ. Rapid improvement of rubeosis iridis from a single bevacizumab (Avastin) injection. *Retina.* 2006;26(3):354-356.

54. Higashide T, Ohkubo S, Sugiyama K. Long-term outcomes and prognostic factors of trabeculectomy following intraocular bevacizumab injection for neovascular glaucoma. *PLoS One*. 2015;10(8):e0135766.

55. Miki A, Oshima Y, Otori Y, Matsushita K, Nishida K. One-year results of intravitreal bevacizumab as an adjunct to trabeculectomy for neovascular glaucoma in eyes with previous vitrectomy. *Eye (Lond)*. 2011;25(5):658-659.

56. Kobayashi S, Inoue M, Yamane S, Sakamaki K, Arakawa A, Kadonosono K. Long-term outcomes after preoperative intravitreal injection of bevacizumab before trabeculectomy for neovascular glaucoma. *J Glaucoma*. 2016;25(3):281-284.

57. Hyung SM, Kim SK. Mid-term effects of trabeculectomy with mitomycin C in neovascular glaucoma patients. *Korean J Ophthalmol*. 2001;15(2):98-106.

58. Kitnarong N, Sriyakul C, Chinwattanakul S. A prospective study to evaluate intravitreous ranibizumab as adjunctive treatment for trabeculectomy in neovascular glaucoma. *Ophthalmol Ther*. 2015;4(1):33-41.

59. Assaad MH, Baerveldt G, Rockwood EJ. Glaucoma drainage devices: pros and cons. *Curr Opin Ophthalmol*. 1999;10(2):147-153.

60. Sidoti PA, Dunphy TR, Baerveldt G, et al. Experience with the Baerveldt glaucoma implant in treating neovascular glaucoma. *Ophthalmology*. 1995;102(7):1107-1118.

61. Mermoud A, Salmon JF, Alexander P, Straker C, Murray AD. Molteno tube implantation for neovascular glaucoma. Long-term results and factors influencing the outcome. *Ophthalmology*. 1993;100(6):897-902.

62. Park UC, Park KH, Kim DM, Yu HG. Ahmed glaucoma valve implantation for neovascular glaucoma after vitrectomy for proliferative diabetic retinopathy. *J Glaucoma*. 2011;20(7):433-438.

63. Tang M, Fu Y, Wang Y, et al. Efficacy of intravitreal ranibizumab combined with Ahmed glaucoma valve implantation for the treatment of neovascular glaucoma. *BMC Ophthalmol*. 2016;16:7.

64. Zhou M, Xu X, Zhang X, Sun X. Clinical outcomes of Ahmed glaucoma valve implantation with or without intravitreal bevacizumab pretreatment for neovascular glaucoma: a systematic review and meta-analysis. *J Glaucoma*. 2016;25(7):551-557.

65. Shen CC, Salim S, Du H, Netland PA. Trabeculectomy versus Ahmed glaucoma valve implantation in neovascular glaucoma. *Clin Ophthalmol*. 2011;5:281-286.

66. Im YW, Lym HS, Park CK, Moon JI. Comparison of mitomycin C trabeculectomy and Ahmed valve implant surgery for neovascular glaucoma. *J Korean Ophthalmol Soc*. 2004;45:1515-1521.

67. Beckman H, Waeltermann J. Transscleral ruby laser cyclocoagulation. *Am J Ophthalmol*. 1984;98:788-795.

68. Oguri A, Takahashi E, Tomita G, Yamamoto T, Jikihara S, Kitazawa Y. Transscleral cyclophotocoagulation with the diode laser for neovascular glaucoma. *Ophthalmic Surg Lasers*. 1998;29(9):722-727.

69. Bloom PA, Tsai JC, Sharma K, et al. "Cyclodiode." Transscleral diode laser cyclophotocoagulation in the treatment of advanced refractory glaucoma. *Ophthalmology*. 1997;104(9):1508-1519; discussion 1519-1520.

70. Eid TE, Katz LJ, Spaeth GL, Augsburger JJ. Tube-shunt surgery versus neodymium:YAG cyclophotocoagulation in the management of neovascular glaucoma. *Ophthalmology*. 1997;104(10):1692-1700.

71. Uram M. Ophthalmic laser microendoscope ciliary process ablation in the management of neovascular glaucoma. *Ophthalmology*. 1992;99(12):1823-1828.

72. Lima FE, Magacho L, Carvalho DM, Susanna R Jr, Avila MP. A prospective, comparative study between endoscopic cyclophotocoagulation and the Ahmed drainage implant in refractory glaucoma. *J Glaucoma*. 2004;13(3):233-237.

73. Bietti G. Surgical intervention on the ciliary body; new trends for the relief of glaucoma. *J Am Med Assoc*. 1950;142(12):889-897.

74. Feibel RM, Bigger JF. Rubeosis iridis and neovascular glaucoma. Evaluation of cyclocryotherapy. *Am J Ophthalmol*. 1972;74(5):862-867.

75. Krupin T, Johnson MF, Becker B. Anterior segment ischemia after cyclocryotherapy. *Am J Ophthalmol*. 1977;84(3):426-428.

76. Sautter H, Demeler U. Antiglaucomatous ciliary body excision. *Am J Ophthalmol*. 1984;98(3):344-348.

16

GLAUCOMA SURGERY

Jessica J. Moon, MD and Cynthia Mattox, MD

Anti-Vascular Endothelial Growth Factor in Filtering Surgery

Glaucoma is one of the leading causes of irreversible blindness worldwide.[1] The term describes a group of diseases that are characterized by a specific optic neuropathy,[2] with the strongest risk factor for development being elevated intraocular pressure (IOP). IOP is maintained by the production of aqueous humor with drainage through the trabecular meshwork in the anterior chamber angle or the uveoscleral outflow pathway. Glaucoma therapy is targeted at reducing IOP and slowing the progression of glaucoma. Conventional first-line therapy in glaucoma involves topical medications or laser trabeculoplasty. When this conservative therapy fails, glaucoma surgery can be performed to control the IOP.[3]

Trabeculectomy

Trabeculectomy was first described in 1968 by Cairns and has remained the gold standard of glaucoma surgery.[4] It is a surgical procedure in which a guarded fistula is created to allow aqueous humor to drain from the anterior chamber into the subconjunctival space. The goal is to bypass the trabecular meshwork, allowing the aqueous humor to exit through the formed bleb to provide a controlled way of lowering IOP. It is the most effective procedure for reducing the IOP in glaucoma.[5,6] However, failure of trabeculectomy due to excessive postoperative scarring remains a significant challenge. Unlike in other surgeries, a completely healed wound is not desirable in a trabeculectomy. Subconjunctival scarring at the site of the bleb can cause adhesions to the episcleral

Duker JS, Liang MC, eds.
*Anti-VEGF Use in
Ophthalmology (pp. 177-195).*
© 2017 Taylor & Francis Group.

tissue and lead to resealing of the bleb, ultimately preventing filtration and leading to an elevated IOP.[7]

Wound healing in trabeculectomy is driven by 2 key pathways, fibroblasts and angiogenesis, and both are modulated by vascular endothelial growth factor (VEGF). Tenon fibroblasts are the main effector cells in scar formation. After surgery, Tenon fibroblasts proliferate, causing excess collagen and elastin deposition.[7] Histologic studies have shown that maximum proliferation of subconjunctival fibroblasts occurs on the third to fifth postoperative day.[8] High VEGF levels are linked to increased fibroblast proliferation, leading to increased collagen deposition and subsequent encapsulation of blebs.[9] Angiogenesis is another important aspect of wound healing in trabeculectomy. New vessels need to grow into the center of the healing site to bring in nutrients and supply oxygen. These vessels bring in mediators that support the rapid growth of new cells to replace the injured cells and thus promote scar deposition. It is known that increased bleb vascularity is associated with a poor prognosis in trabeculectomy.[10]

Current Therapy in Trabeculectomy

The current standard of modulating scar formation in trabeculectomy targets the fibroblast pathway and not the angiogenesis pathway. This therapy involves using antifibrotics to inhibit fibroblasts in wound healing. The 2 main agents used are 5-fluorouracil (5-FU) and mitomycin C (MMC). The agent 5-FU was first introduced in the early 1980s as an antimetabolite that interfered with pyrimidine metabolism. It blocks a crucial step in thymidine nucleotide synthesis and inhibits DNA replication, leading to cell death.[11] MMC was first introduced in 1986 as an antibiotic agent derived from *Streptomyces caespitosus*.[12] Unlike 5-FU, MMC is technically not an antimetabolite but an antifibroblast. It is capable of inhibiting DNA replication, mitosis, and protein synthesis therefore inhibiting fibroblasts.[11] Clinicians tend to favor MMC because of its prolonged effect when compared with 5-FU.

The use of these antifibrotics has improved the success of trabeculectomies.[7] Unfortunately, even with these treatments, the "Tube Versus Trabeculectomy" study found that the probability of failure in patients with prior surgery treated with trabeculectomy with MMC was 46.9% after 5 years of follow-up.[13] Furthermore, a major drawback of antifibrotics is their nonspecific mechanism of action. 5-FU and MMC work well because they inhibit fibroblasts, but they also have the unintended consequence of causing widespread death of other cells. This leads to a high complication rate involving cystic avascular blebs, infection, leakage, and hypotony with maculopathy. Infections range from blebitis to endophthalmitis.[14-16]

These side effects have led to a search for other options with an increasing focus on the role of VEGF in wound modulation. In 1994, before commercial VEGF antibodies were available, angiogenesis inhibitors were found to have inhibitory effects on fibroblast proliferation and migration in vitro.[17] Since then, more evidence has appeared showing that anti-VEGF agents inhibit wound healing.[18,19] In fact, delayed wound healing is listed as a warning on the manufacturer's prescribing information for bevacizumab (Avastin).

Vascular Endothelial Growth Factor in Glaucoma

Multiple studies have shown that aqueous VEGF levels are consistently elevated in eyes with glaucoma. This was first shown in 1998; the aqueous mean concentration of VEGF was higher in eyes with primary open-angle glaucoma (POAG) and higher yet in those with neovascular glaucoma (NVG).[20] The source of VEGF production in glaucoma is not clear. VEGF is expressed and produced by the corneal endothelium, iris pigment epithelium, retinal pigment epithelium, ganglion cells, astrocytes, Müller cells, and choroidal fibroblasts.[21] Not much is known about the production of VEGF in the conjunctiva or Tenon's, but VEGF is elevated in the Tenon's as well as in the aqueous. The size of VEGF (7.56 nm) is smaller than the pores of the trabecular meshwork and the openings of Schlemm's canal (0.5 μm to 0.76 μm), so VEGF may be diffusing from the aqueous cavity into the subconjunctival space even in the absence of a filtration bleb. VEGF is not elevated in plasma so it is postulated that VEGF is produced by local ocular tissue.[22]

It is also unknown how glaucoma upregulates VEGF but elevated IOP may have a role in increasing VEGF production. One study used rat models with induced ocular hypertension to demonstrate elevated VEGF levels in the retinal ganglion cells.[23] Another group demonstrated that aqueous VEGF levels were increased after trabeculectomy in rabbit models and remained elevated until day 30.[9] The baseline elevation of VEGF found in the aqueous and Tenon's of patients with glaucoma may predispose them to an even further degree of scarring after trabeculectomy.

Animal models have shown that anti-VEGF agents suppress the upregulation of VEGF after trabeculectomy.[9] A single intraoperative injection of bevacizumab into the subconjunctival space and anterior chamber lowered VEGF levels compared to control eyes on postoperative day 4. There was a reduced density of blood vessels at the filtration site, decreased total area of collagen with trichrome stain, and a larger bleb area in the treated eye. There were no notable differences in IOP, however.[9] Another group examined 42 trabeculectomy rabbits randomized to receive 7 subconjunctival injections of either 1.25 mg bevacizumab, 5 mg 5-FU, or balanced salt solution. The bevacizumab group had an improvement in bleb survival as well as a larger bleb height and area with less scarring on histological examination. However, they were also unable to show any changes in the IOP outcome, which is a major limitation of these animal models.[24]

Which Anti-Vascular Endothelial Growth Factor Agent to Use

There are various isoforms of VEGF that can be targeted. In vitro analysis after trabeculectomy showed that $VEGF_{121}$ and $VEGF_{165}$ increased vascular endothelial cells whereas $VEGF_{189}$ increased fibroblast growth.[25] This indicates that $VEGF_{121}$ and $VEGF_{165}$ may have a larger role in blood vessel growth while $VEGF_{189}$ may have a larger role in scar formation. Presumably, an anti-VEGF that targets all these isoforms may be more effective in wound modulation than an agent that targets just one isoform.

This theory was tested by comparing pegaptanib, an anti-VEGF selective for $VEGF_{165}$, and bevacizumab, a nonselective anti-VEGF agent. Working in vivo with human and rabbit Tenon fibroblasts and in vitro with rabbit models, they found bevacizumab to be more effective, suggesting the importance of inhibiting both neovascularization and fibrosis, rather than neovascularization alone. Further studies have moved on to focus either on bevacizumab or ranibizumab, both nonselective VEGF inhibitors. At this point, it is unclear which anti-VEGF agent is better. Ranibizumab is a mature antibody that was designed to have a significantly stronger binding affinity than bevacizumab.[26] However, the half-life of bevacizumab is longer than that of ranibizumab. The half-life of intravitreal bevacizumab in the vitreous is 4.32 days while the half-life of ranibizumab is 2.88 days.[27,28] In comparison, the half-life of pegatanib is 3.91 days.[29]

Bevacizumab

There have been several randomized, controlled trials looking at the use of bevacizumab as an adjunctive treatment in trabeculectomies (Table 16-1). The results have been variable and inconclusive. The studies also varied in the route of administration and timing of the administration with no clear consensus on the better choice.

Route of Administration

The best route of administration is unknown. Topical, subconjunctival, and intravitreal administration of bevacizumab has been studied in rabbits.[30] The highest concentration of bevacizumab in the ocular tissues was detected with the intravitreal route and the lowest concentration with topical administration. However, subconjunctival injection was found to have a longer half-life than intravitreal injection, thought to be due to the high scleral permeability of bevacizumab causing a longer sustained-release mechanism. The only studies thus far looking at intravitreal bevacizumab with trabeculectomies have been in patients with NVG.

Subconjunctival Bevacizumab

The majority of studies examining bevacizumab have used subconjunctival bevacizumab intraoperatively during trabeculectomy.[8,31-35] A randomized, double-blind, controlled clinical trial of 38 patients compared intraoperative MMC alone, 3 subconjunctival injections of bevacizumab without MMC, and 1 application of a bevacizumab-soaked sponge intraoperatively. The bevacizumab-soaked sponge had no advantage over MMC; however, the subconjunctival injections of bevacizumab were equally effective as MMC in reducing the IOP but with fewer side effects; the MMC group had one case of bleb leak and one case of hypotony maculopathy while the bevacizumab group did not have any.[31]

Another prospective trial compared 34 eyes randomized to receive either 1 dose of 2.5 mg subconjunctival bevacizumab intraoperatively or 1 dose of MMC intraoperatively. Bevacizumab was effective but not as effective as MMC in controlling IOP (34% vs 56% reduction of IOP, respectively). Additionally, the bevacizumab group required more antiglaucoma medications after surgery for IOP control.[32]

In a more recent study, MMC in conjunction with subconjunctival bevacizumab was found to be superior to bevacizumab alone. Forty-two patients with POAG were randomized to receive 2.5 mg subconjunctival bevacizumab intraoperatively with or without MMC application. Seventy-one percent of eyes in the MMC group met a target IOP of 12 mmHg without antiglaucoma medication while only 33% of eyes in the bevacizumab-alone group met the target at the 1-year follow-up. Interestingly, this study reported

Table 16-1. Anti-Vascular Endothelial Growth Factor in Glaucoma Filtration Surgery

Anti-VEGF Agent	Route of Administration	Timing of Administration	Reference	Outcome
Bevacizumab	Subconjunctival	Intraoperative	• Sengupta et al[31] 2012 • Nilforushan et al[32] 2012 • Kiddee et al[34] 2015 • Sedghipour et al[35] 2011 • Akkan et al[36] 2015	• Bevacizumab as effective as MMC in reducing IOP • MMC more effective than bevacizumab in reducing IOP • No additive benefit of single SCB to MMC in reducing IOP or increasing success rate • No difference in IOP between bevacizumab and placebo • MMC with bevacizumab superior to bevacizumab alone in meeting target IOP
		Postoperative	• Simsek et al[33] 2012 • Tai et al[43] 2015	• 5-FU more effective than bevacizumab • No difference in IOP between bevacizumab and placebo bleb needling as adjunct to MMC
	Intracameral	Intraoperative	• Fakhraie et al[37] 2016 • Vandewalle et al[38] 2014	• Bevacizumab higher success rate than placebo • Bevacizumab + MMC higher success rate than MMC alone
	Topical	Postoperative	• Klos-Rola et al[39] 2013	• Observational case series. Improvement of 75% in bleb vascularity with bevacizumab
Ranibizumab	Intravitreal	Intraoperative	• Kahook[44] 2010	• No difference in IOP compared to MMC only; ranibizumab with less vascular and more broad/diffuse bleb
	Subconjunctival	Intraoperative	• Pro et al[45] 2015	• No difference in IOP compared to MMC only

Anti-VEGF = anti-vascular endothelial growth factor; IOP = intraocular pressure; MMC = mitomycin C; SCB = subconjunctival bevacizumab; 5-FU = 5-flurouracil.

success rates at a much lower IOP than set by other studies that report outcomes at IOP less than 18 mmHg or 21 mmHg, which may not be adequate for advanced glaucoma.[36]

Intracameral Bevacizumab

There have been 2 studies looking at intracameral bevacizumab administered intraoperatively during trabeculectomy surgery. A prospective clinical trial of 71 patients with either POAG or pseudoexfoliation glaucoma were randomized to receive 1.25 mg intracameral bevacizumab or intracameral balanced salt solution (BSS) at the end of the surgery. No antifibrotics were used in either group. In this study, the bevacizumab group had a higher success rate of 83% compared to the placebo group, which had a success rate of 48.5%. Unfortunately, the bevacizumab group also had a higher rate of bleb leak of 34% while the placebo group had only a 9% bleb leak rate. The study was limited by short-term follow-up of only 10 months.[37]

Another prospective, placebo-controlled trial of 138 patients also randomized patients to receive 1.25 mg intracameral bevacizumab or intracameral BSS at the end of surgery. In contrast, both groups also had MMC applied intraoperatively. At 1 year follow-up, the postoperative IOP was lower than baseline in both groups, but there was no significant difference between the 2 groups. The bevacizumab group, however, did have a higher success rate of 71% vs 51% in the placebo group; success was defined as at least 30% reduction in IOP from baseline, with an IOP ≤18 mmHg and >5 mmHg and no loss of light perception vision. Patients who received bevacizumab also needed fewer IOP-lowering interventions such as needling revision postoperatively.[38]

Topical Bevacizumab

An observational case series in Poland examined 21 eyes with increased vascularity after undergoing MMC augmented trabeculectomy 9.8 ± 4.7 days previously. All patients were given standard steroid therapy and topical 5 mg/5 mL bevacizumab drops administered 5 times daily for 20.9 ± 9.8 days. Around 75% of eyes recovered with decreased injection of the bleb. However, 14% of patients also developed an early bleb leak.[39] For comparison, bleb leaks after trabeculectomy with MMC are reported to occur in 5% to 14.5% of cases;[40,41] bleb leaks after trabeculectomy without the use antifibrotics are relatively uncommon, ranging from 0% to 3%.[41,42]

Timing of Administration

Just as the best route of administration has not been established yet, the best time to administer anti-VEGF agents is also unclear. Many of the previously mentioned studies looked at intraoperative application of bevacizumab with variable benefits. However, a few studies have looked at the postoperative use of bevacizumab in needle bleb revisions.

One study of 58 patients with failed trabeculectomy and ExPRESS shunt blebs requiring needling revisions received subconjunctival MMC in addition to either 1 mg subconjunctival bevacizumab or BSS injected posterior to the bleb after needling. There was no difference in success rates and IOP between the control and treatment groups 6 months post-procedure. However, the authors reported that the groups receiving bevacizumab had significantly less vascularity as well as broader, more diffuse blebs.[43]

A different study comparing needle bleb revision with 5-FU to bevacizumab found 5-FU to be more effective, resulting in a statistically significant higher success rate compared with bevacizumab.[33]

Ranibizumab

There have been only 2 studies using ranibizumab for trabeculectomies (Table 16-1). One examined 10 patients in a prospective, open-label study that compared 0.5 mg intravitreal ranibizumab in addition to MMC use during trabeculectomy to MMC alone. There was no significant difference in IOPs between the 2 groups; however, the group receiving ranibizumab had a broader bleb area and lower vascularity at 6 months. This study was limited by a small sample size and short follow-up period.[44]

The other study was a prospective, open-label trial of 24 patients undergoing trabeculectomy. One group received 0.5 mg subconjunctival ranibizumab and the other group received MMC application. The group treated with ranibizumab had a higher mean IOP at one month but there was no difference in IOP at 1-year follow-up. More patients in the ranibizumab group required additional glaucoma surgery.[45]

These studies have not shown superiority of anti-VEGF agents over the current standard of antifibrotic agents. There are still questions about optimal dose, which anti-VEGF agent to use, best route of administration, as well as timing of application. Further research will need to be conducted in order to elucidate the benefit of anti-VEGF therapy in trabeculectomies.

Anti-Vascular Endothelial Growth Factor in Neovascular Glaucoma

Neovascular Glaucoma

Neovascular glaucoma (NVG) is a notoriously aggressive glaucoma that is challenging to treat and has a poor visual prognosis.[46] NVG was first described by Weiss et al[47] in 1963 as a type of glaucoma associated with new iris and angle vessels causing an increase in IOP.[47] It is a secondary glaucoma that is almost always associated with ischemic ocular conditions; 36% of all cases arise from central retinal vein occlusion, 32% from proliferative diabetic retinopathy, and 13% from ocular ischemic syndrome.[48] Retinal ischemia stimulates angiogenic factors like VEGF that cause new vessels and fibrous tissue to grow over the iris and eventually into the angle.[46] Neovascularization characteristically progresses from the pupil margin to the angle.[49]

Three stages of NVG have been described. The first stage is rubeosis iridis in which there is neovascularization of the iris (NVI) with or without neovascularization of the angle (NVA) in the setting of normal IOP. In stage 2, the angle appears open yet fibrovascular tissue blocks the aqueous drainage system. Finally, in stage 3, contraction of the fibrovascular membrane causes the iris to pull over the trabecular meshwork with varying degrees of peripheral anterior synechiae. This leads to secondary angle closure and further IOP elevation.[49]

It is known that hypoxia can trigger VEGF production leading to angiogenesis. VEGF concentration in the aqueous is 40 times higher in patients with NVG than in POAG and

113 times higher than in patients with cataracts.[20] These elevated VEGF levels in NVG have interesting and very important implications for the use of anti-VEGF therapy in NVG.

Current Standard of Therapy

NVG is extremely difficult to manage. Medical control of IOP with topical aqueous suppressants is challenging and the effects are only temporizing. Ideally, patients with ischemic conditions who are at high risk for developing NVG should be followed closely and examined carefully at each visit looking for signs of neovascularization of the iris and angle. If any NVI or NVA is seen, anti-VEGF intravitreal injections can be performed followed by panretinal photocoagulation (PRP). PRP is the current gold standard of therapy for NVG for long-term control after anti-VEGF treatment.[20] It destroys ischemic retinal tissue and thus reduces the oxygen demand in the retina and subsequently the stimulus for angiogenesis.

If performed early enough during the neovascular process, even in the absence of anti-VEGF agents, PRP can cause visible regression of the vessels both posteriorly and anteriorly. Studies have shown reduced levels of VEGF in patients after PRP.[50] While PRP can be effective for early-recognized NVG, there are multiple drawbacks to relying on PRP alone. Specifically, the effects are delayed, so patients may continue to have pain and elevated IOP. PRP also causes death to healthy retinal cells and subsequent constriction of the visual field. It may also be difficult to perform because of a diminished view in patients with media opacities like vitreous hemorrhage, cataracts, or corneal edema from increased IOP. While PRP may be effective in NVG when the angle is open, its benefit in interrupting the process is less so after there is angle closure.[51] Once the fibrovascular membrane extends across the angle and creates peripheral anterior synechiae, NVG will develop with permanent synechial angle closure causing severe IOP elevation in all but the most ischemic eyes, which paradoxically may have reduced aqueous suppression. At that point, anti-VEGF agents and PRP will not reverse the process and further surgical intervention with glaucoma surgery is needed.[51]

Once medications have failed to control IOP and synechial angle closure is present, glaucoma-filtration surgery is the usual surgical option for eyes with salvageable vision. Glaucoma-drainage implants like the Baerveldt, Molteno, or Ahmed valve aqueous drainage shunts have traditionally been preferred because their success is not as affected by the inflammation present in NVG.[52] Trabeculectomy can be difficult to manage because the inflammation increases the risk of bleb failure. Antifibrotic agents have increased the success rate of trabeculectomy in NVG but there are still challenges.[53] Filtration surgery with either method can be difficult because of the extremely friable neovascular vessels that can bleed even with minor manipulation, causing hyphema and clot especially if no anti-VEGF treatment has been given preoperatively. This not only creates difficulty intraoperatively because of an impaired view but can also lead to postoperative complications with the formation of blood clots surrounding the glaucoma drainage implant tube or sclerostomy.[54]

Studies Involving Anti-Vascular Endothelial Growth Factor Treatment for Neovascular Glaucoma

Injection of an anti-VEGF agent causes regression of the newly formed vessels in NVI and NVA. This regression of anterior segment neovascularization is grossly visible on slit lamp exam and gonioscopy and has been demonstrated in multiple case series.[55-59] Neovascularization can be significantly diminished within the first 48 hours[58,59] and improvement seems to be maintained anywhere from 4 to 10 weeks.[60,61] Regression of visible signs of neovascularization ranges from 70% to 100% depending on the study.[59,62-64]

There are several studies evaluating the effect of intravitreal bevacizumab in NVG on IOP. In a prospective, randomized clinical trial of 26 eyes, NVG eyes treated with 3 monthly intravitreal injections of bevacizumab had a significant reduction of IOP at 1, 3, and 9 months.[65] Most of the studies were unable to truly examine the isolated effect of intravitreal bevacizumab as many of the eyes also received concurrent PRP.[61,62,65,66]

The mechanism of IOP lowering by anti-VEGF therapy in NVG is not completely understood. The most likely explanation is that regression of vessels and decreased permeability of the vessels reduces the early fibrovascular membrane covering the angle and improves drainage through the trabecular meshwork. Once the angle is closed with anterior synechiae, the only IOP effect may be a result of some remaining functional trabecular tissue that may improve with regression of newly formed vessels.[67]

A study of intravitreal bevacizumab in open- vs closed-angled NVG found that efficacy may depend on the extent of synechiae formation and fibrovascular membrane contraction. While intravitreal bevacizumab benefited those with NVI and an open angle, eyes with closed-angle NVG had regression of the neovascularization without a change in IOP and 93% of the patients needed surgery within 2 months following injection.[62]

Combining anti-VEGF treatment with PRP was studied in a retrospective comparison of 23 eyes treated with either same-day intravitreal bevacizumab with PRP to PRP alone. The benefits of combination therapy included a higher frequency of neovascular regression (100% of eyes in the combination group vs 17% of eyes in the PRP-only group) and a more rapid rate of regression (complete regression seen by 12 days in the combination group vs 127 days in the PRP-only group). The IOP was also more significantly reduced in the combination group compared to the PRP-only group. Furthermore, fewer eyes in the combination group needed further surgical intervention compared with the PRP group, although they were followed for only 143 days and 118 days, respectively.[68] Another similar study of 14 eyes confirmed the findings that neovascularization regressed more rapidly in the combination group; however, they did not find a significant difference in mean IOP between the groups. Additionally, it was discovered that despite similar angle anatomy at baseline between the 2 groups, the group that received combination therapy with bevacizumab had significantly more open-angle structures at the 6-month mark and this result persisted at 1 year.[69]

Combination Therapy With Ahmed Valve

Shunting devices are extremely useful for refractory cases of NVG because of their efficiency and lower rates of postoperative complications when compared to trabeculectomy in a severely inflamed eye. The choice between the various aqueous drainage devices such as Baerveldt, Ahmed, or Molteno shunts depends mostly on the surgeon's preference. The treatment of NVG continues to be a challenge even with these devices. In a study evaluating 16 eyes with NVG treated with an Ahmed valve, the concentration of VEGF in failed cases ($n = 8$) showed significantly elevated levels of VEGF when compared with successful cases.[70] This outlines the important role of VEGF in the successful outcome of surgery and has implications for anti-VEGF therapy with valve placement.

Multiple studies have evaluated the use of intravitreal bevacizumab in Ahmed valve implantation[71-75] (Table 16-2[A]). To date, there are no studies looking at the role of anti-VEGF therapy in other shunting devices such as the Baerveldt or Molteno for NVG. All reported studies used 1.25 mg intravitreal bevacizumab differing only in the administration either preoperatively or intraoperatively.

Preoperative Bevacizumab

The results of these studies have been very inconsistent. Two groups showed some benefit of preoperative intravitreal bevacizumab over cases that underwent implantation of an Ahmed valve alone.[71,72] However, other studies demonstrated no difference in success rate or IOP after Ahmed valve placement,[73,74] although there were significantly reduced rates of hyphema.

Another group combined preoperative intravitreal bevacizumab before Ahmed valve placement with concurrent PRP at the time of injection. This triple therapy was compared with patients receiving PRP and Ahmed alone. The results showed that patients treated with intravitreal bevacizumab had a significantly reduced IOP with a 95% success rate compared to a 50% success rate when bevacizumab was not used.[75] Other reports state PRP is the most important intervention in decreasing the need for subsequent surgery, as it significantly reduces the need for further surgery whether or not intravitreal bevacizumab is used.[76]

Intraoperative Bevacizumab

Most studies have not been able to demonstrate a significant improvement in success rate of Ahmed valve surgery with the addition of intraoperative intravitreal bevacizumab. One group found a statistically significant lower IOP at 12 and 15 months, but there was no improvement in surgical failure rates between the 2 groups; failure included the need for additional surgery, light perception vision, and IOP greater than 21 despite additional medication.[77] Another study showed no difference in success rate, IOP, and visual acuity. Of note, the group that received intraoperative intravitreal bevacizumab was using fewer antiglaucoma medications than the control group and had more frequent complete regression of rubeosis iridis (80%) compared to the control group (25%).[63]

Table 16-2. (A) Anti-Vascular Endothelial Growth Factor in Neovascular Glaucoma Surgery: Ahmed Valve

Anti-VEGF Agent	Route of Administration	Timing of Administration	Reference	Outcome
Bevacizumab	Intravitreal	Preoperative	• Sevim et al[71] 2013 • Eid et al[72] 2009 • Kang et al[73] 2014 • Sahyoun et al[74] 2015 • Mahdy et al[75] 2013 • Olmos et al[76] 2016	• Higher success rate with IVB but not statistically significant; reduced hyphema with IVB • Higher success rate with IVB • No difference in success rate or IOP but reduced incidence of hyphema and improved visual outcome with IVB • No difference in success rate, IOP, or visual outcome; reduced incidence of hyphema with IVB • IVB + PRP + Ahmed superior to PRP + Ahmed alone in success rate of surgery • No difference in IOP or visual outcome
		Intraoperative	• Arcieri et al[63] 2015 • Ma et al[77] 2012	• No difference in success rate, IOP, or visual outcome • Lower IOP but no difference in surgical failure rate
Ranibizumab	Intravitreal	Preoperative	• Tang et al[78] 2016	• No difference in IOP, visual outcome, postoperative complications

Anti-VEGF = anti-vascular endothelial growth factor; IOP = intraocular pressure; IVB = intravitreal bevacizumab; PRP = panretinal photocoagulation.

Preoperative Ranibizumab

Most studies found in the literature have focused on the use of intravitreal bevacizumab in Ahmed implantation. Only one study looked at a different anti-VEGF, ranibizumab (Table 16-2[A]). It was a prospective, nonrandomized study of 43 eyes that were followed for 6 to 12 months. The authors compared the effect of 0.5 mg intravitreal ranbizumab 3 to 14 days before Ahmed valve implantation with Ahmed valve therapy alone; there was no statistically significant difference in IOP, visual outcome, postoperative complications, or the number of antiglaucoma medications after surgery.[78]

Combination Therapy With Trabeculectomy in NVG

Trabeculectomy is already regarded as having a challenging and unpredictable postoperative course in noninflammatory glaucoma. In eyes with NVG, that risk is even higher and trabeculectomies typically have poor success rates because inflammation and neovascularization promote scarring of the bleb.

Preoperative Bevacizumab

The 1-year success rate of a trabeculectomy for NVG in previously vitrectomized eyes without any adjunctive anti-VEGF therapy is about 50%.[79] A few studies have evaluated the use of preoperative anti-VEGF therapy for trabeculectomy (Table 16-2[B]). One looked at the addition of preoperative 1.25 mg intravitreal bevacizumab and found a higher success rate of 73% at 1 year.[80] Another found a success rate of 77.8% but also used repeated injections of intravitreal bevacizumab postoperatively.[81] Neither of these studies used a control group.

Most studies found a complete regression of neovascularization at statistically significant higher rates that ranged from 70% to 93%.[82] One author speculated that because bevacizumab induced regression of NVI, this helped quiet the eye preoperatively, which then reduced the risk of intraoperative and postoperative bleeding as well as inflammation, which would ultimately improve survival of the bleb. Similar to the studies using the Ahmed valve, fewer complications with hyphema were seen in those receiving intravitreal bevacizumab prior to trabeculectomy.[76,83]

In a 2011 retrospective case series of 57 eyes that compared eyes receiving preoperative intravitreal bevacizumab and subsequent trabeculectomy/MMC with eyes that received trabeculectomy/MMC only, there was a significant reduction in IOP of the group receiving adjunctive intravitreal bevacizumab only in the immediate postoperative periods (7 to 10 days) but there was no statistically significant difference in the long-term (up to 1 year follow-up).[79]

While most of the research with anti-VEGF therapy in trabeculectomies for NVG has involved bevacizumab, 2 studies evaluated ranbiziumab. A prospective, noncomparative study examined the adjunctive benefit of combining intracameral ranibizumab with subsequent trabeculectomy with MMC 4 weeks after the injection. More than 50% of cases achieved complete success without topical medications to control IOP and about 40% had IOP control but with medications. There was only 1 failed trabeculectomy in this study of 13 eyes.[84] Another study used 0.5 mg intravitreal ranibizumab 1 week before a

Table 16-2. (B) Anti-Vascular Endothelial Growth Factor in Neovascular Glaucoma Surgery: Trabeculectomy

Anti-VEGF Agent	Route of Administration	Timing of Administration	Reference	Outcome
Bevacizumab	Intravitreal	Preoperative	• Takihara et al[79] 2011 • Miki et al[80] 2011 • Marey and Ellakwa[81] 2011 • Saito et al[83] 2010	• Reduced hyphema and IOP in early post-operative period but no effect on long-term success • Noncomparative study. Success rate of 73% after one year • Noncomparative study. Success rate of 77.8% • Reduced hyphema and increased surgical success rates
Ranibizumab	Intracameral	Preoperative	• Elmekawey and Khafagy[84] 2014	• Noncomparative study. Success rate >50% without additional meds and additional 40% success with meds
	Intravitreal	Preoperative	• Kitnarong et al[85] 2015	• Noncomparative study. Significant decrease in IOP and >80% success rate

Anti-VEGF = anti-vascular endothelial growth factor; IOP = intraocular pressure.

trabeculectomy with MMC. There was significant reduction of IOP afterward with more than 80% of the eyes having a successful outcome.[85]

To date, there are no prospective, randomized controlled trials of outcomes of anti-VEGF treatment for NVG in either trabeculectomy or aqueous drainage devices. Despite this, the rapid regression of neovascularization, improvement in inflammation, and reduced rates of hyphema have led pre- and intraoperative anti-VEGF therapy to become a standard adjuvant for managing neovascular glaucoma.

Pediatric Glaucoma Surgery

Background

Congenital glaucoma is a devastating cause of blindness in children worldwide. The incidence is low, 1 in 10,000 births; however, it is a challenging disease to treat.[86] Congenital and infantile glaucoma is treated surgically; medications are used temporarily to control IOP prior to surgery as they are ineffective and not tolerated well long term. Goniotomy and trabeculotomy are typically the first-choice procedures for primary congenital glaucoma because of their efficacy and low complication rates.[87] If this does not succeed, trabeculectomy in combination with antimetabolites or aqueous drainage device surgery is the next procedure of choice. There have also been studies showing good success rates of combined trabeculotomy/trabeculectomy.[88]

Trabeculectomy

Trabeculectomy in children is associated with a lower success rate and higher complication rate compared with the same procedure in adults. To improve success rates, adjunctive antimetabolites can be used. MMC is the most widely used agent during surgery in the pediatric population, but it is impractical to use multiple injections after surgery given the age group.[89] The success rate of these procedures varies depending on the study, ranging from 35% to 85%, and depends on the patient's age, number of previous surgeries, and antimetabolite use.[90-93]

While there have been multiple studies examining the effects of adjunctive anti-VEGF therapy for trabeculectomies in adults, there is only one reported study looking at the effects in children. The authors conducted a prospective study looking at 24 eyes in 12 patients with bilateral pediatric glaucoma. One eye of each patient had a trabeculectomy combined with application of MMC with a subsequent 2.5 mg subconjunctival injection of bevacizumab intraoperatively. The other eye had trabeculectomy with MMC application only. At 1 year, there was a statistically significant difference in the mean IOP; the group receiving adjunctive subconjunctival bevacizumab had a significantly lower IOP. The complication rate was comparable between the 2 groups.[94]

Ahmed Drainage Device

Aqueous drainage device surgery has been gaining popularity in the pediatric population. The success rate of tube shunt surgery in children is variable, ranging from 31.3% to 97.2%, and literature has promoted the use of Ahmed glaucoma drainage devices over the use of other procedures such as trabeculectomy.[95,96] To date, there is only one reported study looking at the intraoperative use of subconjunctival bevacizumab around the Ahmed valve tube. In this study, 20 eyes received an Ahmed valve alone without any adjunctive therapy, 20 eyes received an Ahmed valve with intraoperative bevacizumab, and 20 eyes received the valve with MMC application. After 12 months, there was a statistically significant increase in the success rate of eyes that received either MMC or bevacizumab compared with Ahmed alone. There was no statistically significant difference between the MMC and bevacizumab groups. Thirty percent of eyes in the MMC group, however, developed devastating complications of tube or scleral erosion, so bevacizumab appeared to be a safer choice in this cohort.[97]

In conclusion, the use of anti-VEGF agents is still novel in its application for pediatric glaucoma surgery. Limited reports have demonstrated success but more research is needed.

References

1. Dandona L, Dandona R. What is the global burden of visual impairment? *BMC Med.* 2006;4:6.

2. Casson RJ, Chidlow G, Wood JP, Crowston JG, Goldberg I. Definition of glaucoma: clinical and experimental concepts. *Clin Exp Ophthalmol.* 2012;40(4):341-349.

3. Cohen LP, Pasquale LR. Clinical characteristics and current treatment of glaucoma. *Cold Springs Harb Perspect Med.* 2014;4(6).

4. Cairns JE. Trabeculectomy. Preliminary report of a new method. *Am J Ophthalmol.* 1968;66(4):673-679.

5. Burr J, Azuara-Blanco A, Avenell A. Medical versus surgical interventions for open angle glaucoma. *Cochrane Database Syst Rev.* 2005;2:CD004399.

6. Hitchings R. Initial treatment for open-angle glaucoma—medical, laser, or surgical? Surgery is the treatment of choice for open-angle glaucoma. *Arch Ophthalmol.* 1998;116(2):241-242.

7. Lama PJ, Fechtner RD. Antifibrotics and wound healing in glaucoma surgery. *Surv Ophthalmol.* 2003;38:314-316.

8. Grewal DS, Jain R, Kumar H, Grewal SP. Evaluation of subconjunctival bevacizumab as an adjunct to trabeculectomy a pilot study. *Ophthalmology.* 2008;115(12):2141-2145.e2.

9. Li Z, Van Bergen T, Van de Veire S, et al. Inhibition of vascular endothelial growth factor reduces scar formation after glaucoma filtration surgery. *Invest Ophthalmol Vis Sci.* 2009;50(11):5217-5225.

10. Canor LB, Mantravadi A, WuDunn D, Swamynathan K, Cortes A. Morphologic classification of filtering blebs after glaucoma filtration surgery: the Indiana Bleb Appearance Grading Scale. *J Glaucoma.* 2003;12(3):266-271.

11. Salmon SE, Sartorelli AC. Cancer chemotherapy. In: Katsung BG, ed. *Basic and Clinical Pharmacology.* 3rd ed. Norwalk, CT: Appleton and Lange; 1987:676, 680-681.

12. Chen CW, Huang HT, Sheu MM. Enhancement of IOP control effect on trabeculectomy by local application of anti-cancer drug. *Acta Ophthalmol Scand.* 1986;25:1487-1491.

13. Gedde SJ, Schiffman JC, Feuer WJ, et al. Treatment outcomes in the Tube Versus Trabeculectomy (TVT) study after five years of follow-up. *Am J Ophthalmol.* 2012;153(5):789-803.

14. Georgoulas S, Dahlmann-Noor A, Brocchini S, Khaw PT. Modulation of wound healing during and after glaucoma surgery. *Prog Brain Res.* 2008;173:237-254.

15. Jampel HD, Solus JF, Tracey PA, et al. Outcomes and bleb-related complications of trabeculectomy. *Ophthalmology.* 2012;119(4):712-722.

16. Saeedi OJ, Jefferys JL, Solus JF, Jampel HD, Quigley HA. Risk factors for adverse consequences of low intraocular pressure after trabeculectomy. *J Glaucoma.* 2014;23(1):e60-e68.

17. Wong J, Wang N, Miller JW, Schuman JS. Modulation of human fibroblast activity by selected angiogenesis inhibitors. *Exp Eye Res.* 1994;58(4):439-451.

18. Almhanna K, Pelley RJ, Thomas Budd G, Davidson J, Moore HC. Subcutaneous implantable venous access device erosion through the skin in patients treated with anti-vascular endothelial growth factor therapy: a case series. *Anticancer Drugs.* 2008;19(2):217-219.

19. Kim TI, Chung JL, Hong JP, Min K, Seo KY, Kim EK. Bevacizumab application delays epithelial healing in rabbit cornea. *Invest Ophthalmol Vis Sci.* 2009;50(10):4653-4659.

20. Tripathi RC, Li J, Tripathi BJ, Chalam KV, Adamis AP. Increased level of vascular endothelial growth factor in aqueous humor of patients with neovascular glaucoma. *Ophthalmology.* 1998;105(2):232-237.

21. Hu DN, Ritch R, Liebmann J, Liu Y, Cheng B, Hu MS. Vascular endothelial growth factor is increased in aqueous humor of glaucomatous eyes. *J Glaucoma.* 2002;11(5):406-410.

22. Lopilly Park HY, Kim JH, Ahn MD, Park CK. Level of vascular endothelial growth factor in tenon tissue and results of glaucoma surgery. *Arch Ophthalmol.* 2012;130(6):685-689.

23. Ergorul C, Ray A, Huang W, Darland D, Luo ZK, Grosskreutz CL. Levels of vascular endothelial growth factor-A165b (VEGF-A165b) are elevated in experimental glaucoma. *Mol Vis.* 2008;14:1517-1524.

24. Memarzadeh F, Varma R, Lin LT, et al. Postoperative use of bevacizumab as an antifibrotic agent in glaucoma filtration surgery in the rabbit. *Invest Ophthalmol Vis Sci.* 2009;50(7):3233-3237.

25. Van Bergen T, Vandewalle E, Van de Veire S, et al. The role of different VEGF isoforms in scar formation after glaucoma filtration surgery. *Exp Eye Res.* 2011;93(5):689-699.

26. Pieramici DJ, Rabena MD. Anti-VEGF therapy: comparison of current and future agents. *Eye (Lond).* 2008;22(10):1330-1336.

27. Bakri SJ, Snyder MR, Reid JM, Pulido JS, Singh RJ. Pharmacokinetics of intravitreal bevacizumab (Avastin). *Ophthalmology.* 2007;114(5):855-859.

28. Bakri SJ, Snyder MR, Reid JM, Pulido JS, Ezzat MK, Singh RJ. Pharmacokinetics of intravitreal ranibizumab (Lucentis). *Ophthalmology.* 2007;114(12):2179-2182.

29. Apte RS, Modi M, Masonson H, Patel M, Whitfield L, Adamis AP. Pegaptanib 1-year systemic safety results from a safety-pharmacokinetic trial in patients with neovascular age-related macular degeneration. *Ophthalmology.* 2007;114(9):1702-1712.

30. Nomoto H, Shiraga F, Kuno N, et al. Pharmacokinetics of bevacizumab after topical, subconjunctival, and intravitreal administration in rabbits. *Invest Ophthalmol Vis Sci.* 2009;50(10):4807-4813.

31. Sengupta S, Venkatesh R, Ravindran RD. Safety and efficacy of using off-label bevacizumab versus mitomycin C to prevent bleb failure in a single-site phacotrabeculectomy by a randomized controlled clinical trial. *J Glaucoma.* 2012;21(7):450-459.

32. Nilforushan N, Yadgari M, Kish SK, Nassiri N. Subconjunctival bevacizumab versus mitomycin C adjunctive to trabeculectomy. *Am J Ophthalmol.* 2012;153(2):352-357.e1.

33. Simsek T, Cankaya AB, Elgin U. Comparison of needle revision with subconjunctival bevacizumab and 5-fluorouracil injection of failed trabeculectomy blebs. *J Ocul Pharmacol Ther.* 2012;28(5):542-546.

34. Kiddee W, Orapiriyakul L, Kittigoonpaisan K, Tantisarasart T, Wangsupadilok B. Efficacy of adjunctive subconjunctival bevacizumab on the outcomes of primary trabeculectomy with mitomycin C: a prospective randomized placebo-controlled trial. *J Glaucoma.* 2015;24(8):600-606.

35. Sedghipour MR, Mostafaei A, Taghavi Y. Low-dose subconjunctival bevacizumab to augment trabeculectomy for glaucoma. *Clin Ophthalmol.* 2011;5:797-800.

36. Akkan JU, Cilsim S. Role of subconjunctival bevacizumab as an adjuvant to primary trabeculectomy: a prospective randomized comparative 1-year follow-up study. *J Glaucoma.* 2015;24(1):1-8.

37. Fakhraie G, Ghadimi H, Eslami Y, et al. Short-term results of trabeculectomy using adjunctive intracameral bevacizumab: a randomized controlled trial. *J Glaucoma.* 2016;25(3):e182-e188.

38. Vandewalle E, Abegão Pinto L, Van Bergen T, et al. Intracameral bevacizumab as an adjunct to trabeculectomy: a 1-year prospective, randomised study. *Br J Ophthalmol.* 2014;98(1):73-78.

39. Klos-Rola J, Tulidowicz-Bielak M, Zarnowski T. Effects of topical bevacizumab application on early bleb failure after trabeculectomy: observational case series. *Clin Ophthalmol.* 2013;7:1929-1935.

40. Gedde SJ, Schiffman JC, Feuer WJ, et al. Three-year follow-up of the tube versus trabeculectomy study. *Am J Ophthalmol.* 2009;148(5):670-684.

41. Bindlish R, Condon GP, Schlosser JD, D'Antonio J, Lauer KB, Lehrer R. Efficacy and safety of mitomycin-C in primary trabeculectomy: five-year follow-up. *Ophthalmology.* 2002;109(7):1336-1341.

42. Three-year follow-up of the Fluorouracil Filtering Surgery Study. *Am J Ophthalmol.* 1993;115(1):82-92.

43. Tai TY, Moster MR, Pro MJ, Myers JS, Katz LJ. Needle bleb revision with bevacizumab and mitomycin C compared with mitomycin C alone for failing filtration blebs. *J Glaucoma.* 2015;24(4):311-315.

44. Kahook MY. Bleb morphology and vascularity after trabeculectomy with intravitreal ranibizumab: a pilot study. *Am J Ophthalmol.* 2010;150(3):399-403.e1.

45. Pro MJ, Freidl KB, Neylan CJ, Sawchyn AK, Wizov SS, Moster MR. Ranibizumab versus mitomycin C in primary trabeculectomy—a pilot study. *Curr Eye Res.* 2015;40(5):510-515.

46. Hayreh SS. Neovascular glaucoma. *Prog Retin Eye Res.* 2007;26(5):470-485.

47. Weiss DI, Shaffer RN, Nehrenberg TR. Neovascular glaucoma complicating carotid-cavernous fistula. *Arch Ophthalmol.* 1963;69:304-307.

48. Brown GC, Magargal LE, Schachat A, Shah H. Neovascular glaucoma. Etiologic considerations. *Ophthalmology.* 1984;91(4):315-320.

49. Kahook, MY. Neovascular glaucoma. In: Yanoff M, Duker J, eds. *Ophthalmology.* 3rd ed. Philadelphia, PA: Mosby; 2009:1178-1182.

50. Chalam KV, Brar VS, Murthy RK. Human ciliary epithelium as a source of synthesis and secretion of vascular endothelial growth factor in neovascular glaucoma. *JAMA Ophthalmol.* 2014;132(11):1350-1354.

51. Simha A, Braganza A, Abraham L, Samuel P, Lindsley K. Anti-vascular endothelial growth factor for neovascular glaucoma. *Cochrane Database Syst Rev.* 2013;10:CD00792.

52. Park UC, Park KH, Kim DM, Yu HG. Ahmed glaucoma valve implantation for neovascular glaucoma after vitrectomy for proliferative diabetic retinopathy. *J Glaucoma.* 2011;20(7):433-438.

53. Takihara Y, Inatani M, Fukushima M, Iwao K, Iwao M, Tanihara H. Trabeculectomy with mitomycin C for neovascular glaucoma: prognostic factors for surgical failure. *Am J Ophthalmol.* 2009;147(5):912-918, 918.e1.

54. Olmos LC, Lee RK. Medical and surgical treatment of neovascular glaucoma. *Int Ophthalmol Clin.* 2011;51(3):27-36.

55. Avery RL. Regression of retinal and iris neovascularization after intravitreal bevacizumab (Avastin) treatment. *Retina.* 2006;26:352-354.

56. Davidorf FH, Mouser JG, Derick RJ. Rapid improvement of rubeosis iridis from a single bevacizumab (Avastin) injection. *Retina.* 2006;26:354-356.

57. Kahook MY, Schuman JS, Noecker RJ. Intravitreal bevacizumab in a patient with neovascular glaucoma. *Ophthalmic Surg Lasers Imaging.* 2006;37:144-146.

58. Canut MI, Alvarez A, Nadal J, Abreu R, Abreu JA, Pulido JS. Anterior segment changes following intravitreal bevacizumab injection for treatment of neovascular glaucoma. *Clin Ophthalmol.* 2011;5:715-719.

59. Oshima Y, Sakaguchi H, Gomi F, Tano Y. Regression of iris neovascularization after intravitreal injection of bevacizumab in patients with proliferative diabetic retinopathy. *Am J Ophthalmol.* 2006;142(1):155-158.

60. Bakri SJ, Snyder MR, Reid JM, Pulido JS, Singh RJ. Pharmacokinetics of intravitreal bevacizumab (Avastin). *Ophthalmology.* 2007;114(5):855-859.

61. Iliev ME, Domig D, Wolf-Schnurrbursch U, Wolf S, Sarra GM. Intravitreal bevacizumab (Avastin) in the treatment of neovascular glaucoma. *Am J Ophthalmol.* 2006;142(6):1054-1056.

62. Wakabayashi T, Oshima Y, Sakaguchi H, et al. Intravitreal bevacizumab to treat iris neovascularization and neovascular glaucoma secondary to ischemic retinal diseases in 41 consecutive cases. *Ophthalmology.* 2008;115(9):1571-1580, 1580.e1-1580.e3.

63. Arcieri E, Paula JS, Jorge R, et al. Efficacy and safety of intravitreal bevacizumab in eyes with neovascular glaucoma undergoing Ahmed glaucoma valve implantation: 2-year follow-up. *Acta Ophthalmol.* 2015;93(1):e1-e6.

64. Ghosh S, Singh D, Ruddle JB, Shiu M, Coote MA, Crowston JG. Combined diode laser cyclo-photocoagulation and intravitreal bevacizumab (Avastin) in neovascular glaucoma. *Clin Exp Ophthalmol.* 2010;38(4):353-357.

65. Yazdani S, Hendi K, Pakravan M. Intravitreal bevacizumab (Avastin) injection for neovascular glaucoma. *J Glaucoma.* 2007;16(5):437-439.

66. Kotecha A, Spratt A, Ogunbowale L, et al. Intravitreal bevacizumab in refractory neovascular glaucoma: a prospective, observational case series. *Arch Ophthalmol.* 2011;129(2):145-150.

67. Yazdani S, Hendi K, Pakravan M, Mahdavi M, Yaseri M. Intravitreal bevacizumab for neovascular glaucoma: a randomized controlled trial. *J Glaucoma.* 2009;18(8):632-637.

68. Ehlers JP, Spirn MJ, Lam A, Sivalingam A, Samuel MA, Tasman W. Combination intravitreal bevacizumab/panretinal photocoagulation versus panretinal photocoagulation alone in the treatment of neovascular glaucoma. *Retina.* 2008;28(5):696-702.

69. Vasudev D, Blair MP, Galasso J, Kapur R, Vajaranant T. Intravitreal bevacizumab for neovascular glaucoma. *J Ocul Pharmacol Ther.* 2009;25(5):453-458.

70. Kim YG, Hong S, Lee CS, et al. Level of vascular endothelial growth factor in aqueous humor and surgical results of Ahmed glaucoma valve implantation in patients with neovascular glaucoma. *J Glaucoma.* 2009;18(6):443-447.

71. Sevim MS, Buttanri IB, Kugu S, Serin D, Sevim S. Effect of intravitreal bevacizumab injection before Ahmed glaucoma valve implantation in neovascular glaucoma. *Ophthalmologica.* 2013;229(2):94-100.

72. Eid TM, Radwan A, el-Manawy W, el-Hawary I. Intravitreal bevacizumab and aqueous shunting surgery for neovascular glaucoma: safety and efficacy. *Can J Ophthal.* 2009;44(4):451-456.

73. Kang JY, Nam KY, Lee SJ, Lee SU. The effect of intravitreal bevacizumab injection before Ahmed valve implantation in patients with neovascular glaucoma. *Int Ophthalmol.* 2014;34(4):793-799.

74. Sahyoun M, Azar G, Khoueir Z, et al. Long-term results of Ahmed glaucoma valve in association with intravitreal bevacizumab in neovascular glaucoma. *J Glaucoma.* 2015;24(5):383-388.

75. Mahdy RA, Nada WM, Fawzy KM, Alnashar HY, Almosalamy SM. Efficacy of intravitreal bevacizumab with panretinal photocoagulation followed by Ahmed valve implantation in neovascular glaucoma. *J Glaucoma.* 2013;22(9):768-772.

76. Olmos LC, Sayed MS, Moraczewski AL, et al. Long-term outcomes of neovascular glaucoma treated with and without intravitreal bevacizumab. *Eye (Lond).* 2016;30(3):463-472.

77. Ma KT, Yang JY, Kim JH, et al. Surgical results of Ahmed valve implantation with intraoperative bevacizumab injection in patients with neovascular glaucoma. *J Glaucoma.* 2012;21:331-336.

78. Tang M, Fu Y, Wang Y, et al. Efficacy of intravitreal ranibizumab combined with Ahmed glaucoma valve implantation for the treatment of neovascular glaucoma. *BMC Ophthalmol.* 2016;16(1):7.

79. Takihara Y, Inatani M, Kawaji T, et al. Combined intravitreal bevacizumab and trabeculectomy with mitomycin C versus trabeculectomy with mitomycin C alone for neovascular glaucoma. *J Glaucoma.* 2011;20:196-201.

80. Miki A, Oshima Y, Otori Y, Matsushita K, Nishida K. One-year results of intravitreal bevacizumab as an adjunct to trabeculectomy for neovascular glaucoma in eyes with previous vitrectomy. *Eye (Lond).* 2011;25(5):658-659.

81. Marey HM, Ellakwa AF. Intravitreal bevacizumab with or without mitomycin C trabeculectomy in the treatment of neovascular glaucoma. *Clin Ophthalmol.* 2011;5:841-845.

82. Chen CH, Lai IC, Wu PC, et al. Adjunctive intravitreal bevacizumab-combined trabeculectomy versus trabeculectomy alone in the treatment of neovascular glaucoma. *J Ocul Pharmacol Ther.* 2010;26(1):111-118.

83. Saito Y, Higashide T, Takeda H, Ohkubo S, Sugiyama K. Beneficial effects of preoperative intravitreal bevacizumab on trabeculectomy outcomes in neovascular glaucoma. *Acta Ophthalmol.* 2010;88(1):96-102.

84. Elmekawey H, Khafagy A. Intracameral ranibizumab and subsequent mitomycin C augmented trabeculectomy inneovascular glaucoma. *J Glaucoma.* 2014;23(7):437-440.

85. Kitnarong N, Sriyakul C, Chinwattanakul S. A prospective study to evaluate intravitreous ranibizumab as adjunctive treatment for trabeculectomy in neovascular glaucoma. *Ophthalmol Ther.* 2015;4(1):33-41.

86. Dickens CJ, Hoskins HD. Diagnosis and treatment of congenital glaucoma. In: Ritch R, Shields MB, Krupin T, eds. *The Glaucomas.* St. Louis, MO: Mosby; 1989.

87. Chen TC, Chen PP, Francis BA, et al. Pediatric glaucoma surgery: a report by the American Academy of Ophthalmology. *Ophthalmology.* 2014;121(11):2107-2115.

88. Mullaney PB, Selleck C, Al-Awad A, Al-Mesfer S, Zwaan J. Combined trabeculectomy and trabeculotomy as an initial procedure in uncomplicated congenital glaucoma. *Arch Ophthalmol.* 1999;117(4):457-460.

89. Giampani J Jr, Borges-Giampani AS, Carani JC, Oltrogge EW, Susanna R Jr. Efficacy and safety of trabeculectomy with mitomycin C for childhood glaucoma: a study of results with long term follow-up. *Clinics (Sao Paulo).* 2008;63(4):21-26.

90. Beauchamps GR, Parks MM. Filtering surgery in children: barriers to success. *Ophthalmology.* 1979;86:170-180.

91. Inaba Z. Long-term results of trabeculectomy in the Japanese: an analysis by life-table method. *Jpn J Ophthalmol.* 1982;26(4):361-373.

92. Gressel MG, Heuer DK, Parrish RK. Trabeculectomy in young patients. *Ophthalmology.* 1984;91:1242-1246.

93. Debnath SC, Teichmann KD, Salamah K. Trabeculectomy versus trabeculotomy in congenital glaucoma. *Br J Ophthalmol.* 1989;73(8):608-611.

94. Mahdy RA, Al-Mosallamy SM, Al-Aswad MA, Bor'i A, El-Haig WM. Evaluation the adjunctive use of combined bevacizumab and mitomycin c to trabeculectomy in management of recurrent pediatric glaucoma. *Eye (Lond).* 2016;30(1):53-58.

95. Englert JA, Freedman SF, Cox TA. The Ahmed valve in refractory pediatric glaucoma. *Am J Ophthalmol.* 1999;127:34-42.

96. Pirouzian A, Scher C, O'Halloran H, Jockin Y. Ahmed glaucoma valve implants in the pediatric population: the use of magnetic resonance imaging for surgical approach to reoperation. *J AAPOS.* 2006;10(4):340-344.

97. Mahdy RA. Adjunctive use of bevacizumab versus mitomycin C with Ahmed valve implantation in treatment of pediatric glaucoma. *J Glaucoma.* 2011;20(7):458-463.

17

ANTERIOR SEGMENT DISEASES

Alessandro Abbouda, MD; Bijan Khaksari, BA; and
Pedram Hamrah, MD, FRCS

Corneal Neovascularization

Corneal avascularity is fundamental in maintaining a clear cornea and to guarantee optimal vision. The cornea is one of the few avascular tissues in the body. However, several corneal diseases, such as inflammatory conditions, infectious keratitis, pterygium, ocular surface neoplasia, limbal stem cell deficiency, chemical burns, and corneal graft rejection can induce corneal neovascularization.[1] Corneal neovascularization is defined as the development of new vessels originating from the limbus that invade the cornea. It can promote lipid exudation, resulting in lipid keratopathy, and corneal scarring, due to alterations of the stromal collagen architecture and spacing between collagen fibrils.[2]

The lack of avascularity in the normal cornea has been termed *angiogenic privilege.*[2] Several factors have been associated with maintaining corneal angiogenic privilege:

- Corneal dehydration. The relation between corneal edema and neovascularization was mentioned initially in 1949 by Cogan.[3] He noted that in corneal burns, new vessels were found at the site where corneal edema was greatest.
- Preservation of the corneal epithelium. Corneal epithelial cells exhibit anti-angiogenic effects, thus preventing the growth of new vessels.[4,5]
- Extensive corneal innervation, diffusion of aqueous humor across the cornea, and lower corneal temperature.[2]
- Limited levels of pro-angiogenic factors, including low levels of pro-angiogenic matrix metalloproteases (MMPs),[6,7] during hemostasis and wound healing.

Duker JS, Liang MC, eds.
Anti-VEGF Use in
Ophthalmology (pp. 197-209).
© 2017 Taylor & Francis Group.

Table 17-1. Pro- and Anti-Angiogenic Factors Involved in Corneal Neovascularization[9]

Pro-angiogenic Factors	Anti-angiogenic Factors
Vascular endothelial growth factors (VEGF) VEGF-A, VEGF-C	Vascular endothelial growth factor receptors (VEGFR) sVEGFR-1, mVEGFR-3
Fibroblast growth factors FGF1, FGF2 (bFGF)	Pigment epithelium-derived factor (PEDF)
Platelet-derived growth factors (PDGF) PDGF-AA, PDGF-AB	Collagen derivatives Endostatin, Canstatin
Matrix metalloproteinases MT1-MMP, MMP-2	Matrix metalloproteinases Epithelial MT1-MMP, MMP-7
Angiopoietins Ang-1, Ang-2	Angiostatin
Cytokines/chemokines IL-1, IL-8/CXCL8	Cytokines/chemokines IL-1RA, IP-10/CXCL10

IL = interleukin.

- Barrier by limbal stem cells. The parallel orientation of band fibrils and the constant renewal of epithelial cells blocks the development of vessels from the limbus during homeostasis.[2]
- Active expression of anti-angiogenic factors and active suppression of pro-angiogenic factors in the cornea (Table 17-1).[8]

Among pro-angiogenic factors, vascular endothelial growth factor (VEGF) is the most important in the pathogenesis of corneal neovascularization and is the target used for many treatments. Although several different isoforms exist,[10] VEGF-A$_{165}$ is considered to be the dominant pro-angiogenic isoform related to pathologic angiogenesis.[11] VEGF-A is produced by pericytes, smooth muscle cells, and macrophages during inflammation and hypoxia.[12-14] The binding of VEGF-A to its receptor VEGFR-2 promotes pathologic angiogenesis, as well as vascular dilation and enhanced permeability.[15-17]

During corneal insult, pro-angiogenic growth factors cross the tissue, bind to respective receptors on endothelial cells located near the lesion site, and result in proliferation and migration of endothelial cells. Subsequently induced intracellular signaling pathways then generate the production of specific proteolytic enzymes that are capable of degrading the basement membrane collagen of capillaries and venules. Endothelial cells then proliferate and form capillary tubes, forming the backbone of future new vessels. Once proteolytic enzymes degrade stromal collagen, enhancing permeability, the new capillary tubes are able to penetrate the tissue. These capillaries dilate and then branch out, forming vascular loops and connections with neighboring vessels. Finally, specialized smooth muscle cells and pericytes stabilize capillaries by providing structural support. It is only at the end of this last step that the vascular blood flow will commence in the capillary tubes.[15,17]

Therapeutic Drugs for the Treatment of Corneal Neovascularization

Various VEGF inhibitors are currently being investigated for the treatment of corneal neovascularization.

Bevacizumab

Bevacizumab (Avastin) is a full-length, humanized murine monoclonal antibody and has a molecular weight of 149 kD. It recognizes all VEGF-A isoforms.[18] A healthy corneal epithelial barrier precludes its penetration in normal eyes; however, during corneal neovascularization, the integrity of the epithelial tight junction is lost, allowing the antibody to penetrate into the corneal stroma.[19] Several studies have reported the successful use of bevacizumab for corneal neovascularization via different approaches, including topical eye drops and subconjunctival injections.[9,19-28] Both methods of administration have been shown to induce regression of new vessels[27,28] and decrease inflammation, resulting in return of normal corneal function.[27] Reported side effects include corneal epitheliopathy, stromal thinning, and descemetocele with prolonged use.[24,25,28]

Ranibizumab

Ranibizumab (Lucentis) is a humanized recombinant monoclonal antibody fragment that binds to and inhibits all VEGF-A isoforms. The molecular weight of ranibizumab is 48 kD, making it approximately one-third the size of bevacizumab, thus in theory allowing for better corneal penetration. Further, ranibizumab has been affinity-matured and optimized for improved VEGF-A binding potential. These characteristics may allow ranibizumab to treat corneal neovascularization more effectively than bevacizumab.[29]

Pegaptanib Sodium

Pegaptanib sodium (Macugen) is an RNA aptamer that is directed against $VEGF_{165}$. This VEGF isoform is primarily responsible for pathological corneal neovascularization and increased vascular permeability. Currently, no clinical studies using pegaptanib sodium have been performed in patients with corneal neovascularization.

Aflibercept

Aflibercept (Eylea) is a humanized recombinant fusion protein with a molecular weight of 115 kDa that is constructed from the extracellular domains of the human VEGFR-1 and VEGFR-2.[30] It is derived through fusion of the fragment crystallizable regions of human immunoglobulin G1 to the second binding domain of VEGFR-1 and third binding domain of VEGFR-2.[31] Aflibercept acts like a VEGF-trap by binding to circulating VEGF molecules. In contrast to other anti-VEGF agents that solely target VEGF-A, aflibercept also blocks VEGF-B, placental growth factor-1, and placental growth factor-2. The affinity of aflibercept for $VEGF-A_{165}$ is approximately 120 times greater than bevacizumab and approximately 100 times greater than ranibizumab.[32] There are a few murine preclinical studies that have demonstrated its efficacy in treating or inhibiting corneal neovascularization.[33,34]

Figure 17-1. Corneal neovascularization in a patient with *Acanthamoeba* keratitis.

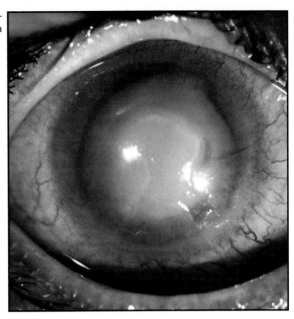

Corneal Neovascularization in Anterior Segment Diseases

The total incidence of corneal neovascular disease in the United States has been estimated to be 1.4 million patients per year, with extended contact lens wearers, corneal transplantation, and infectious keratitis (Figure 17-1) being the most common diseases associated with corneal neovascularization.[35]

Corneal Transplantation and Graft Rejection

Corneal transplantation is the most common organ transplantation performed in the United States and has a higher success rate compared to other forms of solid organ transplantation.[36-38] For uncomplicated low-risk patients, the survival rate is 90% for the first year.[39] However, in high-risk patients, such as in the setting of corneal neovascularization, the survival rate can drop to as low as 20%[40] with significantly increased rates of immune rejection.[41] The number of quadrants with neovascularization in the host has been associated with a higher risk of rejection.[42] In addition, promotion of new vessels into the donor cornea due to sutures and suturing technique, which can act as an inflammatory stimulus, has been associated with increased rate of graft rejection. This is particularly more common if the knots are placed on the limbal or host side, instead of on the donor side.[40]

Recently, the use of anti-angiogenic therapies, in particular anti-VEGF agents, have led to increased success rates in the setting of high-risk corneal transplantation. Anti-angiogenic therapy has been used as an adjunct with topical or subconjunctival applications. Dekaris et al.[20] proposed different treatment protocols according to the number of corneal quadrants involved. In a large prospective clinical trial of 50 patients with 3 years of follow-up, all patients received subconjunctival bevacizumab (0.5 ml of 25 mg/ml). In cases with more than 2 quadrants of corneal neovascularization, patients also received topical bevacizumab (25 mg/ml, 4 times daily, not exceeding 12 weeks). The authors observed decreased neovascularization in 84% of patients and clear corneal grafts in 70% of patients, thus demonstrating successful management in the majority of high-risk cases.[20]

An alternative approach was described by Elbaz et al,[43] who proposed the use of corneal fine-needle diathermy (FND) combined with intrastromal bevacizumab injections in children. The authors inserted FND intrastromally 1 mm from the limbus to the level of the corneal vessels. Unipolar diathermy was used to blanch the vessels without observation of collagen shrinkage. Once the vessels were cauterized, bevacizumab (25 mg/ml) was injected into the stroma in proximity of the vessels. Of 9 treated eyes, 8 eyes obtained complete resolution. The rationale for this approach is to combine the efficacy of bevacizumab for new immature vessels, which is effective prior to vessels acquiring perycites,[44] with the use of FND for more mature vessels that are poorly responsive to topical bevacizumab. However, the use of FND in general has also been shown to induce pro-angiogenic factors.[45]

Another approach was proposed in a prospective case-control series of 27 patients with corneal neovascularization requiring corneal transplantation.[21] The authors pretreated the case group with 3 cycles of subconjunctival and/or intrastromal injections of bevacizumab (5 mg/0.2 ml). In the presence of a large stromal vessel, the authors injected half the dose in the conjunctiva and the other half in the stroma. After an average of six months, all patients underwent corneal transplantation; the case group also received a subconjunctival injection of bevacizumab at the end of the keratoplasty. During a mean follow-up of 26 months, none of the bevacizumab-treated patients demonstrated corneal graft rejection, while 6 out of 13 eyes in the control group demonstrated graft rejection at a mean of 3.8 months, suggesting that treatment of high-risk eyes with corneal neovascularization can improve the survival rate and decrease corneal rejection rate. In addition to the above studies, a multicenter clinical trial is currently underway to assess the safety and efficacy of topical bevacizumab 1% in high-risk corneal transplantation (clinicaltrials.gov identifier NCT01996826).

Both bevacizumab 1% and ranibizumab 1% have been shown to be effective in the treatment of corneal neovascularization as demonstrated by a decrease in the corneal neovascular area as well as vascular caliber.[46-48] However, the lack of change in the invasion area suggests treatment does not reduce vascular length, but rather the caliber alone. Thus, anti-VEGF therapy is more effective in the treatment of new immature vessels, rather than in stable neovascularization with the presence of mature vessels.[46] Preclinical experimental studies comparing ranibizumab to bevacizumab in a rabbit model of corneal neovascularization have shown that subconjunctival injection of either therapy results in the inhibition of new vessel growth in an equivalent fashion.[48] Similar to data in patients, the effect of the anti-VEGF therapy was dependent on the timing of initial therapy after induction of angiogenesis.[26,48]

In addition to corneal neovascularization in the setting of full-thickness penetrating keratoplasty, corneal neovascularization can develop in the stromal interface after deep anterior lamellar keratoplasty procedures. Bevacizumab treatment has also been successfully applied for the treatment of corneal neovascularization in these cases.[9,22,23] It has been injected perilimbally[22] or intrastromally into the interface adjacent to the vessels at doses of 1.25 mg[23] or 2.5 mg.[9]

In summary, anti-angiogenic treatments for corneal neovascularization before and after corneal transplantation has been shown to be safe and effective in inducing regression of vessels and promoting graft survival.

Herpes Simplex Keratitis

The recurrent nature of herpes simplex keratitis makes it the most common infectious cause of corneal blindness in the Western world. The incidence and prevalence of herpes simplex keratitis has been estimated to be around 20.7 and 149 cases/100,000 patients a year, respectively.[49] Corneal neovascularization is a main feature of herpetic stromal keratitis caused by the herpes simplex virus (HSV)-1. Several mechanisms have been associated with angiogenesis and the subsequent corneal scarring and lipid keratopathy in HSV keratitis: upregulation of VEGF-A from HSV-infected epithelial cells and infiltrating macrophages[50] and additional matrix-degrading proteases, such as MMP-9.[51] As such, the inhibition of angiogenesis is advantageous, as it prevents or reduces corneal opacities due to scarring or lipid deposition. An initial case report described the positive outcome of subconjunctival bevacizumab (1.25 mg in 0.05 ml) in an elderly woman with herpes stromal keratitis.[52] The injection resulted in rapid regression of the corneal vessels. Furthermore, no relapse was seen during the 3-month follow-up. Another case report of a young woman with corneal pannus due to HSV keratitis treated with bevacizumab demonstrated no initial change in corneal opacity and vascularization after treatment.[53] However, subsequent treatment with both intrastromal and subconjunctival ranibizumab injections resulted in a significant regression of the vascular area. Several other larger studies have demonstrated the efficacy of anti-VEGF therapy for the treatment of corneal neovascularization in patients with HSV keratitis.[28,43,46] No study to date, however, has directly compared different VEGF inhibitors for corneal neovascularization. In order to justify the increased cost of ranibizumab and other drugs as compared to bevacizumab, it may be necessary to demonstrate their superiority in randomized trials.

Contact Lenses Wear

Corneal neovascularization is relatively common among contact lens wearers. The prevalence is estimated to be between 10% to 30% of cases, with a variable degree of vascularization.[54] Corneal neovascularization in contact lens wearers has been described in 4 levels[55]:

1. Limbal hyperemia with dilation of existing limbal capillaries
2. Penetration of vessels into the superficial cornea with a superficial pannus
3. Deep stromal vessels
4. Intracorneal hemorrhage

Furthermore, limbal stem cell deficiency due to chronic contact lens wear can result in variable levels of corneal neovascularization. Currently, no studies have been conducted assessing the efficacy of anti-VEGF therapies in these patients. However, a case series of 5 patients with corneal neovascularization reported the effective use of the prosthetic replacement of the ocular surface (PROSE) scleral lens as a delivery device for bevacizumab.[56]

Image Analysis of Corneal Neovascularization

The evaluation of corneal neovascularization by direct slit-lamp biomicroscopy does not provide a reliable and scientific methodology that can be applied to clinical trials. While vessels are visible, it is not easy to discern the variation in size, length, and diameter for all vessels. Previously, investigators used software for a more quantitative approach to assess changes in corneal vessels.[28,46] More recently, the application of corneal angiography has been an innovative and effective approach to visualize vessels beyond slit-lamp examination.[57,58] Romano et al[57] reported the application of corneal angiography using both fluorescein angiography and indocyanine green angiography using the Heidelberg system with a 15-degree, 20-degree, or 30-degree lens, and a 32 D or 53 D focus. This application was able to distinguish between presumed active and inactive vessels. Moreover, this technique provided important information about the area of corneal neovascularization, the corneal vessel diameter, as well as vascular tortuosity.[58] Corneal angiography has also been used to demonstrate vascular changes due to fine-needle diathermy.[59]

Furthermore, en-face anterior segment optical coherence tomography (AS-OCT) angiography has allowed visualization of corneal vessels without the use of invasive dye.[60] The quality and resolution of images may not reach the resolution of standard corneal angiography; however, AS-OCT angiography has the ability to visualize blood flow within each layer and may be the gold standard in the years to come. Images obtained by any methodology can be analyzed using the new ImageJ plugin, VesselJ,[61] which was developed to quantify vascular changes. With the increased utility of imaging devices for quantification and assessment of corneal neovascularization and its changes following therapy, centralized anterior segment reading will be required for objective and standardized analysis of vascular alterations.

Pterygium

A pterygium is a common ocular surface condition that presents as a wing-shaped fibrovascular lesion over the nasal or temporal cornea, typically extending from the bulbar conjunctiva. It can be associated with inflammation, superficial corneal neovascularization (Figure 17-2), alterations of limbal epithelial cells, squamous metaplasia, and proliferation of fibroblasts. Patients may have chronic discomfort, conjunctival hyperemia, corneal astigmatism, and, in advanced cases, significant vision loss. As such, the main purpose of pterygium excision is to remove the abnormal tissue from both the cornea and conjunctiva to rehabilitate vision and prevent recurrence.[62]

Several surgical approaches, such as conjunctival autograft and amniotic membrane transplantation in conjunction with excision, have been advocated to reduce recurrence in these patients. The incidence of recurrence with the conjunctival autograft technique is reported to be 5.3%, whereas patients treated with the bare sclera technique have recurrence rates as high as 89%. Notably, the recurrence rate after placement of a conjunctival autograft with glue has been reported to be 9.8%,[62] and the recurrence rate with amniotic transplantation is 20% higher than that for conjunctival autograft.[63]

Figure 17-2. Pterygium with early corneal neovascularization.

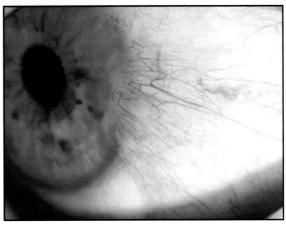

Alternative pharmacological approaches have been investigated to decrease the recurrence rate. The most commonly used is intraoperative 0.02% mitomycin C (MMC) or 5-fluorouracil (5-FU) at the site of pterygium removal in order to prevent recurrent fibrosis. The recurrence rate in MMC-treated eyes has been reported at 8%, compared to an 18% recurrence rate with 5-FU application.[64] Although the adjunctive antifibrotic therapy can allow for a reduction in the incidence of recurrence,[65] MMC has also been reported to cause significant complications, such as limbal cell deficiency, loss of endothelial cells, corneal decompensation, and scleral melting and perforations.[66] Thus, additional pharmacological therapies are required for the treatment of pteryia.

The application of anti-VEGF agents has only recently been introduced for the treatment of this disease and has had variable outcomes. In a randomized clinical trial treating 60 patients with intralesional bevacizumab (1.25 mg/0.05 ml in 20 eyes, 2.5 mg/0.1 ml in 20 eyes, and 3.75 mg/0.15 ml in 20 eyes), bevacizumab only partially and transiently decreased conjunctival vascularization in the pterygium tissue.[67] In addition, a recent meta-analysis showed no significant effect on the prevention of pterygium recurrence.[68] Intraoperative bevacizumab (1.25 mg/0.01 ml or 2.5 mg/0.1 ml) was not found to be effective in reducing the rate of recurrence in several other studies as well.[69,70] However, others have found a significant benefit to the use of anti-VEGF agents. In 1 study, a single 2.5 mg/ml subconjunctival injection of bevacizumab in conjunction with surgical conjunctival autograft procedure was shown to be more effective in preventing recurrence compared to the control group at 1-year follow-up.[71] Moreover, the use of 3 consecutive bevacizumab injections every 2 weeks, beginning at the time of surgery, demonstrated significant reduction in corneal and conjunctival neovascularization in another study.[72] Additional positive results, demonstrating decreased incidence of pterygium recurrence in patients with impending recurrent pterygia, was shown in those who had one or more subconjunctival bevacizumab injections (2.5 mg/0.1 ml).[70] A significant decrease in pterygium size has also been reported.[71]

These diverse outcomes could be due to variable surgical techniques and the application of bevacizumab to both new and recurrent pterygium cases. Anti-VEGF therapy may have a synergistic effect when combined with the best surgical procedure, although recurrence rates in conjunctival autograft cases are already rather low. Similar to that of corneal neovascularization, stable mature vessels may not respond as well as new

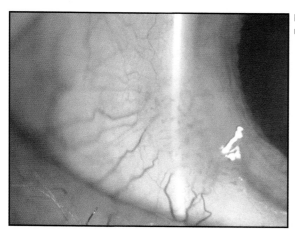

Figure 17-3. Ocular surface squamous neoplasia.

immature vessels, and this may add another variable to treatment outcomes. In general, pterygia remain an enigma and differences in pathogenesis between primary and recurrent pterygia might exist. While the use of bevacizumab is safe and well tolerated by pterygium patients,[72] additional randomized clinical trials in primary pterygium excision with standardized surgical techniques are required to decrease possible bias and elucidate the true utility and efficacy of anti-VEGF therapy in this disease.

Ocular Surface Squamous Neoplasia

Ocular surface squamous neoplasia (OSSN) represents a spectrum of diseases that range from dysplasia to invasive squamous cell carcinoma involving the conjunctival, limbal, and/or corneal epithelium (Figure 17-3). It remains the most common non-pigmented neoplasm of the conjunctiva.[73] The incidence of OSSN is highest among males, particularly in younger age groups.[74] Among the most significant predictive factors for recurrence after excision are the appearance and location of OSSN.[73] In addition to excisional biopsy, several therapeutic pharmacological approaches have been considered effective for the treatment of OSSN, including 5-FU, MMC, and interferon alpha-2b therapy.[73] The use of interferon alpha-2b has shown to be highly favorable in controlling the recurrence of OSSN, albeit, the cost of this drug remains very high.[75]

More recently, the use of anti-VEGF drug therapies has demonstrated favorable results as an adjunct treatment of OSSN, without showing any topical or systemic side effect. One study demonstrated that the application of topical bevacizumab (5 mg/ml) 4 times daily, for a period of 8 weeks, in patients with OSSN resulted in a significant decrease in lesion size that allowed easier excision of the lesion with reduced scar formation. Interestingly, in some patients, the lesion disappeared, which was also confirmed by impression cytology.[76] Another report advocated the use of bevacizumab injection (2.5 mg/0.1 ml), administered at two-week intervals in patients with OSSN, and demonstrated that this treatment was able to decrease the size and vascularity of OSSN.[77] However, in this study, bevacizumab was effective only on the corneal side and not on the conjunctival side. In contrast, a separate study reported that injections with ranibizumab in OSSN were effective in inducing regression on both the conjunctival and corneal side of OSSN.[78] As there are limited data in the literature, larger longitudinal case-control studies or randomized trials need to be conducted to better evaluate the efficacy of anti-VEGF therapy in OSSN patients. Currently, application of anti-VEGF therapy can be considered prior to surgery to reduce lesion size and morbidity of larger excisions.[76-78]

Conclusion

Corneal neovascularization and other anterior segment pathologies can result in significant vision loss and blindness. However, the assessment, imaging, analysis, and therapy of anterior segment neovascularization is far behind that of the posterior segment. The coming years will likely demonstrate significant advances in all of these areas, especially that of the anterior segment.

References

1. Beebe DC. Maintaining transparency: a review of the developmental physiology and pathophysiology of two avascular tissues. *Semin Cell Dev Biol.* 2008;19(2):125-133.

2. Azar DT. Corneal angiogenic privilege: angiogenic and antiangiogenic factors in corneal avascularity, vasculogenesis, and wound healing (an American Ophthalmological Society thesis). *Trans Am Ophthalmol Soc.* 2006;104:264-302.

3. Cogan DG. Vascularization of the cornea; ats experimental induction by small lesions and a new theory of its pathogenesis. *Arch Ophthal.* 1949;41(4):406-416.

4. Sholley MM, Gimbrone MA Jr, Cotran RS. The effects of leukocyte depletion on corneal neovascularization. *Lab Invest.* 1978;38(1):32-40.

5. Nakayasu K, Hayashi N, Okisaka S, Sato N. Formation of capillary-like tubes by vascular endothelial cells cocultivated with keratocytes. *Invest Ophthalmol Vis Sci.* 1992;33(11):3050-3057.

6. Ferrara N, Gerber HP. The role of vascular endothelial growth factor in angiogenesis. *Acta Haematol.* 2001;106(4):148-156.

7. Berman MB. Regulation of corneal fibroblast MMP-1 secretion by cytochalasins. *Cornea.* 1994;13(1):51-57.

8. Cursiefen C. Immune privilege and angiogenic privilege of the cornea. *Chem Immunol Allergy.* 2007;92:50-57.

9. Hashemian MN, Zare MA, Rahimi F, Mohammadpour M. Deep intrastromal bevacizumab injection for management of corneal stromal vascularization after deep anterior lamellar keratoplasty, a novel technique. *Cornea.* 2011;30(2):215-218.

10. Neufeld G, Cohen T, Gengrinovitch S, Poltorak Z. Vascular endothelial growth factor (VEGF) and its receptors. *FASEB J.* 1999;13(1):9-22.

11. Harper SJ, Bates DO. VEGF-A splicing: the key to anti-angiogenic therapeutics? *Nat Rev Cancer.* 2008;8(11):880-887.

12. McCourt M, Wang JH, Sookhai S, Redmond HP. Proinflammatory mediators stimulate neutrophil-directed angiogenesis. *Arch Surg.* 1999;134(12):1325-1331; discussion 1331-1332.

13. Shweiki D, Itin A, Soffer D, Keshet E. Vascular endothelial growth factor induced by hypoxia may mediate hypoxia-initiated angiogenesis. *Nature.* 1992;359(6398):843-845.

14. Witmer AN, Vrensen GF, Van Noorden CJ, Schlingemann RO. Vascular endothelial growth factors and angiogenesis in eye disease. *Prog Retin Eye Res.* 2003;22(1):1-29.

15. Ferrara N, Gerber HP, LeCouter J. The biology of VEGF and its receptors. *Nat Med.* 2003;9(6):669-676.

16. Bates DO, Hillman NJ, Williams B, Neal CR, Pocock TM. Regulation of microvascular permeability by vascular endothelial growth factors. *J Anat.* 2002;200(6):581-597.

17. Hood JD, Meininger CJ, Ziche M, Granger HJ. VEGF upregulates ecNOS message, protein, and NO production in human endothelial cells. *Am J Physiol.* 1998;274(3 Pt 2):H1054-H1058.

18. Ferrara N, Hillan KJ, Gerber HP, Novotny W. Discovery and development of bevacizumab, an anti-VEGF antibody for treating cancer. *Nat Rev Drug Discov.* 2004;3(5):391-400.

19. Dastjerdi MH, Sadrai Z, Saban DR, Zhang Q, Dana R. Corneal penetration of topical and subconjunctival bevacizumab. *Invest Ophthalmol Vis Sci.* 2011;52(12):8718-8723.

20. Dekaris I, Gabrić N, Drača N, Pauk-Gulić M, Miličić N. Three-year corneal graft survival rate in high-risk cases treated with subconjunctival and topical bevacizumab. *Graefes Arch Clin Exp Ophthalmol.* 2015;253(2):287-294.

21. Fasciani R, Mosca L, Giannico MI, Ambrogio SA, Balestrazzi E. Subconjunctival and/or intrastromal bevacizumab injections as preconditioning therapy to promote corneal graft survival. *Int Ophthalmol.* 2015;35(2):221-227.

22. Foroutan A, Fariba B, Pejman B, et al. Perilimbal bevacizumab injection for interface neovascularization after deep anterior lamellar keratoplasty. *Cornea.* 2010;29(11):1268-1272.

23. Jarrin E, Ruiz-Casas D, Mendivil A. Efficacy of bevacizumab against interface neovascularization after deep anterior lamellar keratoplasty. *Cornea.* 2012;31(2):188-190.

24. Kim SW, Ha BJ, Kim EK, Tchah H, Kim TI. The effect of topical bevacizumab on corneal neovascularization. *Ophthalmology.* 2008;115(6):e33-e38.

25. Koenig Y, Bock F, Horn F, Kruse F, Straub K, Cursiefen C. Short- and long-term safety profile and efficacy of topical bevacizumab (Avastin) eye drops against corneal neovascularization. *Graefes Arch Clin Exp Ophthalmol.* 2009;247(10):1375-1382.

26. Lin CT, Hu FR, Kuo KT, et al. The different effects of early and late bevacizumab (Avastin) injection on inhibiting corneal neovascularization and conjunctivalization in rabbit limbal insufficiency. *Invest Ophthalmol Vis Sci.* 2010;51(12):6277-6285.

27. Saravia M, Zapata G, Ferraiolo P, Racca L, Berra A. Anti-VEGF monoclonal antibody-induced regression of corneal neovascularization and inflammation in a rabbit model of herpetic stromal keratitis. *Graefes Arch Clin Exp Ophthalmol.* 2009;247(10):1409-1416.

28. Cheng SF, Dastjerdi MH, Ferrari G, et al. Short-term topical bevacizumab in the treatment of stable corneal neovascularization. *Am J Ophthalmol.* 2012;154(6):940-948.e1.

29. Stevenson W, Cheng SF, Dastjerdi MH, Ferrari G, Dana R. Corneal neovascularization and the utility of topical VEGF inhibition: ranibizumab (Lucentis) vs bevacizumab (Avastin). *Ocul Surf.* 2012;10(2):67-83.

30. Aflibercept: AVE 0005, AVE 005, AVE0005, VEGF Trap-Regeneron, VEGF Trap (R1R2), VEGF Trap-Eye. *Drugs R D.* 2008;9(4):261-269.

31. Economides AN, Carpenter LR, Rudge JS, et al. Cytokine traps: multi-component, high-affinity blockers of cytokine action. *Nat Med.* 2003;9(1):47-52.

32. Papadopoulos N, Martin J, Ruan Q, et al. Binding and neutralization of vascular endothelial growth factor (VEGF) and related ligands by VEGF Trap, ranibizumab and bevacizumab. *Angiogenesis.* 2012;15(2):171-185.

33. Park YR, Chung SK. Inhibitory effect of topical aflibercept on corneal neovascularization in rabbits. *Cornea.* 2015;34(10):1303-1307.

34. Dohlman TH, Omoto M, Hua J, et al. VEGF-trap aflibercept significantly improves long-term graft survival in high-risk corneal transplantation. *Transplantation.* 2015;99(4):678-686.

35. Lee P, Wang CC, Adamis AP. Ocular neovascularization: an epidemiologic review. *Surv Ophthalmol.* 1998;43(3):245-269.

36. Niederkorn JY. The immune privilege of corneal allografts. *Transplantation.* 1999;67(12):1503-1508.

37. Niederkorn JY. The immunology of corneal transplantation. *Dev Ophthalmol.*1999;30:129-140.

38. Niederkorn JY. The immune privilege of corneal grafts. *J Leukoc Biol.* 2003;74(2):167-171.

39. Waldock A, Cook SD. Corneal transplantation: how successful are we? *Br J Ophthalmol.* 2000;84(8):813-815.

40. Dana MR, Schaumberg DA, Kowal VO, et al. Corneal neovascularization after penetrating keratoplasty. *Cornea.* 1995;14(6):604-609.

41. Keane MC, Lowe MT, Coster DJ, Pollock GA, Williams KA. The influence of Australian eye banking practices on corneal graft survival. *Med J Aust.* 2013;199(4):275-279.

42. Dana MR. Angiogenesis and lymphangiogenesis—implications for corneal immunity. *Semin Ophthalmol.* 2006;21(1):19-22.

43. Elbaz U, Mireskandari K, Shen C, Ali A. Corneal fine needle diathermy with adjuvant bevacizumab to treat corneal neovascularization in children. *Cornea.* 2015;34(7):773-777.

44. Cursiefen C, Hofmann-Rummelt C, Küchle M, Schlötzer-Schrehardt U. Pericyte recruitment in human corneal angiogenesis: an ultrastructural study with clinicopathological correlation. *Br J Ophthalmol.* 2003;87(1):101-106.

45. Junghans BM, Collin HB. The limbal vascular response to corneal injury. An autoradiographic study. *Cornea.* 1989;8(2):141-149.

46. Ferrari G, Dastjerdi MH, Okanobo A, et al. Topical ranibizumab as a treatment of corneal neovascularization. *Cornea.* 2013;32(7):992-997.

47. Liarakos VS, Papaconstantinou D, Vergados I, Douvali M, Theodossiadis PG. The effect of subconjunctival ranibizumab on corneal and anterior segment neovascularization: study on an animal model. *Eur J Ophthalmol.* 2014;24(3):299-308.

48. Kim EK, Kong SJ, Chung SK. Comparative study of ranibizumab and bevacizumab on corneal neovascularization in rabbits. *Cornea.* 2014;33(1):60-64.

49. Liesegang TJ. Herpes simplex virus epidemiology and ocular importance. *Cornea.* 2001;20(1):1-13.

50. Zheng M, Deshpande S, Lee S, Ferrara N, Rouse BT. Contribution of vascular endothelial growth factor in the neovascularization process during the pathogenesis of herpetic stromal keratitis. *J Virol.* 2001;75(20):9828-9835.

51. Lee S, Zheng M, Kim B, Rouse BT. Role of matrix metalloproteinase-9 in angiogenesis caused by ocular infection with herpes simplex virus. *J Clin Invest.* 2002;110(8):1105-1111.

52. 52. Carrasco MA. Subconjunctival bevacizumab for corneal neovascularization in herpetic stromal keratitis. *Cornea.* 2008;27(6):743-745.

53. Ahn YJ, Hwang HB, Chung SK. Ranibizumab injection for corneal neovascularization refractory to bevacizumab treatment. *Korean J Ophthalmol.* 2014;28(2):177-180.

54. Papas E. Corneal vascularisation and contact lenses [article in English, Spanish]. *Arch Soc Esp Oftalmol.* 2006;81(6):309-312.

55. Liesegang TJ. Physiologic changes of the cornea with contact lens wear. *CLAO J.* 2002;28(1):12-27.

56. Lim M, Jacobs DS, Rosenthal P, Carrasquillo KG. The Boston Ocular Surface Prosthesis as a novel drug delivery system for bevacizumab. *Semin Ophthalmol.* 2009;24(3):149-155.

57. Romano V, Steger B, Zheng Y, Ahmad S, Willoughby CE, Kaye SB. Angiographic and in vivo confocal microscopic characterization of human corneal blood and presumed lymphatic neovascularization: a pilot study. *Cornea.* 2015;34(11):1459-1465.

58. Steger B, Romano V, Kaye SB. Corneal indocyanine green angiography to guide medical and surgical management of corneal neovascularization. *Cornea.* 2016;35(1):41-45.

59. Spiteri N, Romano V, Zheng Y, et al. Corneal angiography for guiding and evaluating fine-needle diathermy treatment of corneal neovascularization. *Ophthalmology.* 2015;122(6):1079-1084.

60. Ang M, Cai Y, Shahipasand S, et al. En face optical coherence tomography angiography for corneal neovascularisation. *Br J Ophthalmol.* 2016;100(5):616-621.

61. Rabiolo A, Bignami F, Rama P, Ferrari G. VesselJ: A new tool for semiautomatic measurement of corneal neovascularization. *Invest Ophthalmol Vis Sci.* 2015;56(13):8199-8206.

62. Sandra S, Zeljka J, Zeljka VA, Kristian S, Ivana A. The influence of pterygium morphology on fibrin glue conjunctival autografting pterygium surgery. *Int Ophthalmol.* 2014;34(1):75-79.

63. Salman AG, Mansour DE. The recurrence of pterygium after different modalities of surgical treatment. *Saudi J Ophthalmol.* 2011;25(4):411-415.

64. Kareem AA, Farhood QK, Alhammami HA. The use of antimetabolites as adjunctive therapy in the surgical treatment of pterygium. *Clin Ophthalmol.* 2012;6:1849-1854.

65. Narsani AK, Nagdev PR, Memon MN. Outcome of recurrent pterygium with intraoperative 0.02% mitomycin C and free flap limbal conjunctival autograft. *J Coll Physicians Surg Pak.* 2013;23(3):199-202.

66. Mearza AA, Aslanides IM. Uses and complications of mitomycin C in ophthalmology. *Expert Opin Drug Saf.* 2007;6(1):27-32.

67. Lekhanont K, Patarakittam T, Thongphiew P, Suwan-apichon O, Hanutsaha P. Randomized controlled trial of subconjunctival bevacizumab injection in impending recurrent pterygium: a pilot study. *Cornea*. 2012;31(2):155-161.

68. Hu Q, Qiao Y, Nie X, Cheng X, Ma Y. Bevacizumab in the treatment of pterygium: a meta-analysis. *Cornea*. 2014;33(2):154-160.

69. Razeghinejad MR, Hosseini H, Ahmadi F, Rahat F, Eghbal H. Preliminary results of subconjunctival bevacizumab in primary pterygium excision. *Ophthalmic Res*. 2010;43(3):134-138.

70. Bahar I, Kaiserman I, McAllum P, Rootman D, Slomovic A. Subconjunctival bevacizumab injection for corneal neovascularization in recurrent pterygium. *Curr Eye Res*. 2008;33(1):23-28.

71. Nava-Castañeda A, Olvera-Morales O, Ramos-Castellon C, Garnica-Hayashi L, Garfias Y. Randomized, controlled trial of conjunctival autografting combined with subconjunctival bevacizumab for primary pterygium treatment: 1-year follow-up. *Clin Exp Ophthalmol*. 2014;42(3):235-241.

72. Nava-Castañeda A, Ulloa-Orozco I, Garnica-Hayashi L, Hernandez-Orgaz J, Jimenez-Martinez, Garfias Y. Triple subconjunctival bevacizumab injection for early corneal recurrent pterygium: one-year follow-up. *J Ocul Pharmacol Ther*. 2015;31(2):106-113.

73. Shields CL, Shields JA. Tumors of the conjunctiva and cornea. *Surv Ophthalmol*. 2004;49(1):3-24.

74. Dandala PP, Malladi P, Kavitha. Ocular surface squamous neoplasia (OSSN): a retrospective study. *J Clin Diagn Res*. 2015;9(11):NC10-NC13.

75. Shields CL, Kaliki S, Kim HJ, et al. Interferon for ocular surface squamous neoplasia in 81 cases: outcomes based on the American Joint Committee on Cancer classification. *Cornea*. 2013;32(3):248-256.

76. Asena L, Dursun Altınörs D. Topical bevacizumab for the treatment of ocular surface squamous neoplasia. *J Ocul Pharmacol Ther*. 2015;31(8):487-490.

77. Faramarzi A, Feizi S. Subconjunctival bevacizumab injection for ocular surface squamous neoplasia. *Cornea*. 2013;32(7):998-1001.

78. Finger PT, Chin KJ. Refractory squamous cell carcinoma of the conjunctiva treated with subconjunctival ranibizumab (Lucentis): a two-year study. *Ophthal Plast Reconstr Surg*. 2012;28(2):85-89.

Financial Disclosures

Dr. *Alessandro Abbouda* has no financial or proprietary interest in the materials presented herein.

Dr. *Sophie J. Bakri* has not disclosed any relevant financial relationships.

Dr. *Caroline R. Baumal* is an advisory board member and speaker for Allergan (2016).

Dr. *Audina M. Berrocal* is a consultant for Thrombogenics, Genentech, Clarity, and Alcon; and is supported by NIH Center Core Grant P30EY014801, Research to Prevent Blindness Unrestricted Grant, and Department of Defense (DOD- Grant#W81XWH-09- 1-0675).

Dr. *David Brown* has received research grant funding from Alcon/Novartis, Allegro, Allergan, Apellis, Astellas, Avalanche/Adverum, Clearside, Genentech/Hoffman-La Roche, Iconic, NEI/NIH, Ohr, Ophthotech, PRN, Regeneron/Bayer, Regenix Bio, Santen, SciFlour Life Sciences, Second Sight, Thrombogenics, Tyrogenics; is a consultant and resides on the scientific advisory boards for Adverum, Alcon/Novartis, Allegro, Allergan, Carl Zeiss Meditec, Coda Therapeutics, Clearside Biomedical, Envisia, Janssen, Johnson & Johnson, Genentech/Roche, Heidelberg Engineering, Notal Vision, Ohr, Ophthotech, OPTOS/Nikon, Optovue, Pfizer, Regeneron/Bayer, Regenix Bio, Santen, Stealth Biotherpeutics, Thrombogenics, Tyrogenix; and is a co-patent owner of OPTOS "dewarping" algorithms.

Dr. *Michael N. Cohen* has no financial or proprietary interest in the materials presented herein.

Emily D. Cole has no financial or proprietary interest in the materials presented herein.

Dr. *Sabin Dang* has no financial or proprietary interest in the materials presented herein.

Dr. *Shilpa Desai* has no financial or proprietary interest in the materials presented herein.

Dr. *Jay S. Duker* is a consultant for Allergan, Aura, Biosciences, Bayer, and Ironwood Pharma; is a consultant and receives research support from Carl Zeiss Meditech, Optovue, and Topcon; is a Hemera Biosciences stock holder; and is on the board of directors for Eleven Biotherapeutics and the pSivida Corporation.

Dr. Manik Goel has no financial or proprietary interest in the materials presented herein.

Dr. Darin R. Goldman has no financial or proprietary interest in the materials presented herein.

Dr. Pedram Hamrah has no financial or proprietary interest in the materials presented herein.

Dr. Jeffrey S. Heier has the following disclosures: Acucela Inc: Consultant, Investigator, Grants, Other Financial Benefit; AERPIO Aerpio Therapeutics: Consultant, Other Financial Benefit; Alcon Laboratories, Inc: Investigator, Grants; Allergan, Inc: Consultant, Investigator, Grants, Other Financial Benefit; Avalanche Biotechnologies, Inc: Consultant, Other Financial Benefit; Bausch + Lomb: Consultant, Other Financial Benefit; Bayer Healthcare Pharmaceuticals: Consultant, Other Financial Benefit; Dutch Ophthalmic USA: Consultant, Other Financial Benefit; Endo Optiks Inc: Consultant, Other Financial Benefit; Forsight Labs, LLC: Consultant, Grants; Genentech, Inc: Consultant, Investigator, Grants, Other Financial Benefit; Heidelberg Engineering: Consultant, Other Financial Benefit; Janssen Pharmaceuticals, Inc: Consultant, Other Financial Benefit; Kala Pharmaceuticals, Inc: Consultant, Investigator, Grants, Other Financial Benefit; Kanghong Sagent Pharmaceutical: Consultant, Other Financial Benefit; Kato Pharmaceuticals: Investigator, Grants; LPATH, Inc: Investigator, Grants; Neurotech Pharmaceuticals: Consultant, Other Financial Benefit; Notal Vision: Consultant, Other Financial Benefit; Novartis Pharmaceuticals Corporation: Consultant, Investigator, Grants, Other Financial Benefit; OHR Pharmaceutical Inc: Consultant, Investigator, Grants, Other Financial Benefit; Ophthotech Corporation: Investigator, Grants; QLT Ophthalmics, Inc: Consultant, Investigator, Grants, Other Financial Benefit; Quantel Medical: Consultant, Other Financial Benefit; Regeneron Pharmaceuticals, Inc: Consultant, Investigator, Grants, Other Financial Benefit; Saten Pharmaceutical Company, LTD: Consultant, Other Financial Benefit; Stealth Peptides Incorporated: Consultant, Investigator, Grants, Other Financial Benefit; Thrombogenics, Inc: Consultant, Investigator, Grants, Other Financial Benefit; Vision Medicines, Inc: Consultant, Other Financial Benefit; XCOVERY: Consultant, Other Financial Benefit; Xoma Corporation: Consultant, Other Financial Benefit.

Dr. Anthony Joseph has no financial or proprietary interest in the materials presented herein.

Bijan Khaksari has no financial or proprietary interest in the materials presented herein.

Dr. Kendra Klein has no financial or proprietary interest in the materials presented herein.

Dr. Nikisha A. Kothari is supported by NIH Center Core Grant P30EY014801, Research to Prevent Blindness Unrestricted Grant, and Department of Defense (DOD- Grant#W81XWH-09- 1-0675).

Dr. Michael D. Lewen has no financial or proprietary interest in the materials presented herein.

Dr. Michelle C. Liang has no financial or proprietary interest in the materials presented herein.

Dr. Maya H. Maloney has no financial or proprietary interest in the materials presented herein.

Dr. Angeline Mariani Derham has no financial or proprietary interest in the materials presented herein.

Dr. Cynthia Mattox is a consultant for Allergan, Alcon, Transcend and Aerie; and receives research support from Allergan and Transcend.

Dr. Jessica J. Moon has no financial or proprietary interest in the materials presented herein.

Dr. Nora Muakkassa has no financial or proprietary interest in the materials presented herein.

Dr. Eduardo A. Novais has no financial or proprietary interest in the materials presented herein.

Dr. Ehsan Rahimy is a consultant for Allergan.

Elham Rahimy has no financial or proprietary interest in the materials presented herein.

Dr. Elias Reichel has not disclosed any relevant financial relationships.

Dr. Lana M. Rifkin is a speaker for AbbVie, Inc and an investigator for Clearside Biomedical, EYEGATE, and Aldeyra.

Dr. Joel S. Schuman has equity and consulting interests in and royalty income from IP, licensed to Ocugenix, LLC; royalty income from Elsevier; royalty income from the Massachusetts Eye and Ear Infirmary; royalty income from IP, licensed to Zeiss Optical; and rights in IP, assigned to the University of Pittsburgh. He is on the advisory board position and has equity in Opticent Health and IOP Medical Ltd. He also has consulting interests in Annexon Inc, Pfizer, SLACK Incorporated/Vindico Medical Education, Alcon Laboratories, Aerie, and Shire Pharmaceuticals.

Dr. Chirag P. Shah is a sub-investigator on trials sponsored by Genentech and Regeneron.

Dr. Michael D. Tibbetts has no financial or proprietary interest in the materials presented herein.

Dr. Nadia K. Waheed is a consultant for Iconic Therapeutics, Genentech, Optovue, Regeneron, Carl Zeiss Meditec, Topcon, and Nidek.

Dr. Andre J. Witkin has no financial or proprietary interest in the materials presented herein.

Index

Printed in the United States
by Baker & Taylor Publisher Services